To my dear friend, N...

Communication Disorders Across Languages
Series Editors: Dr Nicole Müller and Dr Martin Ball, *University of Louisiana at Lafayette, USA*

While the majority of work in communication disorders has focused on English, there has been a growing trend in recent years for the publication of information on languages other than English. However, much of this is scattered through a large number of journals in the field of speech pathology/communication disorders, and therefore, not always readily available to the practioner, researcher and student. It is the aim of this series to bring together into book form surveys of existing studies on specific languages, together with new materials for the language(s) in question. We also envisage a series of companion volumes dedicated to issues related to the crosslinguistic study of communication disorders. The series will not include English (as so much work is readily available), but will cover a wide number of other languages (usually separately, though sometimes two or more similar languages may be grouped together where warranted by the amount of published work currently available). We envisage being able to solicit volumes on languages such as Norwegian, Swedish, Finnish, German, Dutch, French, Italian, Spanish, Russian, Croatian, Japanese, Cantonese, Mandarin, Thai, North Indian languages in the UK context, Celtic languages, Arabic and Hebrew among others.

Other Books in the Series
Communication Disorders in Spanish Speakers: Theoretical, Research and Clinical Aspects
José G. Centeno, Raquel T. Anderson and Loraine K. Obler (eds)

Other Books of Interest
Bilingual Children's Language and Literacy Development
Roger Barnard and Ted Glynn (eds)
Culture-Specific Language Styles: The Development of Oral Narrative and Literacy
Masahiko Minami
Developing in Two Languages: Korean Children in America
Sarah J. Shin
Language and Aging in Multilingual Contexts
Kees de Bot and Sinfree Makoni
Making Sense in Sign: A Lifeline for a Deaf Child
Jenny Froude
Phonological Development in Specific Contexts: Studies of Chinese-Speaking Children
Zhu Hua
Phonological Development and Disorders in Children: A Multilingual Perspective
Zhu Hua and Barbara Dodd (eds)
Understanding Deaf Culture: In Search of Deafhood
Paddy Ladd

For more details of these or any other of our publications, please contact:
Multilingual Matters, Frankfurt Lodge, Clevedon Hall,
Victoria Road, Clevedon, BS21 7HH, England
http://www.multilingual-matters.com

Research in Logopedics

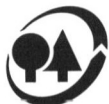

COMMUNICATION DISORDERS ACROSS LANGUAGES
Series Editors: Nicole Müller and Martin Ball

Research in Logopedics
Speech and Language Therapy in Finland

Edited by
Anu Klippi and Kaisa Launonen

MULTILINGUAL MATTERS LTD
Clevedon • Buffalo • Toronto

Library of Congress Cataloging in Publication Data
Research in Logopedics: Speech and Language Therapy in Finland / Edited by Anu
Klippi and Kaisa Launonen.
Communication Disorders Across Languages
Includes bibliographical references and index.
1. Speech therapy–Finland. 2. Language disorders–Treatment--Finland. I. Klippi, Anu.
II. Launonen, Kaisa. III. Series.
[DNLM: 1. Language disorders–therapy–Finland. 2. Language
therapy–methods–Finland. 3. Speech disorders–therapy–Finland. 4. Speech
therapy–methods–Finland. WL 340.2 R432 1988]
RC423.R45 1988
362.194′8550094897–dc22   1987050429

British Library Cataloguing in Publication Data
A catalogue entry for this book is available from the British Library.

ISBN-13: 978-1-84769-058-6 (hbk)

Multilingual Matters Ltd
UK: Frankfurt Lodge, Clevedon Hall, Victoria Road, Clevedon BS21 7HH.
USA: UTP, 2228 Military Road, Tonawanda, NY 13950, USA.
Canada: UTP, 5199 Dufferin Street, North York, Ontario M3H 5T8, Canada.

The policy of Multilingual Matters/Channel View Publications is to use papers that
are natural, renewable and recyclable products, made from wood grown in
sustainable forests. In the manufacturing process of our books, and to further support
our policy, preference is given to printers that have FSC and PEFC Chain of Custody
certification. The FSC and/or PEFC logos will appear on those books where full
certification has been granted to the printer concerned.

Typeset by Techset Composition Ltd.
Printed and bound in Great Britain by MPG Books Ltd.

Contents

The Contributors

Liisa Ahopalo, Paciuksenkaari 27 A 20, 00270 Helsinki.

Kaisu Heinänen, Logopedics, Faculty of Humanities, University of Oulu.

Marja-Liisa Helasvuo, School of Finnish and General Linguistics, University of Turku.

Kerttu Huttunen, Logopedics, Faculty of Humanities, University of Oulu.

Anu Klippi, Department of Speech Sciences, University of Helsinki.

Anna-Maija Korpijaakko-Huuhka, Department of Speech Communication and Voice Research, University of Tampere.

Pirjo Korpilahti, Logopedics, Department of Psychology, University of Turku.

Pirjo Kulju, Department of Teacher Education, University of Tampere.

Kaisa Launonen, Department of Speech Sciences, University of Helsinki.

Eila Lonka, Department of Speech Sciences, University of Helsinki.

Leila Paavola, Logopedics, Faculty of Humanities, University of Oulu.

Seija Pekkala, Department of Speech Sciences, University of Helsinki.

Tuula Savinainen-Makkonen, Logopedics, Faculty of Humanities, University of Oulu.

Anne Suvanto, Logopedics, Faculty of Humanities, University of Oulu, and Private Practice (Speech & Language Therapy), Oulu.

Ritva Takkinen, Department of Languages/Finnish Sign Language, University of Jyväskylä.

Eeva Sala, Department of Otorhinolaryngology – Head and Neck Surgery, Turku University Hospital, Turku.

Susanna Simberg, Logopedics, Faculty of Arts, Åbo Akademi University.

Part 1

Introduction

Chapter 1

Challenges to Logopedics and Speech-Language Therapy in Finland

KAISA LAUNONEN and ANU KLIPPI

Finland: Special Characteristics

Finland is located in the northeast corner of Europe and is a part of the European Union. Culturally, it is situated between the Eastern influence of Russia and the Western influence of Scandinavia, especially of Sweden. Until 1809, Finland was part of Sweden and, after that, part of the Russian Empire for a little more than a hundred years. Therefore, Swedish and later Russian were the languages of administration before Finland gained its independence in 1917. Today, Finland is officially a bilingual country, the official languages being Finnish and Swedish. The population is predominantly Finnish-speaking, with a 6% minority speaking Swedish. The rights of people speaking Sami (a language spoken by some 30,000–50,000 people in Lapland, in the northern parts of Finland, Norway and Sweden), to use and develop their mother tongue, is guaranteed by law. Furthermore, the number of Russian-speaking people in Finland has been growing since the 1990s, as well as other minority language groups, such as Estonian, Somali and English. However, Finland has been, until quite recently, culturally a very homogeneous society and proud of its unique culture and special role at the frontier between Eastern and Western Europe. As part of the European Union, and along with the increasing mobility of people, internationalisation and multiculturalism are now rapidly increasing in Finland. The change from a monocultural to a multi-cultural and multilingual society is a big challenge in modern Finland (see also Bornman & Launonen, 2005).

Modern Finland can be defined as an education society, and it is well known for its high level of education. In the PISA comparisons (Programme for International Student Assessment) between 28 OECD countries, the skills of Finnish 15-year-old students were ranked highest in literacy (in 2000) and in mathematics (in 2003). The official age to start school is seven years, but all children are entitled to one year of pre-school, which most children also attend. The nine-year comprehensive school is free of charge. Of each cohort, 56% continue to three-year upper secondary school, and 35% to vocational schools. The network of higher education is dense, and 64% of each cohort begin university every year. Men and women receive equal education, and the proportion of women beginning university is higher than men. Furthermore, the principles of the Nordic welfare society ensure that the needs of special groups are met. Children with disabilities start school one year earlier than other children, and they study according to an individual curriculum, planned in collaboration with their parents, teachers and other significant professionals. Most children with special needs are integrated in mainstream schools, either individually with their peers, or as groups in special classes. Some special schools still exist for children with severe motor or sensory impairments.

In addition to the high quality of public education, another characteristic feature of Finnish society is the social and health care system maintained by the government. Finland has municipal public day-care, which most families use, at least during the pre-school year of their children. Finnish maternity and child welfare clinics are highly regarded, and take care of women during their pregnancy and administer children's annual health check-ups before school age (at school age they are administered by school health care, which is also part of municipal health care). As part of the annual health check-ups, the speech and language skills of children are screened by educated nurses, with screening tools developed by speech and language therapists. If needed, the child is referred for a thorough speech and language assessment by a speech and language therapist. Concerns expressed by parents or day care personnel are also sufficient cause for referral to a speech and language therapist for evaluation. These services are free of charge for the families, as is also intervention, when the need is determined by a speech and language therapist and confirmed by a physician. However, there are currently insufficient numbers of speech and language therapists to cover the need in Finland, which means that not all get the intervention they need, at a time when they would benefit from it the most.

The Development of Theory and Practice of Logopedics in Finland

The education of speech and language therapists in Finland was started at the University of Helsinki in the Department of Phonetics (since 2004 the Department of Speech Sciences) in 1947. In the early years, the education led to a Bachelor's degree, and after graduating, students had six months of clinical studies and practical, training mainly in hospitals or rehabilitation centres. During the 1970s, the clinical studies were organised more systematically and graduates in speech and language therapy, with a B.A. degree from the Faculty of Arts, attended a nine-month clinical course organised by the Ministry of Health. In 1980, the education programme was completely reorganised. All the students in speech and language therapy took a Master's degree in logopedics, which included the clinical training (Klippi & Korpijaakko-Huuhka, 1998). This structure is mainly valid still today, even though all the university programmes and degrees were reformed in 2005, as part of the joint European improvement of higher education (Bologna process; http://www.dfes. gov.uk/bologna/; see also CPLOL, 1999; Wigforss *et al.*, 1997, 1998, 1999). The present programme in logopedics consists of a minimum of five years of study, leading to a Master's degree and including theoretical, methodological and clinical studies, and a Master's thesis. After taking the degree, an individual is qualified to apply for the right to practice as a licensed professional in speech and language therapy. This licence is granted to health care professionals by the National Authority for Medicolegal Affairs.

At the University of Oulu, education for speech and language therapists (logopedics) began in 1984. For a long time student numbers were small, around 15 new students annually in Helsinki and 20 in Oulu. Later, the numbers gradually increased, while still quite small: around 20 in Helsinki and around 30 in Oulu (2007). A new programme of logopedics started in 2005 as a network of three universities: the Universities of Tampere and Turku, and the Swedish speaking Åbo Akademi University. Thus, in fall 2006, the number of new students in logopedics was 80 in Finland. The number of practicing speech and language therapists is about 1000 (2007), serving a total population of 5.3 million in Finland.

The Finnish system of academic degrees has traditionally had four levels: bachelor, master, licentiate and doctor. Of those, the licentiate degree seems to be disappearing as a purely academic degree (with the exception of medical studies, where it remains the basic degree for professionals in medicine). It is, however, also a developing degree in certain fields, such as logopedics and psychology, where it is used as the specialist degree for speech and language therapists and psychologists. The specialist programme for professional psychologists already has a longer history, but the first specialist programme for speech and language therapists started in 2004 as a network programme of the Universities of Helsinki and Oulu, with two areas of specialisation: developmental and acquired neurological communication disorders. After the conclusion of the first four-year education at the end of 2007, there are plans for a new course, with the aim of making the programme permanent. The other specialisation areas will be voice and hearing disorders.

At the European level, and even globally, the quality of the education of Finnish speech and language therapists can be considered very high.

However logopedics as an academic subject with a research profile of its own (Klippi, 1996; Lehtihalmes, 1996) is a very young discipline. From the very beginning the professional aspects of education in logopedics were well taken care of, but in the early years, the methodological competence of professionals in the field did not yet support the development of the research of logopedics. It was not until the late 1990s that the first post-graduate students with a background in logopedics (and all of them with professional experience from clinical work, as well) received their doctoral degree. Since then, the growth has been stable and by the end of 2006, altogether 23 doctoral degrees within logopedics had been completed. Most of the contributors in this book are among the pioneers of logopedic research in Finland.

With the short history of Finnish research in logopedics and only a few people working in the field, most of the literature used in the education of Finnish speech and language therapists is in English. This gives the Finnish professionals the privilege of being able to follow the latest international literature from the very beginning of their studies. However, this could also easily lead to the unfortunate situation where the knowledge base of the Finnish speech and language therapists would be too heavily based on studies in languages other than the one in which they work. Therefore, it is the responsibility of Finnish researchers to produce Finnish literature, both for the students and professionals in the field, and for the Finnish general public. This, added to the obligation of researchers in all countries to share their findings internationally in the lingua franca of the scientific world, English, doubles the writing load of researchers working in such small language areas as Finnish. The readers of this book will find, however, that the number of Finnish references is relatively high, particularly in some chapters. This has been possible partly because many of the authors of this book have acted as supervisors for high quality Master's theses, which they have been able to refer to in their chapters, as examples of the developing academic research in Finland.

At present, the programme of studies in logopedics has a strong research orientation from the beginning. All students write both Bachelor's and Master's theses before getting their degree. This means that all speech and language therapists start their clinical work equipped with an experience of doing research, albeit small studies under super-vision. They are also encouraged to maintain a research orientation in their later clinical work. Not all professionals in the field are able or even willing to do so, but in some fields, for example augmentative and alter-native communication, Finnish clinical speech and language therapists are very visible even in international scientific conferences, where they give presentations based on their clinical data or development projects. These presentations have also contributed to the Finnish studies referred to in this book.

The Structure and Contents of the Book

This book has been divided into four thematic main parts, with a short introduction to the Finnish language (Helasvuo), and to the assessments methods used by the Finnish speech and language therapists (Huttunen, Paavola and Suvanto). The chapter by Huttunen *et al.* also discusses the need to develop assessment methods for the professionals to be able, even better than today, to recognise communication problems and serve the needs of Finns with communication disorders.

The first thematic part is comprised of three chapters focusing on speech and language development and its disorders (Korpilahti and Heinänen), including aspects of alternative communication used by people with the most complex communication needs (Launonen). The second thematic part focuses on acquired speech and language disorders. It looks at neurological communication disorders from the perspective of two studies on the communication of people with aphasia (Korpijaakko-Huuhka; Klippi and Ahopalo), and contains a review of semantic impairment in Alzheimer's disease (Pekkala).

Three chapters on different aspects of communication and language in children with hearing disorders constitute the third thematic part of the book. They cover issues on sign language acquisition (Takkinen), cochlear implants in children (Lonka), and speech intelligibility of children with hearing impairments (Huttunen). A single chapter of part five on the screening of voice disorders (Simberg and Sala) provides an example not only of voice disorders and therapy, but also of preventative aspects in the work of speech and language therapists.

It is impossible in one single volume to give a comprehensive picture of communication disorders, their study and their treatment in any country or in any language. The editors of this book wish to provide the readers with interesting examples of and insights into the communication challenges in a language that differs substantially from those used in the majority of published reports in the field of language and communication disorders.

References

Bornman, J. and Launonen, K. (2005) Monikulttuurinen kompetenssi ja sen vaikutukset puheterapiatyöhön [Multicultural competence: Implications for the speech-language therapy]. *Puhe ja kieli [Speech and Language]* 25, 243–255.

CPLOL (1999) *1988–1998 10 Years of Activities*. Paris: Standing Liaison Committee of Speech and Language Therapists or Logopedists of European Union.

Klippi, A. (1996) Puheterapiatutkimus – Logopedian ydin [Research on speech and language therapy – Core of logopedics]. In *Puheterapian uudet suunnat. Logopedinen tutkimus ja kuntoutus tänään [New Directions in Speech and Language Therapy. Logopedic Research and Intervention Today]* (pp. 7–17). Helsinki: Puheterapeuttien Kustannus.

Klippi, A. and Korpijaakko-Huuhka, A.-M. (1998) Theory, practice and research: Creating synergy in education of speech therapists. *Conference Proceedings of the 24th Congress of the International Association of Logopedics & Phoniatrics.* August 1998, Amsterdam, the Netherlands, 935–938.

Lehtihalmes, M. (1996) Kommunikaatiohäiriöiden perustutkimus tarpeen [Basic research on communication disorders is needed]. *Aktuumi 1/1996,* 12–16.

Wigforss, E., Beck, J., Camilleri, B., Chaintrain, H., Leterme, M., Klippi, A., Lehtihalmes, M., Schneider, P. and Vieregge, W. (1997) Speech and language therapy. In G. Bloothooft, W. van Dommelen, C. Espain, P. Green, V. Hazan, M. Huckvale and E. Wigforss (eds) *The Landscape of Future Education in Speech Communication Sciences. 1. Analysis* (pp. 73–93). Utrecht: OTS Publications.

Wigforss, E., Beck, J., Chaintrain, H., Docherty, G., Howard, S., Klippi, A., Leahy, M. and Lehtihalmes, M. (1998) The integration of speech communication sciences in speech and language therapy curricula. In G. Bloothooft, W. van Dommelen, P. Espain, V. Hazan, M. Huckvale and E. Wigforss (eds) *The Landscape of Future Education in Speech Communication Sciences. 2. Proposals* (pp. 63–80). Utrecht: OTS Publications.

Wigforss, E., Leahy, M., Beck, J., Chaintrain, H., Docherty, G., Howard S., Huber, W., Klippi, A., Lehtihalmes, M. and Springer, L. (1999) Recommendations for speech communication disorders curricula. In G. Bloothooft, W. van Dommelen, K. Fellbaum, V. Hazan, M. Huckvale, M. Leahy and E. Wigforss (eds) *The Landscape of Future Education in Speech Communication Sciences. 3. Recommendations* (pp. 67–97). Utrecht: OTS Publications.

Chapter 2
Aspects of the Structure of Finnish

MARJA-LIISA HELASVUO

Introduction

Finnish is spoken by some 5 million speakers, mainly in Finland; there are small minorities of Finnish speakers in Sweden, Russia and the United States. Finnish is a member of the Finno-Ugric language family. Its closest relatives include Estonian, while Hungarian is a more distant relative ('Uralic languages', 2006). It is typical of these languages that they show inflectional morphology consisting mostly of suffixes. It is assumed that the Uralic protolanguage had a case system with six cases (Häkkinen, 1985), but in many Finno-Ugric languages the number of cases is much higher (e.g. in Hungarian, there are 17–26 cases depending on where the line is drawn between inflection and derivation).

This chapter presents some characteristic features of the grammar of Finnish, its morphology and syntax. It aims to provide sufficient background for the understanding of the structural features of Finnish that are discussed in the subsequent papers.

The chapter also discusses the phoneme inventory, syllable structure and length, and some morphophonological processes that are typical of Finnish, such as consonant gradation. Finnish has a rich morphology, both in the area of derivation and in inflection. It has an elaborate case system with some 15 cases. Syntactic arguments are coded with the help of case marking and verbal inflection. Predicate verbs agree with the subject according to person and number. Finnish word order is often described as being relatively free. It has been shown, however, to be discourse-conditioned: although all kinds of grammatical permutations are in principle possible, they convey differences in the thematic organisation or focus structure.

Phonology and Morphophonology

This section gives an overview of the vowel and consonant systems in Finnish, and of syllable structure and stress patterns.

Table 2.1 The Finnish vowel system

	Front vowels		*Back vowels*	
		Rounded		Rounded
Close vowels	i	y		u
Mid vowels	e	ø		o
Open vowels	æ		ɑ	

The Finnish vowel system consists of eight vowels as illustrated in Table 2.1. There is a phonemic distinction between long and short vowels, cf. e.g. *kari* 'rock' vs. *kaari* 'arch', *etsi* [search-PAST-3SG] 'searched' vs. *etsii* [search-PRES-3SG] 'searches'.

The occurrence of vowels within one word is constrained by vowel harmony so that back vowels may combine with back vowels and front vowels with front vowels. This means that a given word may contain only back or only front vowels. However, the front vowels /i/ and /e/ are indifferent to vowel harmony and may thus combine with back or front vowels (for more discussion, see Sulkala & Karjalainen, 1992: 378). Vowels may further combine to form diphthongs. There are 18 diphthongs: /ei, øi, æi, oi, ɑi, ey, øy, æy, eu, ou, ɑu, yi, ui, iy, iu, ie, yø, uo/ (Hakulinen *et al.*, 2004: 54[1]).

The consonant system is illustrated in Table 2.2. There are 13–17 consonants in the Finnish phoneme inventory. There are certain sounds whose position in the consonant system is not quite stable (these are given in parentheses in Table 2.2). They occur mainly in loan words and in non-standard Finnish (Hakulinen *et al.*, 2004: 40). Again, there is a phonemic distinction between long and short consonants, cf. e.g. *kato* 'disappearance' vs. *katto* 'roof', *takaan* [assure-PRES-1SG] 'I assure' vs. *takkaan* [fireplace-ILL] 'into the fireplace'.

Table 2.2 The Finnish consonant system

	Labial	*Dental*	*Alveolar*	*Palatovelar*	*Glottal*
Stops	p (b)	t d		k (g)	
Nasals	m	n		ŋ	
Fricatives	(f)	s	ʃ		h
Liquids		l r			
Semivowels	v			j	

Source: Hakulinen *et al.*, 2004: 38.

Table 2.3   Syllable types in Finnish

Syllable type	Examples
CV	ka.la 'fish', he.del.mä 'fruit'
CVC	vil.kas 'lively'
CVCC	kars.ki 'harsh'
CVV	työ 'work', le.pää 'to rest'
CVVC	pää.tää 'to decide', a.va.ruus 'space'
V	a.voin 'open', lu.ke.a 'to read'
VC	ar.vo 'value', no.pe.us 'speed'
VCC	ark.ki 'piece of paper'
VV	aa.mu 'morning', au.ke.aa 'opens'
VVC	aal.to 'wave'

Source: Hakulinen *et al.*, 2004: 45.

There has to be at least one vowel (short or long) or a diphthong to form a syllable in Finnish. Table 2.3 illustrates the different syllable types. After each syllable type there is an example word with the illustrated syllable type given in bold face.

There are some syllable types that are only possible in loan words and in slang which are not listed in Table 2.3. They include CCV (e.g. **pro**.*sent.ti* 'percentage'), CCVC [e.g. **klit**.*su* 'cellar (slang)'], among others.

There is a close correspondence between phonemes and graphemes in Finnish. Among consonants, the palatovelar nasal /ŋ/ lacks a graphemic counterpart of its own, but instead is marked either with g or ng.

Word stress is constant so that the primary stress normally falls on the first syllable of a word and, if the word has at least four syllables, the secondary stress falls on every second syllable (i.e. the third, fifth, etc.). Thus, the second syllable is normally unstressed in Finnish, and so is the last syllable of a word (see Sulkala & Karjalainen, 1992: 381).

There are many morphophonological alternation processes in Finnish, and among them, consonant gradation is perhaps one of the best described ones. Gradation implies weakening of a strong-grade form in certain environments. Phonetically the primary conditioning factor is whether the next syllable is closed or open. In gradation a double stop (a geminate) is reduced to a single one (see Example 1) or a single stop is assimilated or deleted (Example 2) if the next syllable is closed.

(1)   *nukku-u* [sleep-PRES+3SG] 'sleeps': *nuku-n* [sleep-PRES+1SG] 'I sleep'
(2)   *ilta* 'evening': *illa-n* [evening-GEN] 'of the evening'

In Example (1), *nukun* 'I sleep' is in the weak grade, because the syllable following the geminate stop is closed (-*kun*). In (2), the last syllable *lan* is closed thus enforcing a weak-grade form. Therefore, the stop *t* is assimilated with the preceding liquid.

Morphology

Finnish is characterised by rich morphology: it has extensive nominal and verbal inflectional and derivational systems. This section takes a closer look at the case system and the personal inflection on verbs.

Finnish has 15 cases (see Table 2.4 below). In principle all nouns are inflected for case, and furthermore, participial forms of verbs show case inflection. Infinitival forms of verbs can also be inflected for case, but case inflection is more restricted in infinitives. Table 2.4 shows that the nominative has no ending, whereas all the other cases have distinct case endings. The case system is often divided into three groups, namely the grammatical cases, the local cases and others, which are in some ways more marginal.

The grammatical cases are used to mark phrases that function in the syntactic roles of the clause core (subjects, objects and predicate nominals; for more discussion, see next section). There has been considerable controversy over the analysis of the core cases; Table 2.4 represents the views of a recent descriptive grammar of Finnish (Hakulinen *et al.*, 2004). The main difference between Hakulinen *et al.*'s views and the traditional descriptions is that they have decided to restrict the use of the term accusative to refer only to the inflection of personal pronouns when functioning as objects in the clause (e.g. *minu-t* 'me').[2] Consequently, the genitive is used in a wider meaning than has traditionally been the case: according to Hakulinen *et al.*, the genitive is not only used to mark possessive phrases but also objects (see Hakulinen *et al.*, 2004: 1174–1175).

The local cases can be further divided into internal (inessive, elative, illative), external (adessive, ablative, allative) and general cases (essive, translative). In broad terms, the internal cases indicate being inside something or coming from or going into something, whereas the external cases indicate being on the surface of something, coming from something or going into something. They further exhibit a tripartite division into an 'in-case' (inessive, adessive, essive), a 'to-case' (illative, allative, translative) and a 'from-case' (elative, ablative) for further discussion, see Huumo & Ojutkangas, 2006).

Interestingly enough, in spite of the rich set of choices that the case system offers, the use of the different cases clusters around only a few cases. In Helasvuo's conversational data, over half of the noun phrases were in the nominative (i.e. the unmarked case), with the partitive being the second most frequent case ending (15% of noun phrases) (Helasvuo, 2001: 38–39). With data from newspapers and modern fiction, Hakulinen

Table 2.4 The Finnish case system[3]

	Case	Ending	Example	Translation
I Grammatical cases	Nominative	-	talo	'house'
	Genitive	-n	talo-n	'(of) a/the house'
	Accusative	-t	minu-t	'me'
	Partitive	-A, -tA	talo-a	'(of) a/the house'
II Local cases	Essive	-nA	talo-na	'as/for a/the house'
	Translative	-ksi	talo-ksi	'into a/the house'
	Inessive	-ssA	talo-ssa	'in(side) a/the house'
	Elative	-stA	talo-sta	'from inside a/the house'
	Illative	-Vn, -hVn, -seen	talo-on	'into a/the house'
	Adessive	-llA	talo-lla	'by/on/near a/the house'
	Ablative	-ltA	talo-lta	'from a/the house'
	Allative	-lle	talo-lle	'to a/the house'
IV Other cases	Abessive	-ttA	talo-tta	'without a/the house'
	Comitative	-ine	talo-ine-en	'with a/the house'
	Instructive	-n	käsi-n	'by hand'

Source: Helasvuo, 2001: 37.

et al. (2004: 1179) demonstrate that 30–37% of nouns and case-inflected infinitival verb forms are in the nominative. It is important to note that Helasvuo (2001) counts noun phrases, whereas Hakulinen *et al.* (2004) count the case marking of all elements without considering phrase structure. This partly explains the differences in the results of these studies.

Finite verbs are inflected for tense (present, past, perfect and past perfect), person and number. The tense suffix appears closest to the stem before the markers for person and number. The present tense is unmarked (no marker), while the past tense carries the marker *i* (e.g. *katso-i-n* [look-PAST-1SG] 'I looked'). The perfect and past perfect are expressed by periphrastic forms consisting of the auxiliary *olla* 'be' and the past participle of the main verb (e.g. *ole-n katso-nut* [be-1SG look-PAST PARTICIPLE]

Table 2.5 Verbal person inflection in Finnish

Person	Number	
	Singular	Plural
1st	katso-n 'I look'	katso-mme 'we look'
2nd	katso-t 'you look'	katso-tte 'you (pl.) look'
3rd	katso-o 's/he looks'	katso-vat 'they look'

'I have looked'). The person and number marking on the verb indicates the person (1st, 2nd or 3rd) and number (singular vs. plural) of the subject of the clause. Thus, the main function of the person inflection is to code the subject. The person and number markings are conflated so that there is only one marking that indicates both number and person as can be seen from Table 2.5. In the table, the inflection of the verb *katsoa* 'to look' is given as an example. The person and number endings are distinguished from the stem with a hyphen.

Table 2.5 describes the person inflection in the standard language where the verbal marking simply copies the number and person from the subject. In the colloquial varieties, however, person marking is more complicated. In the third person, the singular marking is usually used for both singular and plural subjects. Furthermore, in the first person plural, it is very common to have the first person plural pronoun *me* 'we' combined with a passive verb form *me katsotaan* 'we look') and the construction carries first person plural meaning. (For more discussion of the person system in Finnish, see Helasvuo, 2001: 64–76 and Helasvuo & Laitinen, 2006.)

There are two processes of word formation in Finnish, namely derivation and compounding. There is an extensive inventory of derivational suffixes which can be used to derive nouns or verbs from other nouns, verbs, adjectives, numerals and pronouns. Also adjectives and particles may be derived but the set of derivational suffixes that produce adjectives and particles is more restricted than that of nouns and verbs. Examples are given in (3).

(3)   noun from noun   *kana-la* 'henhouse' ← *kana* 'hen' + *la*
      verb from noun   *loma-ile* 'be on holiday' ← *loma* 'holiday' + *ile*
      noun from verb   *tuot-e* 'product' ← *tuottaa* 'produce' + *e*
      noun from adjective   *must-ikka* 'blueberry' ← *musta* 'black' + *ikka*
      verb from adjective   *kuum-ene* 'become hot' ← *kuuma* 'hot' + *ene*
      noun from numeral   *yksi-lö* 'individual' ← *yksi* 'one' + *lö*
      verb from numeral   *kahde-ntaa* 'reduplicate' ← *kahde-* 'two' + *nta*

noun from pronoun   *min-uus* 'ego' ← *minä* 'I' + *uus*
adjective from noun   *pilku-llinen* 'dotted' ← *pilkku* 'dot' + *llinen*
particle from adjective *nopea-sti* 'quickly, fast' ← *nopea* 'quick' + *sti*

Finnish is a language that is characterised by extensive inflection and derivation in both verbal and nominal categories. This has profound effects on clausal syntax: each constituent of the clause is inflected in a form that identifies its function in the clause. Even uninflected forms, such as particles, show their syntactic function in the clause through the absence of inflection.

Syntax, Semantics and Discourse Structure

In Finnish, case marking and person inflection play a major role in the coding of syntactic roles, especially the roles of the clause core: objects are distinguished from subjects through case marking, and if there is no nominative subject in the clause, and thus, no need to distinguish the object from the subject, the object can also be in the nominative. Furthermore, verbal agreement morphology codes the subject according to person and number. Because of the extensive morphosyntactic coding of elements, word order allows for different kinds of permutations of elements. The permutations do not affect the grammaticality of the clause, but they do have an effect on the discourse structure, that is, what the theme is in the clause, what is in focus, what is in contrast, etc.

The nominative is used to mark subjects and the genitive is used to mark objects (4). The nominative may also be used to mark objects if there is no nominative subject in the clause (5). The partitive is used to mark subjects (6) and objects (7).

(4) *Liisa*   *aukais-i*   *ove-n.*
     Lisa+NOM   open-PST+3SG   door-GEN
     'Lisa opened the door.'
(5) *Ava-a*   *ovi!*
     open-IMP+2SG   door+NOM
     'Open the door!'
(6) *Poik-i-a*   *seiso-o*   *piha-lla.*
     boy-PL-PTV   stand-3SG   yard-ADE
     'There are boys standing in the yard.'/'Some boys are standing in the yard.'
(7) *Liisa*   *ost-i*   *omeno-i-ta.*
     Lisa+NOM   buy-PST+3SG   apple-PL-PTV
     'Lisa bought (some) apples.'

The meaning differences conveyed by the grammatical cases are abstract in nature, and they relate to definiteness and aspectual distinctions. In broad terms, the partitive is used to convey indefiniteness and unbounded aspect. In (4), the object is definite and the action described is telic and therefore the object is marked with the genitive. In (5) there is no nominative subject and thus the object may stand in the nominative. In (6) there is an indefinite quantity of boys and therefore the phrase 'boys' is marked with the partitive. In (7) *omenoita* 'apples' is in the partitive because it is indefinite.

Definiteness or indefiniteness can thus be expressed through case marking in Finnish. In addition, the demonstrative pronoun *se* 'it' and pronominal adjectives can be used much in the same way as definite and indefinite articles. According to Laury (1997), *se* is grammaticalising into a definite article in Finnish. So far, the use of *se* (Example 8) and the pronominal adjectives (Example 9) to express definiteness distinctions is much more common in the colloquial varieties than in standard Finnish.

(8) *Eeva ost-i*   *se-n*   *talo-n*   *eilen.*
     Eva buy-PST+3SG   it-GEN   house-GEN   yesterday
     'Eva bought the house yesterday.'

(9) *Mä nä-i-n*   *se-llase-n*   *kulkue-en.*
     1SG see-PST-1SG   it-ADJ-GEN   procession-GEN
     'I saw a kind of a procession.'

In (8), *sen talon* 'the house' is a definite expression that refers to something that has been spoken about already or is known to the participants. In (9), *sellasen kulkueen* 'a (kind of a) procession' refers to something new in discourse. The pronominal adjective *sellanen* (in the genitive case: *sellasen*) is an adjectival derivative of the pronoun *se* 'it'.

Finnish word order is often characterised as being relatively free with 'very few genuinely grammatical constraints' (Vilkuna, 1989: 9–10). It is true that syntactic permutations rarely yield ungrammatical orderings; consider (10).

(10) a. *Liisa*   *rakasta-a*   *Matti-a.*
        Lisa+NOM   love-PRES+3SG   Matti-PTV
        'Lisa loves Matti.'
     b. *Matti-a*   *rakasta-a*   *Liisa.*
        Matti-PTV   love-PRES+3SG   Liisa+NOM
        Grammatically: 'Lisa loves Matti.'
        Thematically: 'Matti is loved by Lisa.' (theme: Matti)
     c. *Matti-a*   *Liisa*   *rakasta-a.*
        Matti-PTV   Lisa+NOM   love-PRES+3SG
        Grammatically: 'Lisa loves Matti.'
        Thematically: 'It is Matti who Lisa loves' (contrast: Matti)
     d. *Rakasta-a*   *Liisa*   *Matti-a.*
        love-PRES+3SG   Lisa+NOM   Matti-PTV

Grammatically: 'Lisa loves Matti.'
Thematically: 'Lisa does love Matti (against all odds).'

Examples (10a–d) all share the same grammatical meaning: *Liisa* is the subject who loves *Matti*, the object. The sentences differ in their discourse structure: in (10b) *Matti* is the theme; the sentence could apply in a context where the topic is love, and the sentences tell about who is being loved by whom. In (10c), the placement of *Matti* in the initial position before the theme *Liisa* reveals contrast: it is Matti who Lisa loves (not Pentti). In (10d), the verb *rakastaa* 'loves' is in contrast position and the sentence conveys that the loving is against expectations or in contrast to doing something else (e.g. detesting) (for an in-depth discussion of Finnish word order, see Vilkuna, 1989).

In sum, word order is very flexible and changes in the ordering of elements convey changes in the discourse meaning and not in the grammatical analysis. However, actual language use shows clear tendencies. Several corpus-based studies of Finnish have shown that the subject tends to precede the verb, and the object to come after the verb. In Hakulinen *et al.*'s data from written Finnish, the subject preceded the verb in 61% of the clauses (Hakulinen *et al.*, 1980: 145), and in Huumo's data from literary fiction the percentage was around 77% (Huumo, 1994). In Helasvuo's data from everyday conversation, over 90% of the subjects preceded the verb (Helasvuo, 2001: 77). In other words, in clauses where there is a subject and an object or a predicate nominal/adjective, the ordering is mostly likely SVX.

Appendix: Grammatical Glosses

Nominal categories

ADE	adessive ('on (top of) something')
ADJ	derivational suffix which derives adjectives from nominal elements
GEN	genitive
NOM	nominative
PL	plural
PTV	partitive

Verbal categories

IMP	imperative mood
PRES	present tense
PST	past tense
1SG	first person singular (likewise 2nd and 3rd)
1PL	first person plural (likewise 2nd and 3rd)

Notes

1. Differing from Hakulinen *et al.*, this book uses the International Phonetic Alphabet notation in all symbols.
2. In lexical nouns (such as *talo* 'house') the suffix *t* marks plural. Thus, *talo-t* is not an accusative form, but the nominative plural for *talo* 'house'. The *t*-accusative is only restricted to the marking of personal pronouns.
3. In the column for endings capital A can be realised either as front open vowel æ or the back open vowel ɑ depending on vowel harmony. Capital V stands for any vowel (its realisation depends on the quality of the last vowel of the stem. In the English translations both the definite and the indefinite article are given. Finnish does not have a fully grammaticalised marking for definiteness (see below).

References

Häkkinen, K. (1985) *Suomen kielen äänne- ja muotorakenteen historiallista taustaa [Finnish phonology and morphology in a historical perspective]*. Finska institutionen. Åbo Akademi, Åbo.

Hakulinen, A., Karlsson, F. and Vilkuna, M. (1980) *Suomen tekstilauseiden piirteitä: Kvantitatiivinen tutkimus [Features of Text Sentences in Finnish: A Quantitative Study]*. Publications of the Department of General Linguistics, vol. 6. University of Helsinki, Helsinki.

Hakulinen, A., Vilkuna, M., Korhonen, R., Koivisto, V., Heinonen, T.R. and Alho, I. (2004) *Iso suomen kielioppi [Descriptive Grammar of Finnish]*. Helsinki: Finnish Literature Society.

Helasvuo, M-L. (2001) *Syntax in the Making. The Emergence of Syntactic Units in Finnish Conversation*. Amsterdam: John Benjamins.

Helasvuo, M-L. and Laitinen, L. (2006) Person in Finnish: paradigmatic and syntagmatic relations in interaction. In M-L. Helasvuo and L. Campbell (eds) *Grammar from the Human Perspective: Case, Space and Person in Finnish*. Current Issues in Linguistic Theory. Amsterdam: John Benjamins.

Huumo, T. (1994) Näkökulmia suomen ja viron sanajärjestyseroihin [Perspectives on word order differences in Finnish and Estonian]. In *Lähivertailuja 8. Suomalais-virolainen kontrastiivinen seminaari Hailuodossa 7.–9.5.1994 [Contrastive studies on close relatives 8. Papers from the Finnish-Estonian contrastive seminar in hailuoto May 7–9, 1994]*. Oulun yliopiston suomen ja saamen kielen laitoksen tutkimusraportteja 40. Oulu: University of Oulu.

Huumo, T. and Ojutkangas, K. (2006) Finnish spatial relations: Local cases and adpositions. In M-L. Helasvuo and L. Campbell (eds) *Grammar from the Human Perspective: Case, Space and Person in Finnish*. Current Issues in Linguistic Theory. Amsterdam: John Benjamins.

Laury, R. (1997) *Demonstratives in Interaction. The Emergence of a Definite Article in Finnish*. Amsterdam: John Benjamins.

Sulkala, H. and Karjalainen, M. (1992) *Finnish. Descriptive Grammars*. London: Routledge.

'Uralic languages' (2006) In *Encyclopædia Britannica*. On WWW at http://search.eb.com/eb/article-74935. Accessed 21.6.06.

Vilkuna, M. (1989) *Free Word Order in Finnish: Its Syntax and Discourse Functions*. Helsinki: Finnish Literature Society.

Chapter 3

Tests and Assessment Methods Currently Used and New Ones Desired by Finnish Speech and Language Therapists

KERTTU HUTTUNEN, LEILA PAAVOLA and ANNE SUVANTO

Introduction

Like other countries that provide most of the social and health care services for their population through tax revenues, the Finnish government guides and supervises activities within the field of rehabilitation. In the future, national guidance will especially aim at financing branches of rehabilitation that can be proven efficient (Hesketh & Hopcutt, 1997; Valtioneuvosto, 2002). Among other professionals, speech and language therapists are also challenged to provide evidence of positive outcomes of rehabilitation (Roulstone, 2001). Since a lot of work assignments of speech and language therapists are based on judgements on classifying and measuring disorders in communication and monitoring progress in therapy, there is a great need to develop valid and reliable test instruments (Huang *et al.*, 1997). Validated tests also have many shortcomings, but quick auditory-perceptual assessments in particular are susceptible to many sources of error and bias (Cordes, 1994; Kent 1996). Therefore, justification of the use of perceptual assessment as the final basis in clinical decision-making is questionable. Moreover, using only one assessment method – even if valid and reliable – is hardly ever sufficient. In most cases observation can offer valuable additional information. Careful assessment of speech, language and communication often also requires multi-disciplinary teamwork.

Testing is often an essential part of a high-quality speech and language therapy process. However, in many countries there is a paucity of valid and reliable testing instruments. In small language districts such as

Finland, one alternative to developing new assessment methods is to translate and revalidate foreign ones; however, this is usually problematic due to differences in language structures. Additionally, human resources for developing new methods are scarce. The obvious lack of proper test instruments has led speech and language therapists in Finland to use non-standardised and self-adapted methods. Despite the limited resources, there is a growing interest among speech and language therapists in test translation and development and some projects have, indeed, already been started. This work has usually been conducted by small local groups; it is neither nationally organised nor widely communicated to colleagues.

In Finland, a definite need exists to get a firmer basis for the development of tests in the future and, in the long run, enhance unification of assessment procedures. Therefore, a national survey was carried out to examine which kinds of assessment methods are currently in use and under development, and also to identify key areas of need.

Conducting a Survey on the Use of Tests and the Need of New Ones

The public health care service system in Finland is structured into three levels; primary (health centres mainly funded by municipalities), secondary (regional hospitals providing specialised medical care, mainly funded by federations of municipalities) and tertiary (central hospitals and university hospitals owned by federations of municipalities). Services are also provided by the private sector and the so called third sector (interest groups and patient organisations working in the field of welfare and health care; these organisations are financed by, e.g. Finland's Slot Machine Association). Around two-thirds of Finnish speech and language therapists are employed by the public health care system. Our survey was addressed to speech and language therapists working in secondary and tertiary health care units. This target group was selected because work in these units substantially focuses on assessment – and hence the use of formal tests – when rehabilitation plans are being compiled. The contact information of the speech and language therapists was obtained from the member registry of a national trade union to which just over 80% of the 1000 certified Finnish speech and language therapists belonged to in 2002. Altogether 69 of the approximately 100 speech and language therapists working in central and university hospitals were contacted by telephone. The larger the population number of the central or university hospital district was, the more speech and language therapists were contacted in that district. The aim was to reach at least one speech and language therapist from all the main departments (Phoniatrics and Pedaudiology, Otorhinolaryngology, Paediatrics/Child Neurology, Neurology) of each hospital, presuming the hospital had all these units. Co-ordination and assignment of tasks within the hospital was determined in order to reach workers taking care of both children, adults and a varied range of different patient groups.

On the telephone, the speech and language therapists were asked three open-ended questions:

(1) Which tests are you currently using in your work?
(2) Do you use unpublished, that is, unofficially translated, locally developed or self-developed or adapted informal assessment methods that have a test-like character? This kind of assessment method has, for example, a systematic presentation format and/or constant material. If you use this kind of evaluation method/s, what is it/what are they?
(3) What kinds of tests would you need most in your current work?

During the telephone interview, a basic instrumental list of 60 tests and assessment methods was used as an aid. The interviewees were presented either the whole list or part of it (focusing on, e.g. the assessment of children) and asked which tests they currently had in use and which assessment methods not included in the list they used.

Respondents and Results of the Survey

Of the 69 speech and language therapists contacted, 66 responded. The number of respondents represented 7% of all Finnish certified speech and language therapists and two-thirds of the ones working in secondary and tertiary health care. Two of the respondents also rehabilitated Swedish speaking people, who constitute some 6% of the total Finnish population of 5.3 million. All five university hospital catchment areas each responsible for 700,000 to 1,700,000 inhabitants, were fairly equally represented by the number of respondents. An average of 13 speech and language therapists responded from each of the university hospital responsibility areas and an average of 3.3 from each of the 21 hospital districts included in these five university hospital responsibility areas.

The 66 respondents represented different working units in the following way: 20% worked at an outpatient department of Phoniatrics or at a Pedaudiological department/ward, 26% at an outpatient department of Othorhinolaryngology or at a hearing centre, 24% at an outpatient department or department of Child neurology, 21% at an outpatient department or department of Neurology and 9% in other units (e.g. for people with developmental delay). Altogether 43 (65%) of the respondents (re)habilitated mostly children, 18 (27%) mostly adults and five (8%) children and adults equally.

Currently used tests and assessment methods

A system of classification that was partly sample-based, and partly test theory literature-based was created to illustrate the tests and assessment methods in use (Table 3.1).

The speech and language therapists responding to the query reported that they currently used 14 test or assessment methods, on average

Table 3.1 Classification of tests and assessment procedures used by the respondents (*n* = 66)

Validated and standardised test [e.g. Reynell Developmental Language Scales III (Edwards *et al.*, 1997)]   A test published in Finland (either indigenous, i.e. developed entirely in Finland, or published abroad and translated into Finnish) that is or has been officially for sale. The test is also validated by Finnish data. Information on validity and reliability have been appropriately published, age norms/ reference materials are available and they are based on populations that are large and representative enough (age, sex, communication disorder, domicile, socioeconomic state and educational level of the person tested or his/her guardian, etc.).
Established, widely used assessment methods [e.g. Peabody Picture Vocabulary Test (Dunn & Dunn, 1981) used but not revalidated in Finland]   The material and method of administering the test is established in clinical practice, but no age norms/reference material based on careful research are available. The method is possibly (self-) translated. If there were problems in the classification of the methods, a sample-based criterion was used: if at least 10% of the respondents (seven speech and language therapists) mentioned that they currently used a certain assessment method, it was considered to be in wide use. All the screening tools were included in this class, even though they were well researched, because the scope of screening tests is narrower than that of tests suitable for diagnostic purposes.
Assessment methods in elaboration [e.g. the Finnish version of TOM; Therapy Outcome Measures (Enderby, 1997)]   An assessment method elaborated by, for example, the respondent herself alone or in a working group. It can also be a translation of a foreign test, explored in a limited fashion and currently being tried out (data for age norms/reference material are being collected): elaboration of the assessment method is clearly in progress.
Unspecified assessment procedures (e.g. series of illustrations: photos or self-drawn pictures)   The respondent does not necessarily know where, when or how the assessment procedure has been amassed; the procedure might be an unidentified copy from colleagues or from an unknown source, or it may be self-conceived or a combination from various sources/materials. The idea for the method of appraisal may be adapted from an existing test or several tests and the evaluation method has been loosely applied. Conducting the assessment procedure may differ from assessment to assessment; also the materials used may vary. Exercise materials can be used as methods of appraisal, too.

(range 1–33, SD 7, Md 13). This number also included various unspecified, self-created or self-adapted assessment procedures. One to five tests or assessment methods were used by 15% of the speech and language therapists, and six to 10 tests or assessment methods also by 15%. Most of the respondents (33%) used 11–15 and the rest (17%) used 16–20 different tests or assessment methods. The distribution of the number of tests in use by working unit and caseload profile of the respondents is illustrated in Figures 3.1 and 3.2. Generally, the use of a larger number of tests or assessment methods was associated with work among mainly children (mean 16, SD 7), compared to work among mainly adults (mean 8, SD 3). The tests and assessment methods used most often were those measuring overall language development of children and, particularly, receptive and expressive vocabulary, narration, rapid naming ability and mastery of basic concepts. With adults, aphasia, dysarthria and dysphagia were the disorders most often examined with various methods.

All the respondents used at least one formal test or unspecified assessment procedure. Validated and standardised tests (see the system of classification in Table 3.1) were used by 57 (86%) of the 66 respondents,

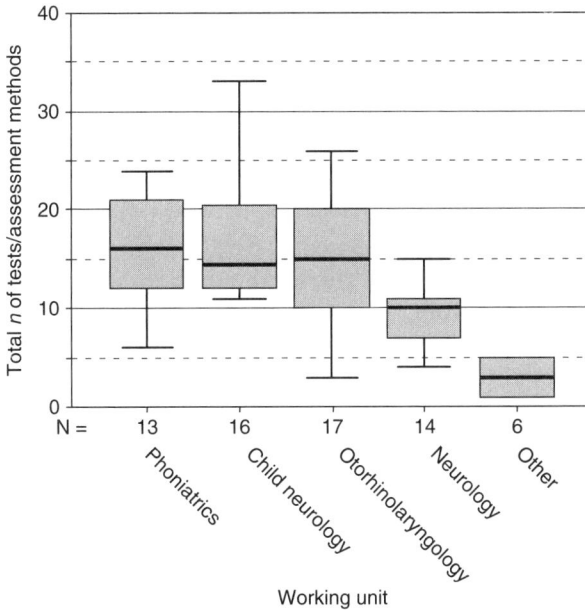

Figure 3.1 Number of tests and assessment methods used by Finnish speech and language therapists (median and quartile values by working unit). The unit 'other' refers to, for example, clinics for people with developmental delay and units providing services on (mainly technical) alternative and augmentative communication

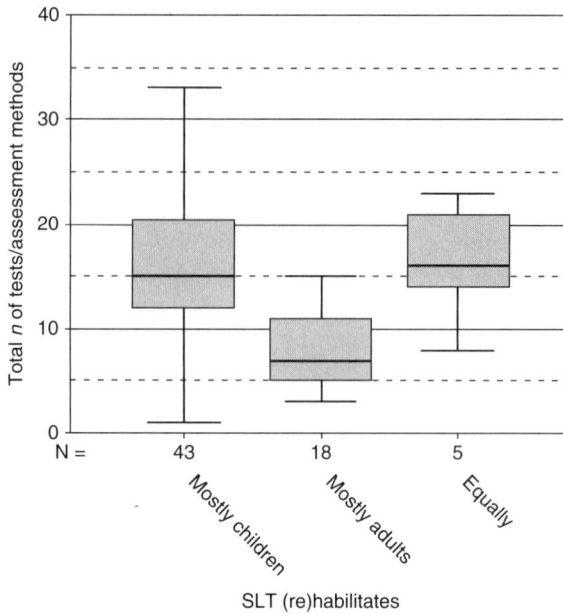

Figure 3.2 Number of tests and assessment methods used by Finnish speech and language therapists (median and quartile values by caseload profile)

63 (95%) used established, widely-used assessment methods, 40 (61%) used assessment methods currently under elaboration, and 55 (83%) used unspecified assessment procedures. The average number of tests belonging to different test or assessment method categories used by the respondents ranged from one to seven; the exact figures can be found in Table 3.2. Established (usually non-validated and non-standardised) tests

Table 3.2 Current use of tests and other assessment procedures (numbers reported per respondent)

	Mean	*Median*	*SD*	*Min*	*Max*
Validated and standardised tests	3.8	3.0	2.5	0	9
Established, widely used assessment methods	6.7	6.0	4.0	0	16
Assessment methods in elaboration	1.0	1.0	1.1	0	4
Unspecified assessment procedures	2.2	2.0	1.9	0	9

were clearly the most prevalent assessments methods used by the respondents. Almost all the assessment methods concerned the impairment level; only a fraction was constructed to measure everyday functional communication abilities. The latter were represented by the few mentions on the use of, for example, Communication Effectiveness Index (CETI, by Lomas *et al.*, 1989) and Functional Independence Measure (FIM and WeeFIM, see, e.g. Granger *et al.*, 1998 and Msall *et al.*, 1994). The International Classification of Functioning, Disability and Health (ICF, World Health Organization, 2001) provides a wide conceptual framework for multi-professional co-operation and emphasise the respectance of the bio-psychosocial unity of a human being also in the assessment of functional status. It is highly desirable that, in the future, the assessment of everyday activities and participation (social aspects of disability) is included in speech therapy.

To name a few tests, two thirds of the speech and language therapists currently used the Boston Naming Test (Kaplan *et al.*, 1976), over half used the Finnish version (Kuusinen & Blåfield, 1974) of ITPA (The Illinois Test of Psycholinguistic Abilities, Kirk *et al.*, 1968) or the (indigenous) Sentence-level test of speech comprehension (Korpilahti, 1996) (Table 3.3). The Finnish version of the Reynell Developmental Language Scales III (Edwards *et al.*, 1997) was published in 2001, and the test has already been implemented in clinical work rather well.

Altogether 94 different established assessment methods (usually not revalidated in Finland) were detailed by the respondents. Only four of these established assessment methods used by at least 10 respondents were conceived for the testing of adults. A common feature of these assessment methods was the fact that despite their typically foreign origin and fairly wide use in Finland, only a few have been examined even at a master's thesis level. Some assessment methods have Finnish norms but even in that case may lack a thorough description of a restandardisation work.

In addition to the established assessment methods for speech and language, altogether 29 speech and language therapists (44% of the respondents) mentioned that they used altogether 45 different methods of assessing cognitive abilities, contact or activities of daily living. For each respondent, the mean number of this kind of assessment method in use was 0.7 (SD 1, range 0–6). For example, the Symbolic Play Test (Lowe & Costello, 1988) was used by 12 and CARS (Childhood Autism Rating Scale) (Schopler *et al.*, 1980) by four respondents.

If the established assessment methods (mostly not revalidated in Finland) were in wide use, so were various unspecified assessment procedures, too. As these 154 different unspecified assessment methods reported to be currently in use were so extremely varied, we do not present this assessment method category in detail. Instead, the results are summarised into four larger groups, separately for children and adults (Table 3.4). Most

Table 3.3 Validated and standardised tests published in Finland currently used by the respondents (n = 66)

	Number of different mentions	% out of the 66 respondents	% out of the validated and standardised tests
Boston Naming Test (Kaplan et al., 1976)	42	63.6	16.7
Illinois Test of Psycholinguistic Abilities (Kirk et al., 1968)*	39	59.1	15.5
Kuullun ymmärtämisen lausetasoinen testi (Korpilahti, 1996) (Sentence-level test of speech comprehension)	37	56.1	14.7
Reynell Developmental Language Scales III (Edwards et al., 1997)	27	40.9	10.8
Nopean sarjallisen nimeämisen testi (Ahonen et al., 1999) (Test for rapid serial naming)	24	36.4	9.6
MacArthur Communicative Development Inventories (MCDI I or II) (Fenson et al., 1991)	23	34.8	9.2
Boston Diagnostic Aphasia Test (Goodglass & Kaplan, 1983)	22	33.3	8.8
Morfologiatesti (Lyytinen, 1988) (Morphology test)	20	30.3	8.0
ALLU – Ala-asteen lukutesti (Lindeman, 2000) (Reading test for the primary school)	13	19.7	5.2
Kuvasanavarastotesti 3–6-vuotiaille (Ruoppila, 1963) (Picture vocabulary test for 3 to 6-year-olds)	3	4.5	1.2
Perusopetuksen kirjoittamisen, kuullun ja luetun ymmärtämisen testit 1–6 luokille (Poussu-Olli & Saarni, 2001) (Writing, listening and reading comprehension test for the primary school classes from 1 to 6)	1	1.5	0.4
Total	**251**	**86.4%**	**100%**

*Many of the respondents announced that they are using only one or two subtests of the ITPA, mostly the subtests of auditory association and auditory sequential memory.

Table 3.4 Use of unspecified assessment procedures grouped in broader classes

	Number of different mentions	*% out of all unspecified assessment procedures (n = 154)*
Assessment methods for children	**99**	**64.3**
Assessment methods for linguistic functions	73	47.4
Assessment methods for speech motor functions, swallowing and voice	11	7.1
Assessment methods for reading and writing	8	5.2
Assessment methods for pragmatics	7	4.5
Assessment methods for adults	**55**	**35.7**
Assessment methods for speech motor functions, swallowing and voice	32	20.8
Assessment methods for linguistic functions	20	13.0
Assessment methods for reading and writing	2	1.3
Assessment methods for pragmatics	1	0.6

of the unspecified assessment procedures were targeted to assess children's auditory memory or narrative abilities, or speech motor functions, swallowing or the voice of adults.

New tests desired

Altogether 154 expressions of desire for new tests were specified by altogether 63 (95%) of the respondents. On average, each respondent reported a need for at least two new tests (SD 1, range 0–6); although 5% of the respondents were satisfied with the tests and assessment methods they were using, and they reported no current need for anything new. Most (63%) of the 63 respondents wishing new tests expressed a need for tests of both children and adults. A vast majority (71%) of the new tests desired were needed for the testing of children (see Table 3.5); for example, for the assessment of children's active and passive vocabulary (24 replies) and comprehensive testing of linguistic abilities of children older than 10 years of age (13 replies). Many speech and language therapists mentioned a need for a new Finnish version of the ITPA (The Illinois Test of Psycholinguistic Abilities) or a whole new test comparable to it. New tools were also desired for the assessment of linguistic concepts and expressive and narrative abilities. The current tests and assessment methods do not suffice for

Table 3.5   Expressed desires for new tests and assessment methods

	Number of different mentions	% out of the 66 respondents
Children's tests	**109**	**65.1**
Assessment methods for linguistic functions	92	63.6
Assessment methods for speech motor functions, swallowing and voice	7	10.6
Assessment methods for reading and writing	9	13.6
Assessment methods for pragmatics	1	1.5
Adults' tests	**45**	**37.9**
Assessment methods for speech motor functions, swallowing and voice	16	19.7
Assessment methods for linguistic functions	15	16.7
Assessment methods for reading and writing	5	7.6
Assessment methods for pragmatics	9	9.1
Total (expressed desires)	**154**	**95%**

specific child populations with sensory impairments or problems with motor development, and new tests were desired to measure these children's linguistic capacity. Tests desired for the assessment of adults were more heterogeneous: new tools were needed to assess for example, voice, dysphagia, dysarthria, mild aphasias and stroke patients in different phases of recovery.

Somewhat contradictorily, some speech and language therapists hoped for new tests which are suitable for a comprehensive examination but, at the same time, would be quick to administer.

Discussion

In the present survey, the response rate (coverage of the universe selected, that is, speech and language therapists working in secondary and tertiary care units) was better than usually reported in similar surveys (Hesketh & Hopcutt, 1997; Huang *et al.*, 1997). This might be due to the way of collecting the data; that is, conducting the survey by telephone interview. However, a relatively short contact via telephone might have resulted in a restricted number of tests or assessment methods being recalled (although rather many colleagues quickly checked the set of tests they had in their working facilities). In spite of this, at least the number of validated and standardised instruments used by Finnish speech and language therapists was in line with reports from elsewhere (Huang *et al.*, 1997).

Speech and language therapists need valid and reliable assessment methods to accurately demonstrate the need for and outcome of intervention (Hicks, 1998). Evidence-based, cost-effective practice and proper allocation of funds for rehabilitation inevitably require sound and efficient outcome measurement tools. Furthermore, at the level of an individual patient, the use of uniform and valid assessment methods helps to make comparisons of testing results when a person is (re)habilitated or followed-up by several professionals one after the other.

Our national survey showed that Finnish speech and language therapists, serving a population of slightly over 5 million people who, for the most part, speak a minor Fenno-Ugric language, have rather few validated and standardised tests for their work. Most of the unspecified assessment procedures in use were targeted for assessing children's auditory memory or narrative abilities, or speech motor functions, swallowing or the voice of adults. One could think that a frequent use of unspecified assessment procedures indicates a clear need of formal tests for the above-mentioned areas. This was confirmed by the answers given when need for new tests was asked.

The need for new tests is obvious. Translation and revalidation of foreign tests is one solution, and many tests have already been translated and piloted. For example, assessment of usability of various tests has been done or reference material for age norms or different special populations have been collected during the past 20 years in over 50 master's theses at the Finnish universities educating speech and language therapists (e.g. Joki, 1995; Korhonen & Lappalainen, 2000; Lahtinen, 1997; Takala, 1997). However, the translation process may be hampered by differences in language structures (grammar and phoneme systems) or cultural characteristics. When a translation and revalidation process of a test is started, it is important to have a clear idea of what the essential characteristics of each language are. Sometimes equivalent expressions reflecting the targeted morpho-syntactic structures are hard to find in different languages. Not surprisingly, when using some of the children's tests translated into Finnish, we personally have experienced inconvenience with the somewhat clumsy or too formal linguistic expressions sometimes resulting from the translation process. We also find it important that the same length and difficulty level of the original test would be maintained as closely as possible. If the difficulty level of a test differs from language to another, possibility for the sound comparison of results of scientific research is endangered. Naturally, national norms for, for example, different age groups, may differ from country to country and they need to be clearly introduced. Apart from that, sometimes a part of the difficulty of a test and hence, variance in the test results, derives from the form of the test. If test instructions are ambiguous or admit several interpretations, a person tested, especially a child, may adopt a wrong answering strategy which results in lower scores that do not reflect his or hers actual skill level. We have some concerns that this kind of problems with internal validity may occur when tests are translated and restandardised.

In many cases, pilot versions of the tests translated into Finnish have neither been effectively communicated to colleagues nor refined into their final, validated versions. Especially in small language districts, co-operation within and between different disciplines is needed when conceiving indigenous tests. Encouraging examples, such as the ALLU test (Lindeman, 2000), have shown that unifying the efforts of different groups of professionals in the collection and processing of large data may well lead to a high-quality, valid and reliable testing instrument. Tests for small special populations with rare disorders are usually possible to construct only with sufficient human resources in areas representing dominant languages.

Construction of new tests or translation of foreign ones does not, however, suffice. Speech and language therapists need to be well-grounded in test theory (or at least in the basics of clinical research) in order to recognise the strengths and weaknesses of informal non-validated tests, and to identify properly validated ones as they become available. They also need to have appropriate abilities in reliable administration (John & Enderby, 2000; Raaijmakers *et al.*, 1995) and careful interpretation of test results (Howlin & Kendall, 1991). This poses challenges to the high-quality basic and continuing education of speech and language therapists but, in turn, strengthens the scientific base of the profession and enhances quality improvement of rehabilitation. One also has to remember that together with in-depth mastery of testing procedures, good interactional and observational proficiency is an integral part of the speech and language therapist's professional skills.

Our survey laid down lines for the translation process and conception of entirely new tests in Finland. These kinds of surveys are needed to build nationally accepted approaches for the measurement of intervention outcomes that are suitable for the health care system in question.

References

Ahonen, T., Tuovinen, S. and Leppäsaari, T. (1999) *Nopean sarjallisen nimeämisen testi [Test for Rapid Serial Naming]*. Haukkarannan koulun julkaisusarjat, tutkimusraportit. Jyväskylä: Haukkarannan koulu.

Cordes, A.K. (1994) The reliability of observational data: I. Theories and methods for speech-language pathology. *Journal of Speech and Hearing Research* 37 (2), 264–278.

Dunn, L. and Dunn L. (1981) *Peabody Picture Vocabulary Test – Revised*. Circle Pines: American Guidance Service.

Enderby, P. (1997) *TOM (Therapy Outcome Measures)*. San Diego: Singular Publishing Group.

Edwards, S., Fletcher, P., Garman, M., Hughes, A., Letts, C. and Sinka, I. (1997) *Reynell Developmental Language Scales III. Third Edition. Manual*. Windsor: NFER-Nelson.

Fenson, L., Dale, P.S., Reznick, J.S., Thal, D., Bates, E., Hartung, J.P., Pethick, S. and Reilly, J.S. (1991) *Technical Manual for the MacArthur Communicative Development Inventories*. San Diego: Singular. Translated and adapted Finnish versions: Lyytinen, P. (1999) *MCDI I. Varhaisen kommunikaation ja kielen kehityksen arviointimenetelmä*. Jyväskylä: Jyväskylän yliopiston lapsitutkimuskeskus & Niilo Mäki Instituutti and Lyytinen, P. (1999) *MCDI II. Varhaisen kommunikaation ja kielen kehityksen arviointimenetelmä*. Jyväskylä: Niilo Mäki Instituutti.

Goodglass, H. and Kaplan, E. (1983) *Boston Diagnostic Aphasia Test*. Baltimore: Waverly.

Granger, C.V., Hamilton, B.B., Linacre, J.M., Heinemann, A.W. and Wright, D.B. (1998) Performance profiles of the Functional Independence Measure. *American Journal of Physical Medicine* 79 (3), 235–240.

Hesketh, A. and Hopcutt, B. (1997) Outcome measures for aphasia therapy: It's not what you do, it's the way that you measure it. *European Journal of Disorders of Communication* 32 (3, Special number), 189–202.

Hicks, P. (1998) Outcomes measurement requirements. In C.M. Frattali (ed.) *Measuring Outcomes in Speech-Language Pathology* (pp. 28–49). New York: Thieme.

Howlin, P. and Kendall, L. (1991) Assessing children with language tests – Which tests to use? *British Journal of Disorders of Communication* 26 (3), 355–367.

Huang, R-J., Hopkins, J. and Nippold, M.A. (1997) Satisfaction with standardized language testing: A survey of speech-language pathologists. *Language, Speech and Hearing Services in Schools* 28 (1), 12–23.

John, A. and Enderby, P. (2000) Reliability of speech and language therapists using therapy outcome measures. *International Journal of Language & Communication Disorders* 35 (2), 287–302.

Joki, K. (1995) CELF-R:n suomenkielisen version soveltuvuus 10-vuotiaille lapsille [Applicability of the Finnish version of the CELF-R Test for 10-year old children]. Unpublished Master's thesis, University of Helsinki, Helsinki, Finland.

Kaplan, E., Goodglass, H. and Weintraub, S. (1976) *Boston Naming Test. Experimental Edition*. Boston: Boston Aphasia Research Center, Boston University.

Kent, R.D. (1996) Hearing and believing: Some limits to the auditory-perceptual assessment of speech and voice disorders. *American Journal of Speech and Language Pathology* 5 (3), 7–23.

Kirk, S., McCarthy, J. and Kirk, W. (1968) *The Illinois Test of Psycholinguistic Abilities (ITPA). Revised*. Illinois: University of Illinois Press.

Korhonen, N. and Lappalainen, M. (2000) Communication and Symbolic Behavioral Scales – testi: pilottitutkimus yksivuotiailla, normaalisti kehittyneillä suomenkielisillä lapsilla [Communication and Symbolic Behavioral Scales: A pilot study on 1-year-old, normally developing Finnish speaking children]. Unpublished Master's thesis, University of Oulu, Oulu, Finland.

Korpilahti, P. (1996) *Kuullun ymmärtämisen lausetasoinen testi [A Sentence Level Test for Speech Understanding]*. Helsinki: Language and Communication Care.

Kuusinen, J. and Blåfield, L. (1974) *Psykolingvististen kykyjen testi ITPA: Testaajan opas [The Illinois Test of Psycholinguistic Abilities (ITPA). Examiner's Manual]*. KTL:n julkaisuja 234. Jyväskylä: University of Jyväskylä.

Lahtinen, J. (1997) The Bus Story lasten narratiivisena tutkimusmenetelmänä [The Bus Story as a narrative assessment method for children]. Unpublished Master's thesis, University of Oulu, Oulu, Finland.

Lindeman, J. (2000) *ALLU – Ala-asteen lukutesti. Käyttäjän käsikirja [ALLU – Reading Test for Primary School. User's Manual]*. Turku: University of Turku, Oppimistutkimuksen keskus.

Lomas, P., Pickard, L., Bester, S., Elbard, H., Finlayson, A. and Zoghaib, C. (1989) The Communicative Effectiveness Index: Development and psychometric evaluation of a functional measure for adult aphasia. *Journal of Speech and Hearing Disorders* 54 (1), 113–124.

Lowe, M. and Costello, A.J. (1988) *Symbolic Play Test*. London: NFER-Nelson.

Lyytinen, P. (1988) *Morfologiatesti. Taivutusmuotojen hallinnan mittausmenetelmä lapsille [The Morphology Test. A Measure of the Mastery of Children's Inflectional Forms]*. Reports from the Department of Psychology 298. Jyväskylä: University of Jyväskylä.

Msall, M.E., DiGaudio, K., Rogers, B.T., LaForest, S., Catanzaro, N.L., Campbell, J., Wilczenski, F. and Duffy, L.C. (1994) The Functional Independence Measure for Children (WeeFIM). Conceptual basis and pilot use in children with developmental disabilities. *Clinical Pediatrics (Phila.)* 33 (7), 421–430.

Poussu-Olli, H-S. and Saarni, M. (2001) *Perusopetuksen kirjoittamisen, kuullun ja luetun ymmärtämisen testit 1–6 luokille [Tests for Writing, Speech Understanding and Reading Comprehension for the Primary School Classes from 1 to 6]*. Naantali: Scribeo.

Raaijmakers, M.F., Dekker, J., Dejonckere, P.H. and van der Zee, J. (1995) Reliability of the assessment of impairments, disabilities and handicaps in survey research on speech therapy. *Folia Phoniatrica et Logopaedica* 47 (4), 199–209.

Roulstone, S. (2001) Consensus and variation between speech and language therapists in the assessment and selection of preschool children for intervention: A body of knowledge or idiosyncratic decisions? *International Journal of Language and Communication Disorders*, 36 (3), 329–348.

Ruoppila, I. (1963) *Kuvasanavarastotesti 3–6-vuotiaille [The Picture Vocabulary Test for 3 to 6-Year-Olds]*. KTL:n julkaisuja 10. Jyväskylä: University of Jyväskylä.

Schopler, E., Reichler, R.J. and Renner, B. (1980) *Childhood Autism Rating Scale*. New York: Irvington Publishers.

Takala, E. (1997) The Communicative Effectiveness Index (CETI) afaatikkojen toiminnallisen kommunikaation kuvaajana [The Communicative Effectiveness Index (CETI) as a depictor of functional communication of persons with aphasia]. Unpublished Master's thesis, University of Helsinki, Helsinki, Finland.

Valtioneuvosto (Finnish Government) (2002) *Kuntoutusselonteko 2002. Valtioneuvoston selonteko eduskunnalle [Report on Rehabilitation. Government Report to the Parliament]*. Publications of the Ministry of Social Affairs and Health 6. Helsinki: Ministry of Social Affairs and Health.

World Health Organization (2001) *International Classification of Functioning, Disability and Health*. Geneva: WHO. Translated into Finnish in 2004: ICF – Toimintakyvyn, toimintarajoitteiden ja terveyden kansainvälinen luokitus. Ohjeita ja luokituksia 2004, 4. Helsinki: Stakes.

Part 2

Characteristics of Finnish and the Study of Child Speech and Language Disorders

Chapter 4

Normal and Disordered
Phonological Acquisition in Finnish

PIRJO KULJU and TUULA SAVINAINEN-MAKKONEN

Introduction

Until the 1980s, Finnish child phonology research focused predomi-
nately on case studies and mainly on the acquisition of phoneme inventory.
However, since the introduction of autosegmental phonology in the 1980s,
including the prosodic hierarchy (Selkirk, 1980), child phonologists have
modelled the prosodic or hierarchical development of word structures
(e.g. Demuth, 1995; Nettelbladt, 1983; Stoel-Gammon, 1996). In recent years,
Finnish studies have also focused more on the hierarchical structure of
words. For example, Turunen (2003) presented a hypothetical model on the
acquisition of word structures in Finnish. Furthermore, Savinainen-
Makkonen (1996, 2001) presented several examples of how Finnish word
structures can be acquired. For instance, the following example illustrates
the acquisition path of a trisyllabic word, /æmpæri/ *ämpäri* 'bucket', in
one child (Savinainen-Makkonen, 1996; Turunen, 2003):

Word level (syllable number) not complete:	[æ:pæ] 1;6–1;7
Syllable level (syllable heaviness) not complete:	[æpæi] 1;8
Phonotactics (cons. sequence) not complete:	[æ:pæ.it] 1;9
	(/æmpærit/plural)
Phoneme level (/r/) not complete:	[æm.pæ.li] 1;9
A target-like word structure:	[æm.pæ.ri] 3;6

Thus, when exploring phonological acquisition, the interplay of phonemes, phonotactics and syllables should be taken into account. It is also
essential to note that different languages have different acquisition paths,
that is, even a deviant feature in one language may be part of a normal
process in an another language.

This chapter is an attempt to draw together the information we have on
Finnish children's phonological development from phoneme inventories
and phonotactics, to the acquisition of word length. Presented next is a

description of Finnish studies on children's phonological acquisition. The following section focuses on consonant inventories, as well as on consonant sequences and quantity distinction. In addition, the vowels will be examined from their order of acquisition to their phonotactics from the point of view of diphthongs and Finnish vowel harmony. In these sections dealing with consonants and vowels, we will also attempt to describe the results from studies concerning atypical language development in Finnish. Although the atypical development of the phonological system of a child should be seen as an acquisition of both paradigmatic and syntagmatic units, current knowledge is based mainly on articulation errors, and only scattered remarks have been made on the deviant phonological acquisition of Finnish. We will focus on syllables and the acquisition of word structures from disyllabic first words to multisyllabic words. Finally, we will expand the discussion from early phonology to its relation to early reading skills and introduce the main results concerning the early phonological precursors of dyslexia.

Studies on Finnish Child Phonology

Menn and Stoel-Gammon (1995) distinguish three main types of child language research: diary studies, cross-sectional studies with the purpose of setting norms, and studies with experimental or naturalistic methods in order to explain linguistic characteristics of child phonology. Most of the information on Finnish phonological acquisition has thus far come from case studies of one or two normally developing infants (e.g. Iivonen, 1994; Laalo, 1994; Savinainen-Makkonen, 1996) and from one case study (Leiwo, 1977) of delayed language development. While case studies provide valuable information on individual characteristics, they cannot be generalised to show the average developmental path. The lack of extensive, systematic studies on child phonology has been recently noted in Finland, and studies on larger groups of children have been published. These systematic studies are essential in order to explore atypical phonological development. In other words, once normative limits are known, it is easier to understand what is deviant and to examine deviant language development. Recent studies have focused on the acquisition of different aspects of word structure and they have also provided quantitative information (see Turunen, 2003).

Kunnari's (2000) longitudinal study of 10 normally developing children emphasised the setting of norms. Kunnari investigated the phoneme inventory as well as the syllable structure during the 50-word stage. Savinainen-Makkonen (2001) analysed the speech of seven normally developing children from their first words to the age of 2;6. Her main purpose was to investigate whether Finnish children follow what is generally claimed to be a universal sequence for long words and for word-initial consonants. This longitudinal study by Savinainen-Makkonen and the large body of transcribed data, which is based on spontaneous speech, provides information on developmental paths in acquiring word structures. By contrast, Turunen (2003) conducted a cross-sectional study based on a picture naming task of nearly 200 children, and this work provides normative information and illustrates variation at age 2;6. The aim of Turunen's study was to investigate, in a constraint-based account, how Finnish children aged 2;6 years produced word structures, as well as to compare children at-risk for dyslexia and their controls. The study also investigated the relationship between early phonology and reading skills. In addition, Torvelainen (2005) examined early word structures, especially word length and consonant harmony. Her data from 20 children at-risk for dyslexia, as well as 20 control children, was based on spontaneous speech. In addition to word structures, she focused on variation in children's skills, as well as on the correlation between phonology, morphology, syntax and early reading skills. The studies by Turunen (2003) and Torvelainen (2005) were part of the Jyväskylä Longitudinal Study of Dyslexia-project (JLD). In the JLD-project children have been followed from birth to school age in order to define the possible early precursors of genetic dyslexia.

An example of an experimental study of Finnish child phonology is the cross-sectional study on production and perception of quantity contrast in infants by Richardson (1998). This research is exceptional in the sense that it examined perception at an early age (6 months). Her study also investigated the children at-risk for dyslexia and their controls in the JLD-project. Aoyama (2001) and Kunnari *et al.* (2001) have studied quantity contrast by comparing Finnish and Japanese children. Other than these, few studies have been conducted on Finnish vowel harmony (e.g. Leiwo *et al.*, 2006; Lieko, 1998).

Moreover, there are only few studies concerning atypical development among Finnish-speaking children. Leiwo's (1977) study reported on two boys and he specifically focused on delayed and deviant language acquisition. Furthermore, Vilkman *et al.* (1988) analysed the speech of two Finnish children with fragile X syndrome, and Mäenpää (1990) investigated six Finnish children with developmental apraxia of speech (DAS). Some studies have been published of phonological acquisition with Finnish children with hearing impairments (Huttunen, 2000, in this volume; Olkkola, 2002) and on the articulation disorders of Finnish children with cleft palates (e.g. Haapanen, 2003; Laitinen *et al.*, 1998, 1999). In addition to these studies, Takkinen (2002, in this volume) has reported on acquisition of Finnish sign language.

There are no Finnish standardised tests specifically on articulation and phonology. Beside informal home made single words tests and conversational speech sampling, speech and language therapists have a few published non-standardised tests[1] to assess children's articulation skills.

Acquisition of Consonants

Consonants

Since the Finnish consonant inventory (/p t d k m n ŋ l r s h v j/) is relatively small, it does not itself offer much challenge. The analysis of articulation manner indicates that the inventory of early words consists of stops and nasals, which is in line with the universal tendency. At the 50-word stage, at least half of Kunnari's (2000) 10 children used seven consonants (/p m t n l k h/). Here the mean size of the consonant inventory was 7.9 and the range was six to 10 consonants. This means that the most advanced Finnish children seem to be quite close to the target size of the inventory at the 50-word stage.

Moreover, the position of a consonant in a word affects phoneme acquisition. In Kunnari's (2000, 2003a, 2003b) study, word-medial consonant inventories were higher than the word initial inventories at the 50-word stage. In Turunen's (2003) naming task data,[2] 31% of the (control) children (*n* = 58) produced word initial /r/ in the word /rat:a:t/ *rattaat* 'strollers' at age 2;6, but the percentage was higher, 47%, in word-medial position in the word /pyøræ/ *pyörä* 'bike'. In addition, unlike in English, Finnish children typically also omit consonants in word-initial position (Kunnari, 2000; Savinainen-Makkonen, 2000a; Turunen, 2003). For normally developing children, this omission process does not, however, last very long. The phonemes /r/ and /s/ are among the last consonants that children acquire, and at the age of 2 years 6 months 12% of the Finnish children (*n* = 58) did not produce /r/ (or any substituting consonant) in word-initial position in the word /rat:a:t/. Furthermore, 5% did not produce /s/ (or any substituting consonant) in the word /sukla:/ *suklaa* 'chocolate' and 7% in the word /sakset/ *sakset* 'scissors' (Turunen, 2003). The omission of word initial consonants or assimilation of consonants may be due to constraints requiring consonant harmony, that is, by deleting or harmonising the word initial consonant, the child avoids a form with two different consonants, for example, [apio], [papio] /lapio/ *lapio* 'shovel' (examples from Turunen, 2003).

Finnish children seem to display a wide range of variation in the number of forms they produce with consonant harmony at the age of two. Torvelainen (2005) investigated consonant and vowel harmony in 2-year-old children's (*n* = 40) comprehensible expressions and in expressions in which the target word was unclear (note that half of her subjects were children at-risk for dyslexia with weak phonological skills).[3] Out of comprehensible word productions, 28% were fully harmonised among the weakest fifth of the children, for example, [pup:u] /kup:i/ *kuppi* 'cup'; however, the proportion of fully harmonised productions was only 3% among the most advanced children. The proportion of fully harmonised production was as high as 72% among the weakest children in the productions with an unclear target word. Torvelainen (2005) thus concludes that strong phonotactic constraints at this age are one reason for unclear speech in young children. Several references mention that in normal language development in Finnish, as well as in English, assimilation at a distance have begins to disappear by the age of 2;6 (e.g. Grunwell, 1987: 216; Savinainen-Makkonen, 2001, 2003; Turunen, 2003). Thus, fairly rare examples at age 2;6 are, for instance, the regressive assimilation [tat: a:t] /rat:a:t/ 'strollers' and the progressive assimilation in [py:'py] /pyøræ/ pyörä 'bike' (Turunen, 2003).

The position of the phoneme may also affect the substitution type. For example, as the children's productions of the above-mentioned words /rat:a:t/ and /pyøræ/ were compared at age 2;6 (Turunen, 2003), it was found that the most common substituting consonants for /r/ in /rat:a:t/ were /h/ (21%) and /l/ (21%), while in the word /pyøræ/ the most common substituting consonant was /l/, which occurred in 41% of the productions. As in Italian (Bortolini & Leonard, 1991), the most common phoneme substitute for /r/ is usually /l/. However, children at a later age try to avoid homonyms, so that instead of producing /l/ – and not yet being able to produce a correctly trilled /r/ – they try to use some kind of phonetic variant of /r/, such as an uvular ([ʀ]) or a fricative ([ð]). Young children also generally substitute /s/ with /t/.[4] At a later age phonetic error is more common: interdental [θ]) and lateral ([ɬ]) variants, which are not included in the Finnish consonant inventory, are often substituted for [s].

Only a few Finnish studies focus specifically on the consonant inventory of the later stages in phonological acquisition. In case studies by Iivonen (1986, 1998), Toivainen (1990, 1997) and Savinainen-Makkonen (1996), the last consonants to be mastered were /r/,/d/ and /ŋ/. The apico-alveolar trill, /r/, is acquired late because it is motorically difficult to produce. In Turunen's (2003) cross sectional study based on a naming task, 11% of the 2;6-year-old children ($n = 196$) produced /r/ in all of their productions of the target words including /r/, and 40% did not produce /r/ in any of these words.[5] Whereas English-speaking children acquire the /d/ very early, which attests to its ease of production, it is among the consonants that are acquired late in the Finnish context. This difference comes from distributional regularities of the input: both /d/ and /ŋ/ are highly restricted in adult Finnish.[6] In addition, the functional load of these late consonants is low (Warren, 2001). Besides /r/, the alveolar fricative /s/ is motorically difficult to produce, and these two sounds are the most common reasons for Finnish children to undergo articulation therapy. Turunen (2003) observed that the /s/ was acquired earlier than /r/, since 32% of the children ($n = 196$) produced /s/ in all of their productions of the target words including /s/, and 18% were unable to produce it in any target words. However, it is not necessary to produce/s/ phonetically correctly or accurately to convey meaning, since in Finnish /s/ does not have phonologically close neighbours, such as the [θ] and [ð] in English.

Acquisition of quantity distinction

A special characteristic of Finnish phonology is quantity distinction. In Finnish, short and long quantity form minimal pairs both in vowels and in consonants. This distinction is visually marked in the orthography as a short segment is written with one letter and a long segment with two letters, for example, *kuka – kukka* 'who – flower', *raja – raaja* 'border – limb'.

Lyytinen *et al.* (1995) have pointed out that the perception and production of Finnish quantity distinction should be studied in the area of dyslexia, since it is typical for Finnish dyslexics to make mistakes in marking the distinction orthographically. It has been shown that dyslexia may be related to perception of temporal information (e.g. Tallal, 1980). Richardson (1998) examined Finnish children's ability to perceive durational information as early as at 6 months of age. She also compared children with a familial risk for dyslexia and their controls. Her main result was that the children did categorise the sounds based on duration but the at-risk children needed longer durational time in order to categorise a sound as long.

It has also been shown that the quantity contrast appears early in children's speech production. Both Richardson (1998) and Kunnari *et al.* (2001) have demonstrated that when children utter their first words at one year of age, already six months later, at the age of 18 months, they are able to differentiate singleton from geminate targets in production. In the study by Saaristo-Helin *et al.* (2006) about 78% of the geminates were correctly used by Finnish children (*n* = 17) at the 50-word stage.

Few cross-linguistic studies exist that analyse quantity contrast. Aoyama (2001) has compared the acquisition of nasal quantity contrast between Finnish and Japanese children at the ages of 3–5. Aoyama found that Finnish children mastered the contrast at age 3, whereas differences were found among Japanese children in the same tasks. The Finnish and Japanese children were also compared by Kunnari *et al.* (2001), but at an earlier age. They discovered that Finnish children begin to differentiate singleton from geminate targets in production by the end of the one-word period whereas Japanese children, although also exposed to a language that makes quantitative contrasts in medial consonants, begin to distinguish them later. The fact that quantity frequency is nearly twice as frequent in Finnish as in Japanese, was offered as an explanation. Indeed, geminate words are very common early Finnish targets. At the 50-word stage, more than 40% of the (adult) words targeted by 17 Finnish-speaking children included a geminate (Saaristo-Helin *et al.*, 2006). Including onomatopoeic and baby talk words, the number of geminate forms would be much higher still.

Consonant sequences

Besides the acquisition of individual consonants, consonant sequences[7] have also been the focus of some studies on Finnish child language. Word-initial consonant clusters are quite common in Finnish but they appear only in loanwords, for example, /traktori/ *traktori* 'tractor'. Complex codas, for example, /nurk:a/ *nurkka* 'corner', and word-medial consonant sequences belong to the original Finnish grammar. Based on Karlsson (1983), there are at least 57 word-medial consonant sequences in the original vocabulary, for example, /jærvi/ *järvi* 'a lake'.

Consonant sequences are a challenge in early speech. Saaristo-Helin *et al.* (2006) observed that 17 normally developing children correctly produced only 16% of the targeted consonant sequences (or clusters) at the 50-word stage. Nevertheless, soon after the lexical milestone of 50 words, children seem to start to produce word-medial consonant sequences. An analysis of the data of seven children in three studies (Savinainen-Makkonen, 1996; Iivonen, 1998; Selin, 2005), reveals that the first realisations may appear as early as at the age of 18 months. By the age of 2;6 children have four to 18 correctly produced and stable word-medial consonant sequences in their phonological system. For these seven children, the first correctly produced consonant sequences were /mp/, /nt/ and /ŋk/. As pointed out by Turunen (2003) a child seems to start off with homorganic sequences and then proceeds to more complex sequences (see also Chervela, 1981). However, even more discreet levels of possible acquisition paths were found by Turunen (2003). These levels are illustrated in the productions of the target word /pork:a na/ *porkkana* 'carrot'. The following examples are produced by several children at the age of 2;6:

(1) [po:k:ana]
(2) [poik:ana]
(3) [poŋk:ana]
(4) [polt:ana]
(5) [polk:ana]
(6) [pork:ana]

The target includes a sequence of the dental /r/ and velar geminate consonant /k/. Difficulties to pronounce these two consonants with different places of articulation result in a reduction in the consonant sequence. Typically, the consonant that is deleted in a sequence is the one that is more difficult to produce, often the later acquired sound, which in this case is the /r/. Furthermore, it is typical for children to produce a long vowel instead of a consonant sequence as in (1). In such cases the child preserves the heaviness of the initial stressed syllable by lengthening the vowel and thereby filling the timing unit slot (also e.g. [mæ:kæ] for /mærkæ/ *märkä* 'wet' in Iivonen, 1994). Compensatory lengthening is especially common in consonant sequences with a liquid as the first member of the sequence (Savinainen-Makkonen & Kunnari, 2004; Selin, 2005). In addition, homorganic consonant sequences may be reduced in the same way, for example, [aːkːa] /aŋkːa/ *ankka* 'duck' (Selin, 2005). Nevertheless, a few children produced a diphthong instead of a long vowel as in (2).

Examples (3) and (4) are rarer but they are worth mentioning since the consonant sequence is produced but it is homorganic. One could suggest that this type of productions are more advanced than forms with a lengthened vowel since they do include a consonant sequence. The production type (5) includes a heterorganic consonant sequence but /r/ is substituted by /l/. Children often substitute sounds for the motorically demanding sound, such as /r/ and /s/ in Finnish (Selin, 2005). Example (5) above thus illustrates a common final stage of phonological acquisition before the target-like production in (6). In Turunen (2003), 44% of the (control) children (*n* = 77) produced a target-like form of the word /porkːana/ at age 2;6. These productions thus tentatively illustrate a possible developmental path in acquiring consonant sequences, although the examples are drawn from a cross-sectional database.

The following results further illustrate the general level of the production of word-medial consonant sequences at the age of 2;6 in Finnish. In a naming task data at age 2;6, the word-medial consonant sequence /ks/ in the target word /sakset/ *sakset* 'scissors' was assimilated in 35% of the subjects (*n* = 86), resulting in productions such as [takːet]. However, 9% of the children produced an inaccurate consonant sequence, for example, [satset], and as many as 56% produced a target-like sequence. In some cases, the assimilation also spread to the word-initial consonant, such as [kakːe] (Turunen, 2003).

Unfortunately the development of the medial consonant sequences of 3–5-year-old children has been studied less than in younger children. Iivonen (1998) compared three Finnish children and reported that the few cases of word-initial clusters Finnish children targeted show the same late acquisition time as the English data put forth by Grunwell (1987) and Stoel-Gammon and Dunn (1985). Yet Finnish children seem to acquire medial consonant sequences earlier than English-speaking children acquire the English word-initial and final clusters.

Consonants and disorders

In clinical practice a diagnosis of an articulation disorder is usually differentiated from a phonological disorder. According to Luotonen (1998),[8] as many as 32.5% of 5-year-olds have *articulation errors* in consonants; the proportion of /r/ among the errors is 60% and the proportion of /s/ is 30%. The amount of errors has decreased to 18% among 7-year-olds and out of 9-year-olds only 7% have articulation errors. As seen above, /r/ and /s/ are also among the last consonants that the children acquire.

The differences in consonant acquisition between *late talkers*[9] and controls are apparent; a cross-sectional data of 2;6-year-old late talkers showed that they were significantly weaker than their controls in the production of both /s/ and /r/. For example, of the 22 late talkers who produced the target word /pyøræ/ *pyörä* 'bike', only 23% (five children) produced /r/, whereas 47% of the control group (*n* = 64) produced /r/ in this target.

How are children with *phonological disorders of consonants* different from normally developing ones in the production of consonants? So far we do not have enough studies dealing with Finnish children to get an overall picture of the normal and the atypical patterns. However, disordered children seem to have at least *persisting normal processes*. They may, for example, produce harmonised forms longer than normally developing children. In addition, they seem to use substitutions, for example, /r/ → /l/, longer, whereas (phonetic) distortions, for example, /r/ → [ʀ], occur primarily in the production of the older, normally developing children. Thus, children with phonological disorder of consonants may have a small inventory of consonants and are unable to use sounds contrastively, which results in their using a large number of homonyms. Moreover, some processes may be confirmed as *atypical patterns*. However, studies dealing with atypical children are an absolute prerequisite in order to define these patterns. These processes might be language-specific as is in the case of word-initial consonant omission: although it is atypical in English (Grunwell, 1987; Howell & Dean, 1994), it is a normal process among children acquiring Finnish (Kunnari, 2000; Savinainen-Makkonen, 2000a; Turunen, 2003).

Normal hearing is crucial for speech and language acquisition. Children with *hearing impairment* often have restricted consonant paradigms (Huttunen, 2000, 2001; see also Huttunen in this volume). Likewise young children using cochlear implants (CI) also have smaller inventories than children in the same lexical stage who have normal hearing (Olkkola, 2002; see Lonka in this volume).

Among organically based problems such as the *cleft palate*, articulation disorders are very common. For instance, the inability to close the velopharyngeal port effects nasalisation as well as other articulatory problems. Out of 280 Finnish 6-year-old children with cleft palates, 44% misarticulated either the /r/ (36%), /s/ (23%) or /l/ (18%) (Laitinen *et al.*, 1998). In addition, posterior cross bites have been significantly associated with defective articulation, so that this is considered as an additional risk factor for correct dental articulation in cleft-affected children (Laitinen *et al.*, 1999). Besides surgical treatment and traditional speech therapy, motor activators (intraoral removable palatal plates) have recently been used to stimulate the tongue movements required for speech articulation (see Haavio, 2001, for a more detailed discussion of the development of oral motor habilitation in Finland). Haapanen (2003) found improvement especially among dentoalveolar consonants in her pilot study of children with cleft palates ($n = 36$). Due to oral plate therapy today, the number of simple articulation errors might already be reduced.

Developmental apraxia of speech (DAS) among children acquiring Finnish has been analysed only in one study of six children (Mäenpää, 1990). Speech characteristics of several of these 5–6-year-old children included consonant harmony, consonant reduction and other typical early phonological processes that normally developing children have suppressed at the same chronological age. Although developmental apraxia of speech is a disorder in the programming of articulation movements, including especially difficulties in sequencing speech movements, Mäenpää's (1990) study also revealed a restricted phonemic repertoire for this disorder. A statistically significant difference emerged between children with developmental apraxia of speech and control children in the amount of consonant errors (in simple CV-syllables). In addition to the above-mentioned, the dentals /r, s, l/ as well as /k/ were difficult. Vilkman *et al.* (1988) found the speech difficulties of two Finnish speakers with *fragile X syndrome* (5- and 8-year-olds) in many respects similar to those of speakers with developmental apraxia. Despite their good performance in isolated words in articulation tests, the intelligibility of connected speech was poor. Perseveration, dysfluency and poor performance in repetition tasks were evident. Most consonant substitution errors occurred in dentals (e.g. /s/, /r/). Somewhat surprisingly, a tendency toward spirantisation was common for both speakers.

Acquisition of Vowels

Vowels

Finnish has eight vowel phonemes /a, e, i, o, u, y, æ, ø/. Specific characteristics regarding vowels are quantity distinction and vowel harmony, which is dealt with below. Differences in vowels across linguistic communities emerge already in the end of the first year of life. A comparative spectrographic analysis did not show differences between Finnish and Russian vowel-like sounds produced during the first three months of life (Lyakso & Silvén, 2002). However, by the age of six months, language-specific characteristics started to appear.

As in many other languages, Finnish vowel acquisition has been studied much less than consonants. The main reasons behind this may be the facts that vowels are mastered earlier than consonants, and that even those children with disordered phonology seem to commit fewer errors in vowels than in consonants. Torvelainen (2005) found that in the speech of 2-year-old children ($n = 40$) consonants were fully harmonised in 6% of the words and vowels were harmonised only in 1% of the words; furthermore, the proportion of productions with both consonant and vowel harmony was 4% (see previous section on consonants). Iivonen (1994, 2004) found language-specific features in his case studies on his normally developing sons. Compared to Jakobson's (1941) often cited universal theory, Iivonen's children differed particularly in the production of their first vowels, for example, /i/ was not acquired among the very first vowels. Both Iivonen's (2004) two sons and Itkonen's (1977) son produced all Finnish eight vowels by the age of 2;6, the latest being /y/ and /ø/. In Huttunen's study (2000), the vowels of five normally developing 3-year-olds were very well stabilised.

Diphthongs

Finnish has eighteen diphthongs altogether, as for example in /laiva/ *laiva* 'boat', /leipæ/ *leipä* 'bread', /yø/ *yö* 'night', /tauko/ *tauko* 'pause'. They appear quite early in children's speech, for example, [eiti], [æiti] for /æiti/ *äiti* 'mother' at ages 1;2–1;3 (Savinainen-Makkonen, 1996). Iivonen (1994) reported that the first target-like diphthongs emerged at the age of 1;8–1;9, for example, [aita] /aita/ *aita* 'fence'.

In Turunen's study (2003) of 196 children, only three children (1.5%) did not produce any diphthongs correctly in a naming task at the age of 2;6, whereas as many as 31% (*n* = 60) produced target-like diphthongs in all of their productions. The diphthongs /øy/ and /yø/ with front vowels were studied more specifically in two target words, namely /pøytæ/ *pöytä* 'table' and /pyøræ/ pyörä 'bike'. The results from both words confirmed that at the age of 2;6, approximately 80% of the (control) children were able to produce a target-like diphthong in those specific words, 8–10% produced an inaccurate diphthong and 8–10% did not produce diphthongs in those words. Productions which did not include a diphthong had a long vowel instead, as in [pø:tæ] /pøytæ/ and in [pø:læ] /pyøræ/. This indicates that by compensatory lengthening, the child preserves a heavy stressed syllable, a phenomenon which is also typical in avoiding complex consonant sequences. Inaccurate diphthongs had phoneme substitutions as in [pøipæ] /pøytæ/. In some cases the front vowels were produced as back, as in [puota] /pøytæ/. In the late talker -group the number of target-like diphthongs were lower but still more than half of late talkers produced diphthongs in those words at age 2;6.

Finnish vowel harmony

In Finnish vowel harmony, back vowels (/u/, /o/, /a/) and front vowels (/y/, /ø/, /æ/) cannot occur in the same word, unless they occur in a compound word. However, the phonologically 'neutral' unrounded front vowels (/i/, /e/) can occur with back vowels in a word, whereas the front rounded vowels (/y/, /ø/) cannot.

There are some descriptions how Finnish vowel harmony is acquired (Leiwo, 1977; Leiwo *et al.*, 2006; Lieko, 1998, 2001; Toivainen, 1997). As stated earlier in this chapter, if a child encounters problems in producing vowels, usually the front vowels are produced as back vowels and these substitutions may result in a violation of Finnish vowel harmony (e.g. [nena] for /nenæ/ 'nose', [veikea] for /veikeæ/ 'funny' and [tyhma] for /tyhmæ/ 'stupid', from Lieko, 1998). Finnish morphemes often have either front or back vowels depending on the vowels in word stem, for example, the question particle can be either -*ko* or -*kø*. According to Toivainen (1997), children sometimes used -*ko* with front vowels, thus violating vowel harmony.

Leiwo, *et al.* (2006) studied the production of vowel harmony based on a database of nearly 200 children. Their main result was that Finnish vowel harmony is not violated in general at the age of 2;6. The proportion of vowel harmony errors in a naming task was approximately 2–4%, depending on different target words. As expected, if violations occurred, they were due to problems with the front vowels /y/, /ø/ and /æ/. The back vowels did not cause any problems; they were never produced as front vowels.

The role of the 'neutral' front vowels /i/ and /e/ is interesting in the acquisition of Finnish vowel harmony, since they occur with both front and back vowels. In the study by Leiwo *et al.* (2006) these neutral vowels behaved neutrally and did not cause fronting of back vowels, as one might expect. However, the acquisition process of vowel harmony should also be investigated in younger children, since at age 2;6, the vowel system is quite advanced in children and vowel harmony does not seem to be problematic in normal language development. Leiwo *et al.* (2006) conclude that the problems with Finnish vowel harmony may be related to problems in language development. Thus, they also note that the syntagmatic aspect of vowel acquisition should be studied more systematically in order to develop diagnostic tools for the early diagnosis of language problems.

Vowels and disorders

Although out of 1600 Finnish 5-year-old children as many as 30% had *articulation disorders*, only 1.4% had problems with vowels (Pietarinen, 1987). The few vowel errors that emerged concerned the front vowels /y, æ, ø/ that were generally replaced with their corresponding back pair /u, a, o/, as in the quite rare cases in young normally developing children.

In Leiwo's (1977) study, a 7-year-old boy who had a *delayed profile in language and phonology* misarticulated almost a third of his front vowels /y, æ, ø/. Even more misarticulations were produced by a 7-year-old boy, diagnosed with SLI. Although he was able to produce all the sounds in all word positions, out of 300 productions of /y, æ, ø/, only 15% were correctly produced. In addition, /a/ was often substituted for /e/.

In accordance with studies from other languages (e.g. Maassen *et al.*, 2003), Finnish children with *developmental apraxia of speech* seem to have problems with vowels. Three of Mäenpää's (1990) six dyspraxic children (at age 4;9–6;3) had vowel errors,[10] whereas none of the six control children had them. Contrary to the supposition of the easiness of the corner vowels (/u, a, i/), for children with developmental apraxia of speech, the highest tongue postures may be especially challenging (Mäenpää, 1990). In addition, 5-year-old and 8-year-old children with *fragile X syndrome* in a study by Vilkman *et al.* (1988) had a tendency to omit vowels or substitute them. A few quantity errors of vowels were also found; long vowels were produced as short, not vice versa.

A few studies (e.g. Huttunen, 2000, 2001) focus on the vowel errors produced by Finnish children with hearing impairment. Huttunen (2001) found that 4–6-year-old children ($n = 10$) with moderate hearing impairment had twice as many vowel errors (e.g. front vowels were substituted by back vowels) as normally hearing 3-year-olds ($n = 5$). Another study (Huttunen, 2000) reported that severely and profoundly hearing-impaired children also made errors that violated Finnish vowel harmony. In addition, nasalisation of vowels and quantity errors were evident (see Huttunen in other chapters in this volume).

Although the normal development of vowels has received little attention, and the atypical development has been studied even less, it is evident that out of the Finnish vowels, /y, æ, ø/ are the most challenging.

Acquisition of Syllable Structures and Word Length

Syllable structure

There are 10 basic syllable structures in Finnish (see Helasvuo in this volume). CV is the most frequent (Häkkinen, 1978), and it is also a universally unmarked and common syllable structure. It is also the most common syllable structure in the first words of Finnish children (Kunnari, 2001). In Savinainen-Makkonen's (1998) case study, CV was the most common (39%) at the period of the first 50 words, but the proportion of syllables with coda consonants was as high as 23%. Those syllables were usually in word-initial position, and the coda was part of a geminate. Thus, in nominative forms, productions such as [pa:p:a] /sa:pas~sa:p:a:t/*saapas~ saappaat* 'boot(s)' (age 1;2–1;3, Savinainen-Makkonen, 1998) are common during the early stages of Finnish language acquisition.

The position of a syllable in a word affects its acquisition; some syllables are more prominent than others, and syllables can also be viewed in relation to word stress (Turunen, 2003); Finnish stress is fixed on the first syllable, but the heaviness of the syllable does not depend on stress, in other words, heavy syllables may occur in unstressed positions. An extreme example of this kind of conflict between syllable stress and length is the /a.vain/ *avain* 'key' (V.CVVC), in which the stressed initial syllable includes only the nucleus vowel, and the unstressed syllable is heavy. In *avain*, at the age of 2;6, approximately 50% of the children ($n = 59$) produced the unstressed syllable correctly, 37% produced an intermediate CVC or CVV syllable, and 12% produced a light CV syllable. Trisyllabic forms also occurred, such as [a.va.ne], which may indicate that a child rather produces a trisyllabic form with light syllables than a disyllabic form with a heavy unstressed syllable (Turunen, 2003).

All in all, one of the most common syllable structure processes among the first words of Finnish children, final consonant deletion, is a general process at least during the first 50 words (Kunnari, 2000, 2003a, 2003b; Savinainen-Makkonen, 1998). It is to be noted that of the consonants, only the dental phonemes /t s n l r/ occur word-finally in the native vocabulary of Finnish. However, word-final consonants are essential in inflection, for example, in marking plurality (*kissa:kissat* 'a cat: cats') genitive (*kissa: kissan*) and illative (*kissa:kissaan*). Torvelainen (2005) presents an example in which a child lengthens a light unstressed syllable in a truncated trisyllabic word: [lat:i:] /lat:ia:/ *lat.ti.aa* 'floor (partitive)'. One may thus assume that a child learns to also produce the heavy syllables in word final position at the onset of acquiring multimorphemic expressions. Before moving on to three- and four-syllable words, we will consider the acquisition of the very first words of Finnish children.

The structure of the first words

Children's early words tend to group into phonologically based sets. The child may modify the words to fit into one or two patterns. Especially during the 50-word stage, children may select words with structures they can produce accurately, and avoid other words (Schwartz & Leonard, 1982). Consequently, the phonologically favoured patterns may affect early lexical development.

The effective factor determining the structure which a child will detect most easily may be perceptual saliency. The most recent Finnish studies suggest that for Finnish children, the medial geminate is more salient than the word-initial structures (Savinainen-Makkonen, 2001; Saaristo-Helin, 2003).

This favouring of geminate structure in early words may also be explained by the fact that it represents a large part of the words children target; in the study of Saaristo-Helin *et al.* (2006), 41% of all the words that the 17 Finnish children targeted at the 50-word stage included a medial geminate (e.g. [kuk:a] /kuk:a/ *kukka* 'flower' and /kak:a/ *kakka* 'poo-poo'). An interesting example of the accommodation of diverse adult forms to this preferred early output pattern is found in Joel, the boy in

Savinainen-Makkonen's study (2003). At the age of 1;6, Joel had problems in producing diphthongs; instead of diphthongs, he produced geminates, for example, [æt:i] /æiti/ *äiti* 'mother', [ak:i] /auki/ *auki* 'open'.

Numerous studies in languages other than Finnish have confirmed that in their early words, children truncate disyllabic targets (e.g. Demuth, 1996; Fee, 1996; Ingram, 1989). However, in Finnish the reduction of disyllabic words is uncommon, and the children seem to favour disyllabic words with a geminate (Savinainen-Makkonen, 2000a, 2001; Kunnari, 2002). As many as 96% of the disyllabic words were produced as disyllables by 17 Finnish-speaking children at the 50-word stage (Saaristo-Helin *et al.*, 2006). However, Torvelainen (2005) found that it was typical for the weakest fifth of the children (*n* = 8) at age 2;0 to produce monosyllabic targets in spontaneous speech situations. She points out, however, that the high proportion (45%) of monosyllabic target words among those children may be due to learned communication patterns; for example, the children may give minimal feedback to their mother by saying [jo:] /jo:/ *joo* 'yes'. Torvelainen also concluded that at the age of 2;0, the words that Finnish children (*n* = 40) produce vary in length. While the most advanced fifth of the children (*n* = 8) attempted words with as many as five syllables and the frequencies of their word lengths were the same as in adult (mother) speech, the less advanced children (*n* = 8) attempted only mono- or disyllabic word forms (Torvelainen, 2005).

Acquisition of multisyllabic words

Finnish is an agglutinative language, which basically means that morphemes are added to the word stem, for example, /talo-i-s:a/ 'in the houses' (see Helasvuo in this volume). It is thus apparent that Finnish children acquire long words fairly early, at the onset of producing multi-morphemic expressions. So far, the production of long words has been studied mainly from a phonological perspective in Finnish child language research.

Trisyllabic words

A common phonological process, the truncation of trisyllabic targets, usually applies at the age of 2 in English and in Dutch (see Pater, 1997). This is seen also in most of the Finnish-speaking children at the early stages of word production. In a study of 17 children, almost 60% of the words with three syllables were reduced to disyllabic productions at the 50-word stage (Saaristo-Helin *et al.*, 2006). The study of Savinainen-Makkonen (2000b) showed that many children succeeded in producing trisyllabic targets already by the age of two. Furthermore, four children out of 40 in the study by Torvelainen (2005) actively produced three and four syllable words and did not show any truncation tendencies at the age of 2;0. In Turunen's (2003) picture naming task,[11] approximately 10% of the trisyllabic targets were truncated at the age of 2;6 and only 5% of the children (*n* = 196) produced no trisyllabic forms.

Although most Finnish children produce long words by the age of two, the phonological structure of target words affects the form of the realisation. For example, the proportion of truncated productions was higher in the target /auriŋko/ *aurinko* 'sun' (19%) than in the phonologically more simple word structure /lapio/ *lapio* 'shovel' (9%) (Turunen, 2003). It has been suggested that what is referred to as the prosodic SW-template (strong–weak syllable) or prosodic constraints cause these truncations (e.g. Pater, 1997; Savinainen-Makkonen, 2000b). In short, the child will rather delete a syllable than produce a syllable which does not belong to the foot, which in Finnish is trochaic, for example, /pu.he.lin/> [pu.he] 'telephone' (Turunen, 2003).

Since Finnish is a trochaic language and the main stress is always on the first syllable, one could assume that children preserve the initial two syllables. This is contrary to how it is in English, in which it is suggested, for example, that children usually preserve the stressed first and unstressed word-final syllable (Echols & Newport, 1992; Pater, 1997). Based on several studies (e.g. Laalo, 1994; Savinainen-Makkonen, 2000b; Torvelainen, 2005; Turunen, 2003), the preservation of the two word initial syllables is indeed the main type of truncation in Finnish. There are, however, exceptions to that pattern. If we look at the exact form of truncated productions, they often include conflated syllables, as in [moti] /toma:t:i/ *tomaatti* 'tomato' (Savinainen-Makkonen, 2000c) or [pu:hi] /puhelin/ *puhelin* 'telephone' (Turunen, 2003). It seems that – as Kehoe and Stoel-Gammon (1997) have suggested – prominence effects such as syllable structure and segmental factors play a role. A child may, for example, produce a less sonorant onset consonant, as in the following examples: [penu] /peruna/ *peruna* 'potatoe' (Laalo, 1994) and [ha:ku] /ha:ruk:a/ *haarukka* 'fork' (Iivonen, 1994; see also Pater, 1997). Savinainen-Makkonen (2000bc, 2001) has also pointed out the role of geminates in the production of long words; a child may preserve the geminate in his/her truncated form, for example, [pi:k:a] /pi:rak:a/ *piirakka* 'pie'. The effect of geminate structure was also seen also in the data presented by Torvelainen (2005) on 2-year-olds, for example, [o:k:a] /mo:nika/ *Monika*.

Turunen (2003: 109) found wide variation in the actual realisation of truncated forms. An extreme example of variation was the realisation of /auriŋko/ *aurinko* 'the sun'. Half of the truncated forms (*n* = 31) included the word-initial foot, that is, the first and second syllable, for example, [auri], [auli]. However, the less sonorant onset consonant was also often produced instead of the /r/, as in [a:ŋka] and in [aiko]. These forms illustrate what is referred to as the conspiracy effect, which means that at a certain stage, a child may not be able to produce diphthongs and complex consonant sequences in the same output.

To conclude, Finnish children usually produce the word-initial foot, but sonority of consonants, phonotactics or geminates later in the word may also affect the type of truncated forms.

Four-syllable words
Four-syllable words are also challenging for children between the ages of 1 and 2 years, and they often truncate these to bi- or trisyllabic forms:

[lolo] /joulupuk:i/ *joulupukki* 'Santa Claus' (Iivonen, 1994)
[mulanen] /mu:rahainen/ muurahainen 'ant.' (Savinainen-Makkonen, 2000b)

One could assume that when truncations occur, an unstressed syllable from the feet with secondary stress would be deleted (Bernhardt & Stemberger, 1998; Turunen, 2003). Turunen (2003) showed that indeed an unstressed syllable was deleted, but often also from the first foot:

[ap:es:i], [apsi:ni] /ap:elsi:ni/ *appelsiini* 'orange'
[leŋkone] /lentokone/ *lentokone* 'aeroplane'
[liumæki] /liukumæki/ *liukumäki* 'slide'

Since Finnish is rhythmically trochaic, that is, the word stress follows a strong–weak-pattern, it has been hypothesised that it may be easier for Finnish-speaking children to master four-syllable words with two feet than trisyllabic words with one unparsed syllable. A few case studies support this hypothesis (Räisänen, 1975; Savinainen-Makkonen, 2000b). However, Turunen (2003) reported that the proportion of truncated forms was approximately the same in four-syllable (11%) and in trisyllabic targets (10%) in control children.[12] While 5% of the children ($n = 196$) did not produce any trisyllabic forms of trisyllabic targets, slightly more, 9% of the children, did not produce any four syllable forms in a naming task. The syllable number was correct in all trisyllabic and four syllable words in the productions of 60% of the children. It seems thus that four-syllable words are in general not easier for Finnish children than trisyllabic words, but in careful analyses of individual children, one may find preferences for the four-syllable pattern over the trisyllabic.

The effects of truncation on morphosyntax
There is some evidence of a relationship between phonological trunca-tion patterns and morphosyntax. Torvelainen (2005) found that children who actively attempted to produce multisyllabic words at age 2 were advanced also in morphological and syntactical skills. In addition, the MLU (Mean Length of Utterance) and FIPSyn (Finnish Index of Productive Syntax, see Nieminen & Torvelainen, 2003) scores of spontaneous speech were analysed of five selected children who in the naming task truncated trisyllabic words at the age of 2;6. The results showed that those children indeed scored lower in the MLU and FIPSyn than others. The production

of morphosyntax was, however, not completely blocked since some children used different strategies to overcome the constraint, for example, specific syntactical frames which they had acquired (Turunen *et al.*, 2000). Thus, inflected forms which increase the number of syllables, are therefore not necessarily completely hindered by truncation. Since it seems to be rare that a child deletes morphemes from the end of the word in spontaneous speech, the following example represents an exceptional pattern in a child's speech at age 2;6 (example from Turunen, 2003): [tæ: paista, metsæ] /tæ: paista:, metsæs:æ/ *tää paistaa, metsässä* 'this shines, in the forest'. This 2;6-year-old child produced a light syllable in word *paistaa* 'shines' in which the final /a/ marks the third person. He also truncated the trisyllabic word *metsässä* 'in the forest' by omitting the case ending (inessive). In this situation, the child referred to the forest by using his hand to point and thus he also used gestures in order to supplement communication in the situation.

In short, it is evident that strong prosodic constraints are more detrimental in phonological disorders than segmental problems (Nettelbladt, 1983). The problem in producing long words may hinder the growth of vocabulary and morphosyntax in children with phonological disorders.

Early Precursors of Dyslexia

Finnish orthography has a high grapheme-phoneme correspondence. For this reason, basic decoding skills are acquired quite fast when a child starts receiving reading instruction. Practically all the Finnish children who do not show symptoms of for example, dyslexia, learn to read relatively well already after the first semester of elementary school. There are, however, those who face problems in learning to read even if they develop otherwise normally. Because the exact cause of dyslexia is still unknown, an exclusionary criterion is often used in definitions. Basically dyslexia is a reading disability which can not be attributed to sensory, intellectual, emotional, or socio-economic handicaps or to other known impediments to learning to read (Critchley, 1970; Scarborough, 1990). Since dyslexia appears only in reading and writing, it can not be diagnosed before school age. This has led researchers to investigate its possible early precursors in language development, so that possible rehabilitative or preventive treatments could be assessed before school age. This section introduces the results of a large Finnish project, the Jyväskylä Longitudinal Study on Dyslexia (JLD), which investigates the early precursors of dyslexia in Finnish-speaking children. This description is mainly based on the report by Lyytinen *et al.* (2004) and we will mainly concentrate on the results related to early phonology.

The JLD-project has followed nearly 200 children from birth to school age and 107 of these children have a familial risk for dyslexia. The selection of children was made through a three-stage process which was conducted for families visiting maternity clinics in Central Finland between 1993 and 1996. In short, the at-risk and control children were selected by interviewing and testing the parents (see Leinonen *et al.*, 2001 for a detailed description). According to a report of the project, 45 children have completed the third grade at school and only after a few years will the younger children reach the point when the potential dyslexia diagnosis can be made (Lyytinen *et al.*, 2004). The project is based on a multi-approach assessment, and great effort has been made to reach the most relevant features of development which may be related to later manifestation of dyslexia. The study will look, for example, at the psychophysiology (studied by Event-Related Potential methods), speech perception, attention, motor coordination and language development of the children.

It is agreed that reading disorders have a language-related origin (e.g. Catts, 1989), but the more specific nature of the underlying deficits in language development has not yet been identified. Some researchers suggest that a deficit in speech perception leads to fuzzy phonological representations (e.g. McBride-Chang, 1995). This assumption was also the starting point of the JLD-project (Lyytinen *et al.*, 1995, 2004).

Studies on early precursors of dyslexia in Finnish children were referred to earlier in this chapter, in the context of quantity. Quantity has been the focus in dyslexia studies, since its orthographic marking is typically problematic for Finnish dyslexics. By using a head-turn paradigm, Richardson (1998) and Richardson *et al.* (2003) found that at the age of 6 months, children at-risk for dyslexia had more problems in perceiving durational information than the control children. Similar consonant duration differences were also found by using the ERP method (Leppänen *et al.*, 2002). Since these studies appeared to differentiate the at-risk and control groups, one could suggest that the auditory/language areas of the brain in at-risk infants are differently recruited for speech sound processing (Lyytinen *et al.*, 2004).

The role of quantity was further studied at school age in a preliminary analysis by Nordqvist-Palviainen *et al.* (2004), who explored quantity in writing with a computer tool, Scriptlog (Strömqvist & Karlsson, 2001). This dictation task measured a child's ability to write nonsense words with short and long quantities based on auditory stimuli. The results showed that the transition times (TT) before single or geminate consonants in word medial position were significantly longer than the TT in other positions. The analysis also revealed a significant correlation between TT and literacy measures (reading and spelling accuracy, as well as reading fluency). In addition, the comparison of good ($n = 54$) and poor ($n = 14$) readers showed that the transition times before geminates were significantly longer in the poor reader group, and that poor readers ($n = 13$) also made more spelling errors and editings than good readers ($n = 29$). It thus seems that the processing of medial stops (especially stop geminates) requires more processing time than other letters in the writing process. In addition, the pre-stop interval TT (especially for geminates) were longer, and more spelling errors and editings were made in relation to the stops, in the poor reader group. These findings suggest that the perception and spelling of stops, and especially stop geminates, require extra effort for poor readers. The authors conclude that these preliminary results are in accordance with the results of the JLD infant perception studies (see Richardson, 1998).

According to Lyytinen *et al.* (2004) out of the early language measures, the maximum sentence length, based on parents' reports at the age of 2 years, was the first measure to differentiate between the two groups: children in the control group produced longer utterances. Later, at the age of 3;6, the at-risk children had lower scores than the controls on the tests measuring expressive language skills (Finnish version of the Boston naming test; Kaplan *et al.*, 1983; Laine *et al.*, 1993; and Inflectional Morphology Test; Lyytinen P. *et al.*, 2001), however, the measure of receptive language based on Peabody Picture Vocabulary Test-Revised (Dunn & Dunn, 1981) did not reveal significant group differences at this age. Lyytinen H. *et al.* (2001) also report that later, at 5 years of age, group differences emerged both in expressive and in receptive language measures. In addition, phonological awareness, for example, blending of phonological units, was studied with the help of computer-animated tasks, at age 3;6. The control group had better mastery in phonological awareness than at-risk children (Puolakanaho *et al.*, 2004).

In the JLD-project, it was discovered that the late initiation of talking seems to be more persistent in the at-risk group than in the control group. By the age of 3;6 late talkers[9] in the control group reached the level of their age mates more often than the late talkers in the at-risk group (Lyytinen, P. *et al.*, 2001).

Expressive language was studied by analysing the children's word structures at age 2;6. Scarborough (1990) observed that dyslexic children made more errors than controls in consonant production in spontaneous speech. The aim of Turunen (2003) and Kulju (2003) was to compare the Finnish at-risk and control groups and to investigate the children's word structures from an autosegmental perspective by applying the prosodic hierarchy (see Selkirk, 1980). The data was based on a naming task at 2;6, and phonological scores were calculated based on transcripts from this task. The following phonological parameters were taken into account: production of three and four syllabic words, heavy unstressed syllables, consonant sequences and diphthongs and the individual phonemes /s/ and /r/. Against expectations, no clear differences emerged between the at-risk and control children at 2;6 years in the phonological quality of their productions. It is to be noted, however, that only about half or fewer of the children in the at-risk group are expected to show delays and deficits in language development and ultimately in their reading performance. As seen earlier in this chapter, the more demanding experimental methods (e.g. head turn paradigm) were able to reveal both group differences and significant predictions to later language skills at a very early age (see Lyytinen *et al.*, 2004; Turunen, 2003 for discussion).

The results of a word structure analysis, based on a naming task at age 2;6, were also analysed in relation to later reading skills. Groups of poor, intermediate and good readers were identified at school entry based on Lindeman's (2000) test measuring word recognition skills. A comparison of the three groups revealed significant differences in the early phonological skills: children who eventually became good readers at school entry had been significantly more advanced than the intermediate or poor readers in their production of word length and syllable structures, as well as in the production of some phoneme sequences at 2;6 years. These results indicate a correlation between early reading skills and acquisition of the phonological structure (for details, see Kulju, 2003; Turunen, 2003). Similar results were reported by Torvelainen (2005), who found that the number of unintelligible harmonised words in spontaneous speech at age 2;0 correlate significantly with childrens' reading skills at age 7.

Lyytinen *et al.* (2004) discovered that at school entry at age 7 (before reading instruction), almost two-thirds of the control group children have basic decoding skills, but less than one-third of the at-risk group possessed these skills. It also seems that environmental effects such as shared reading serves as a protective factor to the children at risk for language problems. Taken together, the findings of the JLD-project indicate a strong correlation between early language development and later reading skills. The purpose is to define the early precursors of dyslexia in such a way that early interventions can then focus on those specific linguistic skills that were problematic for the dyslexics. According to Lyytinen *et al.* (2004), some methods are currently being developed, for example, 'training' the perception of sounds, including duration.

Concluding Words

This chapter presents an outline main arguments concerning how Finnish children acquire phonology. In addition, results of research into the early precursors of dyslexia were presented. The existing linguistic studies vary from case studies to more recent studies in groups of children, as well as quantitative analyses. The focus has mainly been on normal phonological development in Finnish, however, there still is a need for more extensive studies on disordered development, both in the area of phonology as well as in morphosyntax. Furthermore, a future challenge is to develop standardized tests on phonological skills and articulation for clinical practice.

Mainly based on the knowledge of normal acquisition, the identification of moderate to severe phonological disorders may be relatively simple for an experienced clinician. However, in order to provide efficient intervention, we should first analyse the phonological system of children thoroughly. An obvious cause of problems, such as a hearing impairment, helps us to plan the appropriate treatment plan, although language-specific features should also be taken into account with these children. However, in the majority of cases, children with phonological disorders have normal hearing and cognitive abilities with no apparent structural abnormality. They represent the major challenge for researchers and speech and language therapists.

The speech and language therapy services in Finland are presently mainly directed at children under school-age with SLI or other moderate or severe speech, language or other communication disorders. Children with communication disorders are offered speech therapy in local health care centres, in day-care units or by private practitioners. Furthermore, children with simple articulation errors are offered consultation with homework, and only few, if any, individual or group speech therapy sessions. Consequently, in Luotonen's study (1998) as much as 18% of all 7-year-olds had moderate articulation errors (mainly in /r, s, d/). School-aged children with phonological disorders continue their speech and language therapy, whereas children with simple articulation errors are not offered speech therapy; instead, they are offered individual or group speech training by specialist trained teachers who work in the school systems.

The language characteristics and difficulties of children with SLI for example, are best understood when compared to those of normally developing children. Indeed, there are several on-going studies dealing with normal and atypical phonological acquisition. Moreover, clinical assessments to evaluate the phonological skills of Finnish children are currently being developed.

Notes

1. Artikulaatiotesti. Äänteenmukainen sanakuvatesti [Picture naming articulation test] (Remes & Ojanen, 1996) and Artikulaation arviointitehtäviä [Assessment of articulation] (Vainio, 1993).
2. The naming task was carried out in the JLD-project at age 2;6 for nearly 200 children with and without a familial risk for dyslexia. Children named the pictures twice and the most advanced production was taken into account. The percentages mentioned in this article are drawn from the database of control children unless mentioned otherwise (see Turunen, 2003, for more specific information).
3. The subjects were children at-risk for dyslexia ($n = 20$) and their controls ($n = 20$). These 20 at-risk children were selected in the JLD-project from a larger group of at-risk children on the basis of several tests measuring phonological skills at age 3;6. The purpose was to form a group of at-risk children with weak phonological skills.

4. This was shown in Turunen's (2003) 2½-year-old's data. For example, in the word /sukla:/ *suklaa* 'chocolate' 65% of the children (*n* = 63) produced the word initial /s/ correctly and out of substitutions, /t/ was the most common, appearing in 18% of the productions.
5. It is to be noted that phonetic variation in the production of /r/ was high; for example, the uvular [R] was accepted. Approximately half of the children were at-risk for dyslexia and statistically /r/ was produced more often in the control group.
6. /d/ occurs in fully native words in standard spoken Finnish but it is absent from local dialects. Neither /d/ nor /ŋ/ occur in word-initial or word-final positions.
7. We differentiate consonant clusters and consonant sequences. Clusters occur within syllables and consonant sequences consist of consonants that appear within different syllables for example, *kan.taa* 'to carry'.
8. Luotonen (1998) reported the amount of articulation errors of 5-, 7- and 9-year-olds (*n* > 1500).
9. The late talker-group (*n* = 34) was a subgroup of a larger database of 200 children which included children at risk for dyslexia (*n* = 20) and their controls (*n* = 14). They were selected on the basis of the Finnish version of the MacArthur Communicative Development inventories and Bayley's expressive score at age 2;0 (Bayley, 1993, Fenson *et al.*, 1994; Lyytinen *et al.*, 2001).
10. The child was asked to imitate all eight Finnish vowels /a e i o u y æ ø /.
11. Children at risk for dyslexia and their controls did not differ significantly in this matter.
12. Children at risk for dyslexia truncated four-syllable target words more often than control children.

References

Aoyama, K. (2001) A psycholinguistic perspective on Finnish and Japanese prosody. *Perception, Production and Child Acquisition of Consonantal Quantity Distinctions.* Boston: Kluwer Academic Publishers.

Bayley, N. (1993) *The Bayley Scales of Infant Development* (2nd edn). San Antonio, TX: Psychological Corporation.

Bernhardt, B. and Stemberger, J.P. (1998) *Handbook of Phonological Development. From the Perspective of Constraint-Based Nonlinear Phonology.* San Diego: Academic Press.

Bortolini, U. and Leonard, L. (1991) The speech of phonologically disordered children acquiring Italian. *Clinical Linguistics and Phonetics* 5, 1–12.

Catts, H. (1989) Defining dyslexia as a developmental language disorder. *Annals of Dyslexia* 39, 50–67.

Chervela, N. (1981) Medial consonant cluster acquisition of Telugu children. *Journal of Child Language* 8, 63–73.

Critchley, M. (1970) *The Dyslectic Child.* London: Heinemann.

Demuth, K. (1995) Markedness and the development of prosodic structure. In J. Beckman (ed.) *Proceedings of the North East Linguistic Society 25* (pp. 13–25). Amherst, MA: GLSA, University of Massachusetts.

Demuth, K. (1996) Stages in the development of prosodic words. In E.V. Clark (ed.) *The Proceedings of the Twenty-seventh Annual Child Language Research Forum* (pp. 39–48). Stanford University: CSLI.

Dunn, L.M. and Dunn, L. (1981) *Peabody Picture Vocabulary Test-Revised.* Circle Pines, MN: American Guidance Service.

Echols, C.H. and Newport, E.L. (1992) The role of stress and position in determining first words. *Language Acquisition* 2, 189–220.

Fee, E.J. (1996) Two strategies in the acquisition of syllable and word structure. In E.V. Clark (ed.) *The Proceedings of the Twenty-seventh Annual Child Language Research Forum* (pp. 29–38). Stanford University: CSLI.

Fenson, L., Dale, P.S., Reznick, J.S., Bates, E., Thal, D. and Pethick, S.J. (1994) Variability in early communicative development. *Monographs of the Society for Research in Child Development* 59 (5, serial no. 242).

Grunwell, P. (1987) *Clinical Phonology* (2nd edn). London: Chapman & Hall.

Haapanen, M-L. (2003) Suunsisäisen irtokojeen käytön aiheet ja hoitovaste puhehäiriöissä [Oral plate therapy in speech disorders – Indications and treatment response]. *Suomen lääkärilehti* 39, 3877–3881.

Haavio, M-L. (2001) Oral motor dysfunction and rehabilitation in Finland. In M. Sillanpää (ed.) *Practices in Orafacial Therapy* (pp. 53–54). Turku: Pallosalama.

Häkkinen, K. (1978) Eräistä suomen kielen äännerakenteen luonteenomaisista piirteistä ja niiden taustasta. [Some phonological phenomenon in Finnish. Backround and characteristics]. Unpublished Licentiate's thesis, University of Turku, Turku, Finland.

Howell, J. and Dean, E. (1994) *Treating Phonological Disorders in Children: Metaphon – Theory to Practice* (2nd edn). London: Whurr.

Huttunen, K. (2000) Early childhood hearing impairment: Speech intelligibility and late outcome. Acta Universitatis Ouluensis B 35. PhD thesis, University of Oulu, Oulu, Finland.

Huttunen, K. (2001) Phonological development in 4–6-year-old moderately hearing impaired children. *Scandinavian Audiology* 30 (53), 79–82.

Iivonen, A. (1986) Lapsen fonologisen kehityksen tutkimusmetodiikka [Research methodology of children's developmental phonology]. In M. Lehtihalmes and A. Klippi (eds) *Logopedis-foniatrinen tutkimus Suomessa* (pp. 17–58). Helsinki: Suomen logopedis-foniatrisen yhdistyksen julkaisuja 19.

Iivonen, A. (1994) Paradigmaattisia ja syntagmaattisia näkökohtia lapsen foneettis-fonologisessa kehityksessä [Paradigmatic and phonotactic aspects in phonetic and phonological development of children]. In A. Iivonen, A. Lieko and P. Korpilahti (eds) *Lapsen normaali ja poikkeava kielen kehitys* (2nd edn) (pp. 34–77). Helsinki: Finnish Literature Society.

Iivonen, A. (1998) Aspects of the phonotactical acquisition in children. In K. Heinänen and M. Lehtihalmes (eds) *Proceedings of the Seventh Nordic Child Language Symposium* (pp. 82–84). Suomen ja saamen kielen ja logopedian laitoksen julkaisuja 13, University of Oulu, Oulu.

Iivonen, A. (2004) Vokaalien kehitys protosanoista kielen mukaiseen järjestelmään [The acquisition of vowels – the development from protowords towards target language]. In S. Kunnari and T. Savinainen-Makkonen (eds) *Mistä on pienten sanat tehty. Lasten äänteellinen kehitys* (pp. 74–78). Helsinki: WSOY.

Ingram, D. (1989) *Phonological Disability in Children* (2nd edn). London: Whurr.

Itkonen, T. (1977) Huomioita lapsen äänteistön kehityksestä [Remarks on the development of child's phonology]. *Virittäjä* 81, 279–308.

Jakobson, R. (1941/1968) *Child Language, Aphasia, and Phonological Universals*. The Hague/Paris: Mouton.

Kaplan, E., Goodglass, H. and Weintraub, S. (1983) *The Boston Naming Test* (2nd edn). Philadelphia: Lea & Febiger.

Karlsson, F. (1983) *Suomen kielen äänne- ja muotorakenne [Phonology and morphology of Finnish]*. Porvoo: WSOY.

Kehoe, M. and Stoel-Gammon, C. (1997) The acquisition of prosodic structure: An investigation of current accounts of children's prosodic development. *Language* 73, 113–144.

Kulju, P. (2003) 2;6-vuotiaiden lasten sanarakenteiden tuottamisesta ja varhaisen fonologian yhteydestä lukihäiriöriskiin ja lukutaidon oppimiseen [On the relationship between early word structures and early phonology with the risk of dyslexia and learning to read in 2,6-year-old children]. *Puhe ja kieli* 23 (4), 173–188.

Kunnari, S. (2000) Characteristics of early lexical and phonological development in children acquiring Finnish. Acta Universitatis Ouluensis. PhD thesis, University of Oulu, Oulu, Finland.

Kunnari, S. (2002) Word length in syllables: Evidence from early word production on Finnish. *First Language* 22, 119–135.

Kunnari, S. (2003a) Consonant inventories: A longitudinal study of Finnish-speaking children. *Journal of Multilingual Communication Disorders* 1 (2), 124–131.

Kunnari, S. (2003b) Suomea omaksuvien lasten ensisanojen konsonantit [Early consonant inventories in children acquiring Finnish]. *Puhe ja kieli* 23 (4), 197–205.

Kunnari, S., Nakai, S. and Vihman, M.M. (2001) Cross-linguistic evidence for acquisition of geminates. *Psychology of Language and Communication* 5, 13–24.

Laalo, K. (1994) Kaksitavuvaihe lapsen kielen kehityksessä [The disyllabic stage in language acquisition]. *Virittäjä* 98, 430–448.

Laine, M., Koivuselkä-Sallinen, P., Hänninen, R. and Niemi, J. (1993) Bostonin nimentätestin suomenkielinen julkaisematon testiversio [Unpublished Finnish pilot version of Boston naming test]. Helsinki: Psykologien kustannus Oy.

Laitinen, J., Haapanen, M-L., Paaso, M., Pulkkinen, J., Heliövaara, A. and Ranta, R. (1998) Occurence of dental consonant misarticulations on different cleft types. *Folia Phoniatrica et Logopaedica* 50, 92–100.

Laitinen, J., Ranta, R., Pulkkinen, J. and Haapanen, M-L. (1999) Associations between dental occlusion and misarticulations of Finnish dental consonants in cleft lip/palate children. *European Journal of Oral Sciences* 107, 109–113.

Leinonen, S., Müller, K., Leppänen, P.H.T., Aro, M., Ahonen, T. and Lyytinen, H. (2001) Heterogeneity in adult dyslexic readers: Relating processing skills to the speed and accuracy of oral text reading. *Reading and Writing: An Interdisciplinary Journal* 14, 265–296.

Leiwo, M. (1977) Kielitieteellisiä näkökohtia viivästyneestä kielenkehityksestä [Linguistic aspects on delayed language acquisition]. Studia Philologica Jyväskyläensia 10. PhD thesis, University of Jyväskylä, Jyväskylä, Finland.

Leiwo, M., Kulju, P. and Aoyama, K. (2006) The acquisition of Finnish vowel harmony. In M. Suominen, A. Arppe. A. Airola, O. Heinämäki, M. Miestamo, U. Määttä, J. Niemi, K.K. Pitkänen and K. Sinnemäki (eds) *A Man of Measure: Festschrift in Honour of Fred Karlsson on his 60th Birthday* (pp. 149–161). The Linguistic Association of Finland, Turku. Special Supplement to SKY Journal of Linguistics, Volume 19.

Leppänen, P.H.T., Richardson, U., Pihko, E., Eklund, K.M., Guttorm, T.K., Aro, M. and Lyytinen, H. (2002) Brain responses to changes in speech sound durations differ between infants with and without familial risk for dyslexia. *Developmental Neuropsychology* 22, 407–422.

Lieko, A. (1998) Vokaaliharmonia lapsen kielessä [Vowel harmony in child language]. *Virittäjä* 101 (3), 417–420.

Lieko, A. (2001) Vokaaliharmonian omaksuminen [Acquisition of Finnish vowel harmony]. *Puhe ja kieli* 21 (1), 13–20.

Lindeman, J. (2000) Ala-asteen lukutesti: käyttäjän käsikirja [Reading test for elementary schools. User's guide]. Oppimistutkimuksen keskus, University of Turku, Turku.

Luotonen, M. (1998) Factors associated with linguistic development and school performance: The role of early otitis media, gender and day care. Acta Universitatis Ouluensis, series D Medica, 453. PhD thesis, University of Oulu, Oulu, Finland.

Lyakso, E.E. and Silvén, S.A.M (2002) Comparative characteristics of early vocalizations in Finnish and Russian infants. *Journal of Sensory System* 16, 65–74.

Lyytinen, H., Leinonen, S., Nikula, M., Aro, M. and Leiwo, M. (1995) In search of the core features of dyslexia: Observations concerning dyslexia in the highly orthographically regular Finnish language. In V.W. Berninger (ed.) *The Varieties of Orthographic Knowledge II: Relationship to Phonology, Reading, and Writing* (pp. 177–204). Dordrecht: Kluwer Academic Publishers.

Lyytinen, H., Ahonen, T., Eklund, K., Guttorm, T.K., Laakso, M-L., Leinonen, S., Leppänen, P.H.T., Lyytinen, P., Poikkeus, A-M., Puolakanaho, A., Richardson, U. and Viholainen, H. (2001) Developmental pathways of children with and without familial risk for dyslexia during the first years of life. *Developmental Neuropsychology* 20, 535–554.

Lyytinen, H., Ahonen. T., Eklund, K., Guttorm, T., Kulju, P., Laakso, M-L., Leiwo, M., Leppänen, P., Lyytinen, P., Poikkeus, A-M., Richardson, U., Torppa, M. and Viholainen, H. (2004) Early development of children at familial risk for dyslexia – follow-up from birth to school age. *Dyslexia* 10 (3), 146–178.

Lyytinen, P., Poikkeus, A-M., Laakso, M-L., Eklund, K. and Lyytinen, H. (2001) Language development and symbolic play in children with and without familial risk for dyslexia. *Journal of Speech, Language and Hearing Research*, 44, 873–885.

Maassen, B., Groenen, P. and Crull, T. (2003) Auditory and phonetic perception of vowels in children with apraxic speech disorders. *Clinical Linguistic & Phonetics* 17 (6), 447–467.

Mäenpää, M. (1990) Kehityksellinen verbaali dyspraksia kuudella esikoulukäisellä lapsella [Developmental verbal dyspraxia: A multi case study of six pre-school children]. Unpublished Master's thesis, University of Helsinki, Helsinki, Finland.

McBride-Chang, C. (1995) Phonological processing, speech perception, and reading disability: Integrative review. *Educational Psychologist* 30, 109–121.

Menn, L. and Stoel-Gammon, C. (1995) Phonological development. In P. Fletcher and B. MacWhinney (eds) *Handbook of Child Language* (pp. 335–359). Oxford: Blackwell.

Nettelbladt, U. (1983) *Developmental Studies of Dysphonology in Children*. Travaux de l'institut de linguistique de Lund. CWK Gleerup.

Nieminen, L. and Torvelainen, P. (2003) Produktiivisen syntaksin indeksi – suomenkielinen versio [Index of productive syntac – a Finnish version]. *Puhe ja kieli* 23 (3), 119–132.

Nordqvist-Palviainen, Å., Richardson, U. and Leiwo, M. (2004, September) Geminates – a Processing Bottleneck in Finnish Orthography. Paper presented at Writing 2004: *9th International Conference of the EARLI Special Interest Group of Writing*, Geneva, Switzerland.

Olkkola, A. (2002) Kuulovammaisten, sisäkorvaistutetta käyttävien lasten varhaisen fonologisen ja leksikaalisen kehityksen piirteitä: Kolmen lapsen tapaustutkimus [Phonological and lexical development in children with cochlear implants: A case study of three children]. Unpublished Master's thesis, University of Helsinki, Helsinki, Finland.

Pater, J. (1997) Minimal violation and phonological development. *Language Acquisition* 6 (3), 201–253.

Pietarinen, A. (1987) Vantaalaisten v. 1980 syntyneiden lasten viisivuotisseulalla mitatut kielelliset häiriöt ja niiden yhteydet kehityksen muihin osatekijöihin

[Speech and language disorders and their connection to other developmental features – Screening test for five-year-old children born in 1980 in Vantaa city]. Unpublished Master's thesis, University of Helsinki, Helsinki, Finland.

Puolakanaho, A., Poikkeus, A-M., Ahonen, T., Tolvanen, A. and Lyytinen, H. (2004) Emerging phonological awareness as a precursor of risk in children with and without familial risk for dyslexia. *Annals of Dyslexia* 54 (2), 221–243.

Remes, K. and Ojanen, A-K. (1996) *Artikulaatiotesti. Äänteenmukainen sanakuvatesti [Picture Naming Articulation Test]*. Helsinki: Early Learning Oy.

Richardson, U. (1998) Familial dysleksia and sound duration in the quantity distinctions of Finnish infants and adults. Studia Philologica Jyväskyläensia 44. PhD thesis, University of Jyväskylä, Jyväskylä, Finland.

Richardson, U., Leppänen, P.H.T., Leiwo, M. and Lyytinen, H. (2003) Speech perception of infants with high familial risk for dyslexia differ at the age of 6 months. *Developmental Neuropsychology* 23, 385–397.

Räisänen, A. (1975) Havaintoja lastenkielestä [Observations on child language]. *Virittäjä* 79, 251–266.

Saaristo-Helin, K. (2003) *Äänteellinen kehitys ensisanojen kaudella: Neljän lapsen tapaustutkimus* [Phonological development in the stage of first words: A case study of four children]. Unpublished Master's thesis, University of Helsinki, Helsinki, Finland.

Saaristo-Helin, K., Savinainen-Makkonen, T. and Kunnari, S. (2006) The phonological mean length of utterance: Methodological challenges from a crosslinguistic perspective. *Journal of Child Language*, 33, 179–190.

Savinainen-Makkonen, T. (1996) Lapsenkielen fonologia systemaattisen kehityksen kaudella [Child phonology at the stage of phonological processes]. Unpublished Licentiate's thesis, University of Helsinki, Helsinki, Finland.

Savinainen-Makkonen, T. (1998) Ensisanojen kauden fonologiaa: Tapaustutkimus [Phonology of the first words: A case study]. In M. Karjalainen (ed.) *Kielen ituja: Ajankohtaista lapsenkielen tutkimuksesta* (pp. 44–83). Suomen ja saamen kielen ja logopedian laitoksen julkaisuja 10. Oulu: Oulun yliopistopaino.

Savinainen-Makkonen, T. (2000a) Word-initial consonant omissions – A developmental process in children learning Finnish. *First Language* 20, 161–185.

Savinainen-Makkonen, T. (2000b) Learning long words – A typological perspective. *Language and Speech* 42 (2), 205–225.

Savinainen-Makkonen, T. (2000c) Learning to produce three-syllable words: A longitudinal study of Finnish twins. In M. Perkins and S. Howard (eds) *New Directions in Language Development and Disorders* (pp. 223–231). New York: Plenum Publishing.

Savinainen-Makkonen, T. (2001) Suomalainen lapsi fonologiaa omaksumassa [Finnish children acquiring phonology]. Publication of the Department of Phonetics no 42. PhD thesis, University of Helsinki, Helsinki, Finland.

Savinainen-Makkonen, T. (2003) Lisänäyttöä geminaattamallin olemassaololle: Tapaustutkimus [Evidence for a geminate template: A case study]. *Puhe ja kieli* 23 (4), 189–196.

Savinainen-Makkonen, T. and Kunnari, S. (2004) Systemaattisen kauden rajoitukset ja fonologiset prosessit [Constraints and phonological processes after the first words stage]. In S. Kunnari and T. Savinainen-Makkonen (eds) *Mistä on pienten sanat tehty: lasten äänteellinen kehitys* (pp. 99–109). Helsinki: WSOY.

Scarborough, H. (1990) Very early language deficits in dyslexic children. *Child Development* 61, 1728–1743.

Schwartz, R. and Leonard, L. (1982) Do children pick and choose: An examination of phonological selection and avoidance in early lexical acquisition. *Journal of Child Language* 9, 319–336.

Selin, O. (2005) *Konsonanttiyhtymien omaksumisen ensiaskeleet: Neljän lapsen tapaustutkimus.* [The early stages of heterosyllabic consonant cluster acquisition: A case study of four children]. Unpublished Master's thesis, University of Helsinki, Helsinki, Finland.

Selkirk, E.O. (1980) The role of prosodic categories in English word stress. *Linguistic Inquiry*, 11, 563–605.

Stoel-Gammon, C. (1996) Phonological assessment using a hierarchical framework. In K.N. Cole, P.S. Dale and D.J. Thal (eds) *Assessment of Communication and Language* (pp. 77–95). Baltimore: Paul Brookes.

Stoel-Gammon, C. and Dunn, J. (1985) *Normal and Disordered Phonology in Children.* Baltimore: University Park Press.

Strömqvist, S. and Karlsson, H. (2001) ScriptLog for Windows – User's Manual. (Tech. Rep.) Department of Linguistics, University of Lund, and Centre for Reading Research, University College of Stavanger. On WWW at http://www.scriptlog.net/.

Takkinen, R. (2002) Käsimuotojen salat: Viittomakielisten lasten käsimuotojen omaksuminen 2–7 vuoden iässä [The secrets of handshapes: The acquisition of handshapes by native signers at the age of two to seven years]. PhD thesis. Helsinki: Kuurojen Liitto ry.

Tallal, P. (1980) Auditory temporal perception, phonics, and reading disabilities in children. *Brain and Language* 36, 182–198.

Toivainen, J. (1990) *Acquisition of Finnish as a First Language: General and Practical Themes.* Turun suomalaisen ja yleisen kielitieteen laitoksen julkaisuja 35, University of Turku, Turku.

Toivainen, J. (1997) Acquisition of Finnish. In D.I. Slobin (ed.) *The Crosslinguistic Study of Language Acquisition* (Vol. 4) (pp. 87–182). Mahwah, NJ: Lawrence Erlbaum.

Torvelainen, P. (2005) 2;0-vuotiaiden lasten fonologisen kehityksen variaatio. Puheen ymmärrettävyyden, sananmuotojen tavoittelun ja tuottamisen sekä sananmuotojen yksikonsonanttisuuden ja – vokaalisuuden tarkastelu [Variation in phonological development of 2-year-old Finnish children: A study of speech intelligibility, targeting and production of word structures and consonant and vowel harmony]. Unpublished Licentiate's thesis, University of Jyväskylä, Jyväskylä, Finland.

Turunen, P. (currently Kulju, P.) (2003) Production of word structure. A constraint-based study of 2;6-year-old Finnish children at-risk for dyslexia and their controls. Jyväskylä Studies in Languages 52. PhD thesis, University of Jyväskylä, Jyväskylä, Finland.

Turunen, P., Korhonen, P. and Nieminen, L. (2000, September) Interaction between phonology, morphology and sentence production in children with strong prosodic constraints. Paper presented at Turku Symposium on First Language Acquisition, Turku, Finland.

Vainio, L. (1993) *Artikulaation arviointitehtäviä* [*Assessment of Articulation*]. Helsinki: Early Learning.

Vilkman, E., Niemi, J. and Ikonen, U. (1988) Fragile X speech phonology in Finnish. *Brain and Language* 34, 203–221.

Warren, S. (2001) Phonological acquisition and ambient language: A corpus based cross-linguistic exploration. PhD thesis, University of Hertfordshire, UK.

Wijnen, F., Krikhaar, E. and Den Os, E. (1994) The (non)realization of unstressed elements in children's utterances: Evidence for a rhythmic constraint. *Journal of Child Language* 21, 59–83.

Chapter 5

Logopedic Research on Communication Difficulties in Childhood

PIRJO KORPILAHTI and KAISU HEINÄNEN

Introduction

In Finland, the follow-up of language development in early childhood is well organised by mother and child welfare clinics. Before school age (7 years) every Finnish child is seen by a specialised nurse once a year, and when necessary, the family is referred to a speech and language therapist for further assessment (Liuksila, 2000). In the past few decades, screening for language development has also been started at day care centres. New screening methods take into account language-specific and cultural aspects and thereby reach better validity and predictive value. The Finnish version of the MacArthur Communicative Developmental Inventory (MCDI; Lyytinen, 1999) has enabled parents to participate in the assessment of language development in early infancy. Many programmes supporting early language and interaction skills have also been started in close co-operation with speech and language therapists (e.g. Överlund, 1996).

Logopedic research on disordered language development is mostly carried out in collaboration with units of child neurology, child psychiatry, or phoniatrics or special schools. One of the most important topics in the history of Finnish logopedic research has been the work by Parre *et al.* (1980), namely the study of speech disorders in high-risk infants. Today, there is a wide range of research groups, which enhances the interest in language impairment from different perspectives. However, most published articles in logopedics come from researchers working at universities or doctoral students enrolled in graduate schools.

Deficient language development can be understood only by comparing its features with typical age-specific development. Finnish, being a highly inflected language, has a very complex structure (see also Helasvuo in this volume), and research on normal development hence also has great value for the study of communication disorders. In logopedic research, Kunnari

(2000) and Savinainen-Makkonen (2001) were the first to study the phono-logical development of Finnish-speaking children; these two studies are discussed in more detail in other chapters of this book (see Kulju and Savinainen-Makkonen in this volume). The same applies to the research by Launonen (1998, this volume) on language development and early intervention of children with Down syndrome. In Finland, there is a solid research tradition in psychology and special education concerning dyslexia and related learning problems. However, these topics are outside the scope of this chapter.

This chapter reviews three strong lines of logopedic research on deficient language development in Finland, all of which are documented in doctoral theses and international scientific publications. We review the following topics: (1) follow-up studies of premature and small-for-date babies, (2) neurocognitive correlates of impaired language skills measured with event-related potentials of the brain (ERPs), and (3) auditory perception of children with autistic spectrum disorders, especially Asperger syndrome.

Development of Language Skills in Preterm Children

In the past few decades, even very small-for-date and premature babies have had good chances of survival, thanks to the high standard of neona-tal intensive care in the central hospitals of Finland. In 1995, the incidence of preterm birth in the Finnish population was 5.6%, and 4.3% of new-borns weighed less than 2500 g (Saarikoski, 1998). Many prematurely born children have severe neurological disorders and impairment of vision or hearing. Serious learning problems at school are found even in children with normal intelligence and only 'soft signs' of deficient develop-ment in early infancy. They may have problems in spatial relationships, sensory integration, attentive skills, mathematics, reading and writing, and often in language skills. Different studies have yielded contradictory results concerning the relationship between preterm birth and deficient language development. However, most researchers believe that preterm birth has long-lasting effects on later development and academic skills (e.g. Jennishe & Sedin, 2001; Wolke & Meyer, 1999). The neonatal period and early infancy have been found to be especially important for language acquisition and later learning skills related to language. The language development of children at risk for deficient language has been discussed in the doctoral theses by Riitesuo (2000), Yliherva (2002), and Jansson-Verkasalo (2003). The early lexical development of prematurely born children is also studied in the PIPARI project at Turku University Hospital (Stolt et al., 2005).

Early communicative and linguistic development is based on neural prerequisites, environmental factors, and early mother–child interaction (e.g. Laakso et al., 1999; Paavola et al., 2005; Saxon, 1997). Preterm babies spend the first months of their lives in neonatal intensive care units and do not have equal possibilities for early mother–child interaction compared to healthy newborns. Follow-up studies are important for understanding the effects of an immature neuronal system and, on the other hand, of the environmental factors related to neonatal status on the child's subsequent development. Riitesuo (2000) studied the speech and language development of preterm infants as part of mental and overall development during the first two years of life. Developmental pathways were followed in the context of perinatal risks, and assessments were mainly carried out at the children's homes. The results were assessed at both corrected and chronological age. Preterm infants were divided into two groups on the basis of gestational age (older preterm infants, i.e. 29–32 weeks, and younger preterm infants, i.e. 24–28 weeks). The results were assessed within the preterm group and compared with the standards of the tests administered. Riitesuo found that the degree of prematurity and the diagnosed problems were reflected in the test results. The older preterm infants began to perform without age correction between the ages of 1 year and 1½ years, depending on the assessment device used. Speech production tended to develop more slowly than other skills. Many of the younger preterm infants continued to perform below the expected levels at the corrected age of two years. The results of the Bayley (1969), Reynell & Huntley (1985), and ASQ (Ages and Stages Questionnaires; Squires *et al.*, 1993) tests had significant positive correlations with each other. As a group, the preterm children with diagnoses of developmental deficiencies ($n = 6$) tended to score lower than the preterm children without diagnoses ($n = 18$), and there was an especially prominent deficiency in gross motor skills.

Jansson-Verkasalo (2003) studied language development in very low birth weight (VLBW) preterm children, many of them with abnormalities in neonatal magnetic resonance imaging (MRI) scans, and matched controls. Language development was assessed at 2, 4 and 6 years. Both language comprehension and production were evaluated. Special interest was focused on the development of auditory processing as a predictor of lexical development. In addition to behavioural measures, auditory event-related potentials (ERPs) were recorded at the ages of 4 and 6 years. ERP measures were based on scalp-recorded brain activation elicited by semi-synthetic syllables modified acoustically from natural speech.

Jansson-Verkasalo noticed that, at the age of 2 years, VLBW children achieved significantly lower scores on language comprehension tests than their matched controls (matching for age, gender and length of mother's education) (Jansson-Verkasalo *et al.*, 2004). VLBW children also used shorter and less mature sentences. Two years later, they had difficulties in language comprehension, naming, and auditory discrimination. These children's language test scores at 2 years correlated significantly with their auditory discrimination scores at 4 years. The VLBW preterm children had difficulties with auditory discrimination, as indexed by behavioural discrimination tests and by the diminished amplitude of mismatch negativity (MMN) and late mismatch negativity (lMMN). These two un-attended ERP components have been found to correlate closely with auditory discrimination (Cheour *et al.*, 2001). Jansson-Verkasalo *et al.* (2003a) found the MMN response to index language impairment in VLBW preterm children. The MMN amplitude, as elicited by vowel duration changes in syllables, was attenuated in the preterm group at the age of 4 and that for consonant change at the age of 6. The low-level ERP activation and poor auditory discrimination at the behavioural level were found to correlate with poor lexical development.

The language development of preterm and small-for-date babies at the age of 8 years was studied by Yliherva (2002) in her doctoral thesis. The children (*n* = 42) came from the Northern Finland Birth Cohort (NFBC) for the years 1985–1986. The main research questions concerned psycholinguistic skills, speech and language comprehension, morphological skills, and lexical development as measured at elementary school. Yliherva *et al.* (2000) did not find any deviance in the auditory modality, but the study showed poorer performance in visual skills in prematurely born school-aged children than in their matched controls. In the subsequent article, Yliherva *et al.* (2001) reported linguistic skills with reference to different neurological statuses. They found that the preterm children with minor neurodevelopmental dysfunctions scored lowest in the Token Test for Children (DiSimoni, 1978). The preterm children with neurological problems scored always poorer in psycholinguistic tests than the full-term children.

Linguistic and motor problems of low birth weight (LBW) children were investigated in the NFBC. There were altogether 279 children with birth weight lower than 2500 g. When examined at the age of 8 years, the LBW children appeared to have experienced more difficulties than normal birth weight children in speech, language, learning, and motor abilities. It seems that particularly LBW boys are at risk for problems at school. There was a clear relationship between speech and motor disabilities in the LBW group. Mother's young age, family size, reconstructed family structure, hearing impairment and male gender were the key determinants of poor speech and language abilities at 8 years of age. In addition, smallness for gestational age was a risk factor for communication problems.

Brain Imaging of Auditory Perception and Impaired Language Development

Language acquisition is related to the maturation of brain structures and neural plasticity (Bates *et al.*, 2003). During language learning, auditory perception is automatised. Children do not only pay attention to the word form, but also become increasingly interested in word meanings. The brain's architecture is changed by language-related experiences (Karmiloff & Karmiloff-Smith, 2001). As a consequence, the child's auditory perception and speech decoding become more focused (Gerken, 1994). This learning is easily disturbed in noisy surroundings, even when neural maturation has been normal. Both inhibitory acts and selectivity of hearing are necessary for language learning.

The neural organisation of language-related brain functions is highly differentiated during language learning (Holopainen *et al.*, 1997a; Korpilahti, 1996). The early phases of language acquisition are mainly unconscious and therefore cannot be measured by direct tests or inspection (Diamond *et al.*, 1994). In recent years, different methods of brain imaging have been used increasingly to study speech and language processing in children. Cortically recorded event-related potentials (ERPs) are useful for early diagnosis of language impairment. Auditory ERPs can be used to inspect neural activation elicited by simple tones, single speech sounds, syllables, words, or even complex structures related to cognition, language and memory (Krause *et al.*, 1998; Lang *et al.*, 1995). When combined with behavioural assessment, auditory ERPs offer an objective window into language and its disorders.

Auditory ERPs have certain advantages compared to other research methods. They are especially useful in the study of language because they are built on precise temporal and spectral information of language processes (Korpilahti 1996; Korpilahti *et al.*, 2001). ERP analyses are based on EEG recordings. This method is non-invasive and widely used in child neurology. Recordings can be carried out even with non-co-operative subjects, for example, preterm children or children with intellectual impairments. ERP analyses are carried out with effective computer programs, so very large amounts of information can be compared with a fair degree of statistical accuracy. This increases the reliability of the results, even though the number of subjects in any one experiment may be quite small.

Collection of normative ERP data is necessary to understand atypical neural maturation and functioning. Korpilahti *et al.* (2001) studied the recognition of words and pseudo-words in healthy preschoolers. They found that the early MMN component, as an index of phonemic discrimination, was elicited by sine tones and complex pseudo-word stimuli. On the other hand, words elicited a stronger late MMN waveform, which was interpreted to reflect word recognition on a gestalt basis. This study supports the view that word perception is not based exclusively on acoustic analyses or the form of the word. Speech contains many kinds of 'encodedness'; for example, the meaning of a word is closely related to the person's knowledge of the language. On the other hand, the auditory perception of children with language impairments reflected decoding of separate acoustic features without neural activation of language units (Korpilahti, 1996).

Central auditory processing disorder (CAPD) is an observed deficiency in mechanisms and processes related to a variety of auditory behaviours (ASHA, 1996). Children with CAPD have difficulties in processing or interpreting auditory stimuli in the absence of a peripheral hearing loss. The estimated incidence of CAPD ranges from 3% to 5%. CAPD can be the primary diagnosis, but these children have often been reported to have learning disabilities, ADHD, or specific language impairment (SLI). Early identification of and intervention in auditory processing disorder can help children to reach better language skills before school age and to avoid secondary learning problems.

Auditory ERPs of the brain act as indices of language impairment (Holopainen *et al.*, 1997a, 1997b, 1998; Korpilahti, 1995, 1996; Korpilahti & Lang, 1994). Korpilahti and Lang (1994) studied un-attended auditory discrimination in severely dysphasic children at school age. They found longer ERP latencies and attenuation of the MMN component in an experiment where sine tones (500/553 Hz) were used as stimuli. Korpilahti (1995) reported impaired auditory discrimination of sound frequencies and syllables to correlate with neurocognitive measures. Holopainen *et al.* (1997b) replicated the ERP study among younger language-impaired children with similar results. Impaired auditory perception was related to a fast stimulus presentation rate and can be interpreted to support Tallal's theory of temporal processing as one of the main problems in language impairment (Tallal *et al.*, 1985).

Language Skills of Children with Autistic Spectrum Disorders

Asperger syndrome (AS) is a neurobiological condition that belongs to the group of high functioning autism spectrum disorders (ASD). It is considered to be less severe than infantile autism, with IQs of 70 or higher (see Frith, 2004; Rapin & Dunn, 2003). Children with AS are often characterised by normal early language development, but impairments in semantics and pragmatics (for a review, see Volkmar & Pauls, 2003). Despite the presence of communicative deficits, logopedic research of auditory deficits in this field is sparse. Jansson-Verkasalo *et al.* (2003b) were able to show atypical encoding of transient sound features in children with AS for tones and syllables. This study reported distorted brain activation (diminished amplitudes and prolonged latencies of the obligatory ERP responses P1 and N2) in children with AS and also delayed MMN responses indicating deficient detection of sound differences, especially over the right hemisphere.

At Oulu University Hospital a large interdisciplinary group has been working on the research theme *Genetic Study of High Functioning Autism and Asperger's Syndrome in Finland*. As part of this large project,

Jansson-Verkasalo *et al.* (2005) and Korpilahti *et al.* (2007) studied auditory perception in children with AS and their parents. ERPs were recorded from 20 children (aged 9–12 years) with diagnosed AS, their parents ($n = 34$), and age-matched controls ($n = 18$) and their parents ($n = 31$). AS was assigned by using the Autism Diagnostic Interview – Revised (ADI-R, Lord *et al.*, 1994; Rutter *et al.*, 2003) and the Autism Diagnostic Observation Schedule – Generic (ADOS-G, Lord *et al.*, 2000, 2003). In children with AS, the range of IQs was 84–150. Children with AS did not have any diagnoses of severe emotional or behavioural co-morbidities, specific language learning disorders (SLI), or tic disorders.

Jansson-Verkasalo *et al.* (2005) reported defects in auditory perception in children with AS and also in their parents. The experiment was based on ERPs elicited by low tones, 280–320 Hz, imitating the frequency spectrum of F_0 in human speech. Both obligatory ERPs and MMN responses were found to differentiate children with AS from controls. Sound encoding, as reflected by exogenous ERPs, was similar in children with AS and their mothers, whereas cortical auditory discrimination as indexed by MMN, was similarly abnormal in children with AS and their fathers. It turned out that the activation of auditory brain processes distinguished the parents of children with AS from the fathers and mothers of normal control children matched for age and socio-economic status.

Korpilahti *et al.* (2007) investigated the detection of affective speech prosody in AS. They aimed to find out if poorly developed skills in understanding the pragmatic aspects, for example, emotional messages, of human communication reflect defective neural activation in auditory modality, and if this impairment is familial in nature. Earlier brain imaging studies have shown the presence of a network, called 'social brain' that connects the frontal and temporal brain regions in a highly integrative way (Frith, 2004). Korpilahti *et al.* (2007) addressed this question in more detail. Affective prosody includes the personal style of speech, and it carries the speaker's feelings and emotional state (Hargrove, 1997). It is related to the changes in the fundamental frequency (F_0) of the speaker's voice. Changes of F_0 give utterances their emotional tone and have effects on both the melody contour and the spectral patterns of speech. Perception of intonation is found to develop much earlier than speech and is important because it enables the child to understand word meanings. Processing of prosodic features is part of the newborn's adaptation to sensory percepts.

Korpilahti *et al.* (2007) studied the automatic detection of emotional prosody in Asperger syndrome. Results from fourteen boys with AS were compared with those from thirteen normally developed boys of the same age. Another aim was to investigate the evidence of phenotypic defects in AS. This was accomplished by comparing the brain activation of the fathers ($n = 12$) in the AS group with that of the control fathers ($n = 12$).

The stimuli consisted of different one-word utterances of *Anna!* (*Give it to me!* in English), spoken either with a tender or a demanding voice. Automatic detection of the affective features of voice was studied with auditory ERP measures. The obligatory N1 wave was analysed to find out the neural spectral encoding and activation, and MMN to study the detection of auditory differences and memory functions (Näätänen, 1992, 1995). The auditory difference detection of the stimuli was inspected in two time windows: the early component, eMMN, representing phonemic difference detection, and the later component, lMMN, indicating detection of differences in 'gestalt bases' (Cheour *et al.*, 2001; Korpilahti *et al.*, 2001). The results indicated that boys with AS had neurofunctionally based difficulties in processing the affective connotations of spoken utterances. Some dysfunction, especially over the right hemisphere, was also observed in the fathers of the boys with AS. It was suggested that deficient affective language processes at the level of brain activation could provide new evidence of the familial and neurobiological basis of Asperger syndrome.

Conclusion

Many research groups in Finland work actively in the field of rehabilitation of language disorders. Intensive training, computer-based intervention programs, and the efficacy of speech and language therapy and training are central topics in logopedic research (Heinänen & Lehtihalmes, 1998; Lehtihalmes, 2003). Effects of rehabilitation are not only assessed by test scores and neurophysiologic measures but also behaviourally and by observing changes in daily life.

The special features of Finnish as an inflected and morphologically very rich language (see Helasvuo in this volume) set notable demands for the assessment methods and tests to be used in logopedic practice (see Huttunen *et al.* in this volume). New tests of oral-motor skills, articulation, phonology, auditory discrimination and language comprehension have been developed for the assessment of speech and language development. On the other hand, there is a great need for comparisons of the research results obtained worldwide. Hence, we should also use tests known internationally (e.g. Reynell Developmental Language Scales, Third Edition, Edwards *et al.*, 1997 and its Finnish standardized version, Kortesmaa *et al.*, 2001). The Children's Communication Checklist (CCC) (Bishop, 1998) was translated into Finnish and adopted into clinical use by Yliherva (2004). This new method helps to diagnose pragmatic disabilities, SLI, and autistic disorders. A multi-professional group is making diagnostic evaluations using the Autism Diagnostic Interview – Revised (ADI-R, Lord *et al.*, 1994; Rutter *et al.*, 2003) and the Autism Diagnostic Observation Schedule – Generic (ADOS-G, Lord *et al.*, 2000, 2003), which are widely used in the study of autism.

This chapter has reviewed Finnish logopedic research strands in deficient language development. The language prerequisites of preterm babies are discussed in many doctoral theses in logopedics. At present, a follow-up study on premature and small-for-date babies (PIPARI project, researcher Suvi Stolt) and their language development is active at the University Hospital of Turku. The mapping of language in human brains has encouraged many new researches into this demanding field. Studies are addressed in collaboration with psychologists and specialists in medicine. In Finland, five doctoral theses in logopedics will be completed in the coming few years using ERPs, MEG and fMRI as research methods. Studies in autism spectrum disorders are also actively continued at the Universities of Oulu and Helsinki.

References

ASHA (1996) Central auditory processing: Current status of research and implications for clinical practice. *American Journal of Audiology* 5, 41–54.

Bates, E., Thal, D., Finley, B. and Clancy, B. (2003) Early language development and its neural correlates. In I. Rapin and S. Segalowitz (eds) *Handbook of Neuropsychology, Vol. 6, Child Neurology* (pp. 2–62). Amsterdam: Elsevier.

Bayley, N. (1969) *The Bayley Scales of Infant Development.* New York: Psychological Corporation.

Bishop, D. (1998) Development of the Children's Communication Checklist: A method for assessing quantitative aspects of communicative impairment in children. *Journal of Child Psychology and Psychiatry* 39, 879–891.

Cheour, M., Korpilahti, P., Martynova, O. and Lang, A.H. (2001) Mismatch negativity and late discriminative negativity in investigating speech perception and learning in children and infants – A review. *Audiology & Neuro-Otology* 6, 2–11.

Diamond, A., Werker, J.F. and Lalonde, C. (1994) Toward understanding commonalities in the development of object search, detour navigation, categorization, and speech perception. In G. Dawson and K.W. Fisher (eds) *Human Behaviour and the Developing Brain* (pp. 380–426). New York: Guilford Press.

DiSimoni, F. (1978) *The Token Test for Children.* Massachusetts: Teaching Resources Corporation.

Edwards, S., Fletcher, P., Garman, M., Hughes, A., Letts, C. and Sinka, I. (1997) *Reynell Developmental Language Scales* (3rd edn). Windsor: The NFER-Nelson.

Frith, U. (2004) Emmanuel Miller lecture: Confusions and controversies about Asperger syndrome. *Journal of Child Psychology and Psychiatry* 45 (4), 672–686.

Gerken, S. (1994) Child phonology: Past research, present questions, future directions. In M.A. Gernsbacher (ed.) *Handbook of Psycholinguistics* (pp. 781–820). San Diego: Singular Publishing Group.

Hargrove, P. (1997) Prosodic aspects of language impairment in children. *Topics in Language Disorders* 17 (4), 76–83.

Heinänen, K. and Lehtihalmes, M. (1998) Lasten kielellisten häiriöiden tutkimuksen haasteita [Challenges to research of child language disorders]. In K. Heinänen and M. Lehtihalmes (eds) *Kielihäiriöisen lapsen tutkiminen – testaamistako? [Assessment of a child with specific language impairmen – testing only?].* Publications of the Finnish Association of Logopedics and Phoniatrics 30, 5–8.

Holopainen, I., Korpilahti, P. and Lang, A.H. (1997a) Mitä tietoa poikkeusärsykev-aste antaa puheen ja kielen kehityksen häiriöissä [Using mismatch negativity in diagnosis of SLI]? *Duodecim* 19, 1865–1871.

Holopainen, I., Korpilahti, P., Juottonen, K., Lang, A.H. and Sillanpää, M. (1997b) Attenuated auditory event-related potential (Mismatch negativity) in children with developmental dysphasia. *Neuropediatrics* 28, 253–256.

Holopainen, I., Korpilahti, P., Juottonen, K., Lang, A.H. and Sillanpää, M. (1998) Abnormal frequency mismatch negativity (MMN) in mentally retarded children and in children with developmental dysphasia. *Journal of Child Neurology* 13 (4), 178–183.

Jansson-Verkasalo, E. (2003) Auditory event-related potentials as indices of language impairment in children born preterm and with Asperger syndrome. Acta Universitas Ouluensis, Humaniora B 54. PhD thesis, University of Oulu, Oulu, Finland.

Jansson-Verkasalo, E., Korpilahti, P., Jäntti, V., Valkama, M., Vainionpää, L., Alku, P., Suominen, K. and Näätänen, R. (2003a) Neurophysiologic correlates of deficient phonological representations and object naming in prematurely born children. *Clinical Neurophysiology* 115, 179–187.

Jansson-Verkasalo, E., Ceponiene, R., Kielinen, M., Suominen, K., Jäntti, V., Linna, S-L., Moilanen, I. and Näätänen, R. (2003b) Deficient auditory processing in children with Asperger Syndrome, as indexed by event-related potentials. *Neuroscience Letters* 338, 197–200.

Jansson-Verkasalo, E., Valkama, M., Vainionpää, L., Pääkkö, E., Ilkko, E. and Lehtihalmes, M. (2004) Language development in very low birth weight preterm children: A follow-up study. *Folia Phoniatrica et Logopaedica* 56, 108–119.

Jansson-Verkasalo, E., Kujala, T., Jussila, K., Mattila, M-L., Moilanen, I., Näätänen, R., Suominen, K. and Korpilahti, P. (2005) Similarities in the phenotype of the auditory neural substrate in children with Asperger syndrome and their parents. *European Journal of Neuroscience* 22, 986–990.

Jennishe, M. and Sedin, G. (2001) Linguistic skills at 6,5 years of age in children who required neonatal intensive care in 1986–1989. *Acta Paediatrica* 90, 22–33.

Karmiloff, K. and Karmiloff-Smith, A. (2001) *Pathways to Language. From Fetus to Adolescent.* Cambridge: Harvard University Press.

Korpilahti, P. (1995) Auditory discrimination and memory functions in SLI: A comprehensive study with neurophysiological and behavioural methods. *Scandinavian Journal of Logopedics and Phoniatrics* 20, 131–139.

Korpilahti, P. (1996) Electrophysiological correlates of auditory perception in normal and language impaired children. Annales Universitats Turkuensis, Medica – Odontologica D 232. PhD thesis, University of Turku, Turku, Finland.

Korpilahti, P. and Lang, A.H. (1994) Auditory ERP components and MMN in dysphasic children. *Electroencephalography and Clinical Neurophysiology* 91, 256–264.

Korpilahti, P., Krause, C.M., Holopainen, I. and Lang, A.H. (2001) Early and late mismatch negativity (MMN) elicited by words and speech-like stimuli in children. *Brain and Language* 76, 332–339.

Korpilahti, P., Jansson-Verkasalo, E., Mattila, M-L., Kuusikko, S., Suominen, K., Rytky, S., Pauls, D.L. and Moilanen, I. (2007) Processing of affective prosody of speech is impaired in Asperger syndrome. *Journal of Autism and Developmental Disorders*, 37, 1539–1549.

Kortesmaa, M., Heimonen, K., Merikoski, H., Warma, M-L. and Varpela, V. (2001) *Reynellin kielellisen kehityksen testi [Finnish version of the Reynell Developmental Language Scales. Third Edition].* Helsinki: Psykologien Kustannus.

Krause, M.C., Korpilahti, P., Pörn, B., Jäntti, J. and Lang, A.H. (1998) Automatic auditory word perception as measured by 40 Hz EEG responses. *Electroencephalography and Clinical Neurophysiology* 107, 84–89.

Kunnari, S. (2000) Characteristics of early lexical and phonological development in children acquiring Finnish. Acta Universitas Ouluensis, Humaniora B 34. PhD thesis, University of Oulu, Oulu, Finland.

Laakso, M-L., Poikkeus, A-M., Katajamäki, J. and Lyytinen, P. (1999) Early intentional communication as a predictor of language development in young toddlers. *First Language* 19, 207–231.

Lang, A.H., Eerola, O., Korpilahti, P., Holopainen, I., Salo, S., Uusipaikka, E. and Aaltonen, O. (1995) Practical issues in the clinical application of the MMN. *Ear and Hearing*, Special Issue 16 (1), 118–130.

Launonen, K. (1998) *Eleistä sanoihin, viittomista kieleen. Varhaisviittomisohjelman kehittäminen, kokeilu ja pitkäaikaisvaikutukset Downin syndrooma -lapsilla [From gestures to words, from signs to language. Development, application, and long-term effects of an Early Signing Programme in the early intervention of children with Down syndrome].* FAMR Research Publications, No. 75. Helsinki: Kehitysvammaliitto ry.

Lehtihalmes, M. (2003) Puheterapian vaikuttavuus – tarua vai totta [Effectiveness of speech therapy – fact or fiction]? In M. Lehtihalmes (ed.) *Kuntoutuksen vaikuttavuus [Effectiveness of rehabilitation].* Publications of the Finnish Association of Speech and Language Research 35, 2–6.

Liuksila, P-R. (2000) Lastenneuvolan viisivuotistarkastus ja sen merkitys lapsen selviytymiselle ensimmäisellä luokalla koulussa [Examination of the five-year-old child at the Child Health Center and its significance for the child's progress in the first grade at school]. Annales Universitats Turkuensis Scripta Lingua Fennica Edita C 161. PhD thesis, University of Turku, Turku, Finland.

Lord, C., Rutter, M. and Le Courteur, A. (1994) Autism Diagnostic Interview – Revised: A revised version of a diagnostic interview for caregivers of individuals with possible pervasive developmental disorder. *Journal of Autism and Developmental Disorders* 24, 659–685.

Lord, C., Risi, S., Lambrecht, L., Cook, Jr, E.H., Leventhat, B.L., DiLavore, P.C., Pickles, A. and Rutter, M. (2000) The Autism Observation Schedule – Generic: A standard measure of social and communication deficits associated with the spectrum of autism. *Journal of Autism and Developmental Disorders* 30 (3), 205–223.

Lord, C., Rutter, M., DiLavore, P.C. and Risi, S. (2003) *Autism Diagnostic Observation Schedule, ADOS.* Los Angeles, CA: Western Psychological Services.

Lyytinen, P. (1999) *Varhaisen kommunikaation ja kielen kehityksen arviointimenetelmä [Finnish edition of MacArthur Communicative and Language Development Inventory (CDI)].* Jyväskylä: Niilo Mäki Institute.

Näätänen, R. (1992) *Attention and Brain Function.* Hillsdale, NJ: Erlbaum.

Näätänen, R. (1995) The mismatch negativity: A powerful tool for cognitive neuroscience. *Ear and Hearing* 16 (1), 6–18.

Överlund, J. (1996; 6th edition 2006) Puhe ja kieli kehittyvät vuorovaikutuksessa [Speech and language develop in interaction]. In K. Launonen and A.-M. Korpijaakko-Huuhka (eds) *Kommunikoinnin häiriöt – syitä, ilmenemismuotoja ja kuntoutuksen perusteita [Disorders of Communication – Causes, Characteristics and Basics of Rehabilitation]* (pp. 19–38). Helsinki: Palmenia.

Paavola, L., Kunnari, S., Moilanen, I. and Lehtihalmes, M. (2005) The functions of maternal verbal responses to prelinguistic infant as predictors of early communicative and linguistic development. *First Language* 25, 173–195.

Parre, M., Donner, M., Helenius, M. and Michelsson, K. (1980) Speech development and its disorders in 5-year-old high-risk children. Paper presented at the *XVIII Congress of International Association of Logopedics and Phoniatrics, IALP*. Washington DC, USA.

Rapin, I. and Dunn, M. (2003) Review article: Update on the language disorders of individuals on the autistic spectrum. *Brain & Development* 25, 166–172.

Reynell, J.K. and Huntley, M. (1985) *Reynell Developmental Language Scales* (2nd edn). Windsor: The NFER-Nelson.

Riitesuo, A. (2000) A preterm child grows: Focus on speech and language during the first two years. Jyväskylä Studies in Education, Psychology and Social Research. PhD thesis, University of Jyväskylä, Jyväskylä, Finland.

Rutter M., Le Couteur, A. and Lord, C. (2003) *ADI-R, Autism Diagnostic Interview-Revised*. Manual. Los Angeles, CA: Western Psychological Services.

Saarikoski, S. (1998) Ennenaikainen synnytys [Preterm birth]. *Duodecim* 21, 2243–2252.

Saxon, T. (1997) A longitudinal study of early mother-infant interaction and later language competence. *First Language* 17, 271–281.

Savinainen-Makkonen, T. (2001) Suomalainen lapsi fonologiaa omaksumassa [Finnish children acquiring phonology]. Publications of the Department of Phonetics 42. PhD thesis, University of Helsinki, Helsinki, Finland.

Squires, J.K., Bricker, D. and Potter, L. (1993) Infant/Child Monitoring Questionnaires, Revised. University of Oregon. Center on Human Development.

Stolt, S., Takila, P., Lehtonen, L., Lapinleimu, H. and Haataja, L. (2005, July) Quantitative and qualitative aspects of early lexicon in prematurely born VLBW and full term Finnish children at two years of age. Paper presented in the *X International Congress for the Study of Child Language*, Berlin, Germany.

Tallal, P., Stark, R.E. and Mellits, D. (1985) The relationship between auditory temporal analysis and receptive language development: Evidence from studies of developmental language disorder. *Neuropsychology* 23, 527–534.

Volkmar, F.R. and Pauls, D. (2003) Autism. *The Lancet* 362, 1133–1141.

Wolke, D. and Meyer, R. (1999) Cognitive status, language attainment, and pre-reading skills of 6-year-old very preterm children and their peers: The Bavarian longitudinal study. *Developmental Medicine and Child Neurology* 41, 94–109.

Yliherva, A. (2002) Ennenaikaisina ja pienipainoisina syntyneiden lasten puheen- ja kielenkehityksen taso kahdeksan vuoden iässä. Pohjoissuomalainen syntymäkohortti 1985–86 [Speech and language abilities of preterm and low birthweight children at 8 years of age in the northern Finland 1-year birth cohort for 1985–86]. Acta Universitas Ouluensis, Humaniora B 44. University of Oulu, Oulu, Finland.

Yliherva, A., Olsén, P., Suvanto, A. and Järvelin M-R. (2000) Language abilities of 8-year-old preterm children among the northern Finland 1-year birth cohort for 1985–1986. *Logopedics Phoniatrics Vocology* 25, 98–104.

Yliherva, A., Olsén, P., Mäki-Torkko, E., Koiranen, M. and Järvelin M-R. (2001) Linguistic and motor abilities of low-birthweight children as assessed by parents and teachers at 8 years of age. *Acta Paediatrica* 90, 1440–1449.

Yliherva, A. (2004) Lasten kommunikaation arviointimenetelmä CCC-2 [Children's Communication Checklist-2]. *Puheterapeutti* (4), 19–20.

Chapter 6
Alternative Communication Form as a Genuinely Shared Language

KAISA LAUNONEN

Introduction

Augmentative and alternative communication has established its position in intervention with people with severe communication disorders around the world. Alternative communication forms have created opportunities for social participation and a better quality of life for people who would earlier have been left on the margin of their society, with very little content and variety in their lives. The main body of research in this field has been built up over the last few decades. The research on issues concerning speech and language pathology, in general, is young in Finland, and has also mainly emerged during that period. Studies on augmentative and alternative communication have played a not insignificant role in this development. As the number of academic researchers is still small in Finland, most of these studies have been Master's theses or reports of development projects carried out by speech and language therapists, alongside their clinical work. Some other professionals, such as occupational therapists and AAC workers, have also been involved in these studies but their number is, nevertheless, small compared to that of speech and language therapists.

In many European countries speech and language therapists do not actively engage in research and practice in the field of augmentative and alternative communication, but rather the field is mainly the responsibility of other professions, such as special education teachers or psychologists. The active role of Finnish speech and language therapists may have arisen, at least partly, from the historical fact that they were first trained in Finland, in the 1960s, to work in institutions for people with learning disabilities ('mental retardation'). People with the most severe communication problems have, thus, been the main responsibility of Finnish speech and language therapists from the very beginning of the history of the profession.

Also, the Finnish health care legislation, which guarantees intervention using public resources for people with severe impairments, may account for the larger number of speech and language therapists dealing with alternative communication issues.

Only a few doctoral theses on topics dealing with augmentative and alternative communication issues have been written in Finland so far (see Launonen, 1998; Rautakoski, 2005; Salminen, 2001). However, even the findings of Master's theses, based on small studies, may remain topical and be utilised in clinical practice, if they are of good quality. This has happened to many theses written on the themes of augmentative and alternative communication, and they have also been developed further into new studies, or at least parts of them. During a reasonably short time, starting in the last decade of the 20th century, an active group of speech and language therapists working in the field of augmentative and alternative communication has been built up in Finland. Many of these colleagues have a genuine research orientation in their clinical work, and attend both international conferences (particularly the International Society for Augmentative and Alternative Communication, ISAAC) and national ones (Sillalla – På bron; 'On the bridge'), presenting their clinical experiments and development projects (see also Huuhtanen, 1992, 2001). The number of speech and language therapists who do post-graduate studies, with the aim of writing a doctoral thesis on a topic of augmentative and alternative communication, has been rising during the first decade of the 21st century.

Alternative Communication Forms in Finland

Manual signs are the most common alternative communication form used in Finland, followed by Pictograms (Maharaj, 1980), pictures and gestures (Launonen, 2002a, 2002b). The Picture Communication Symbols (PCS) (Johnson, 1981) have become increasingly popular during the early 21st century, and have probably attained the popularity of Pictograms, or even surpassed them. As the alternative communication forms presently in use are more or less universal, research and the application of its findings are easily considered to be independent of the language of the speaking community. To some extent this may be true, but this view may also have its risks, if it is taken as given that all the findings in alternative communication studies in certain countries are applicable as such in all others. For one thing, societies differ in their language and minority politics and service systems, which creates differences in language use even if the alternative system may be the same in different countries.

Moreover, probably most people who use alternative communication forms rely in their comprehension mainly on spoken language, which is, and should be, in most cases, used alongside alternative communication.

In addition, for many small children their alternative communication form is only a temporary means of expression, the purpose of which is to support their receptive language and speech development, as part of their early intervention (Martinsen & von Tetzchner, 1996). The body of research on developmental issues in alternative communication is, so far, very limited (but see von Tetzchner & Grove, 2003a), and the relationship between spoken language and the alternative communication form in bimodal language learning is not properly understood. It is clear, however, that the two are closely connected and that, therefore, there are always language-specific features, based on the spoken language of the society, that should be taken into account, both in research and in practice. For the most advanced users of alternative communication systems, the opportunity of comparing and matching their system with the spoken and written language of society is particularly important, because the aim is often to progress from pictorial to written communication, perhaps via Blissymbols (Bliss, 1965). At some phase of this progress, the different forms may even be mixed, so that pictorial signs and written words may together form a sentence.

The alternative communication systems that are most commonly used both in Finland and internationally were mainly developed in English-speaking countries, and also the main body of research in this field is based on English-speaking communities. This presents a challenge for the application of these systems alongside languages such as Finnish, the grammar of which is very different from that of English (see Helasvuo, in this volume). Particularly problematic is the characteristic that morphological endings are attached to the word stem, the form of which often alters when the ending is added. This problem has become evident, for example, in recent projects developing advanced dynamic displays (see Burkhart, 1994; Porter, 2000) for graphic sign users.

From Intervention to Communication: A Shift of Focus

In many countries, including Finland, alternative communication is still often seen more as an intervention tool and less as a real communication form, both by professionals in the field and by people with disabilities and their communication partners (Martinsen & von Tetzchner, 1996; von Tetzchner & Grove, 2003b). This may be due to historical reasons, especially to the fact that the emphasis of language intervention has traditionally been mainly in individual therapy. With the movement towards a socially constructed view of disabilities, growing in many countries (see World Health Organization, 2005), communication disabilities are, however, no longer seen as deficits of individuals only, but as obstacles in the social interaction of their societies in general. Accordingly, the emphasis in communication intervention has turned more towards communities and their interaction. Professionals have started to develop intervention methods that aim at enhancing the communication skills of whole communities with people who need alternative communication forms. These efforts include early intervention with families with children who have high risks of disordered language development (e.g. Launonen, 1998, 2003a), as well as different forms of community based rehabilitation, for example, in daycare, schools and supported employment settings (e.g. Grove & Park, 1996; Hildén *et al.*, 2001; Huuhtanen, 2002b; Martikainen, 2004; Merikoski & Hildén, 2000; Pulli *et al.*, 2002; Widell *et al.*, 2002). The basic ideology behind these ecological approaches is that even alternative communication forms must be genuinely shared by people who need them in their daily interaction. If and when people with communication disabilities are to be regarded as full members of their communities and society at large, the need for an alternative communication form should be seen as a shared need for these people and all their communication partners. According to rough estimates, this need concerns approximately 20,000 Finns of different ages, and their communication partners (von Tetzchner & Martinsen, 1999: 79).

This chapter will discuss opportunities and challenges of ecological approaches in the development of alternative communication forms to genuinely shared languages for people who need them in their daily interaction. The discussion will be mainly based on studies and development projects by Finnish authors. A general framework for the discussion will be the theory of ecological systems by Urie Bronfenbrenner (1979, 1995; Bronfenbrenner & Ceci, 1994). This theory provides a useful framework for presenting and discussing various approaches to the development and use of shared communication forms between people with special communication needs and their environment. In terms of this theory, the opportunities for interaction of an individual can be looked at and evaluated at the levels of his or her micro-, meso-, exo- and macrosystems (Figure 6.1).

Interaction Between Individuals

The *microsystems* of an individual consist of the social communities formed by his or her family, day-care, classroom, work, spare-time activities and friends. He or she is a direct member of these systems, affecting their functioning by his or her own behaviour, as they in turn affect his or her own functions. In terms of communication development this means, first of all, that the more able communication partners of a child provide him or her with a developmentally fit *scaffolding* (Bruner, 1983), enabling the child to communicate and learn new ways of communication at its *zone of proximal development* (Vygotsky, 1978). This effect is not, however, one-way. Behaviour of the child also has a decisive impact on how people

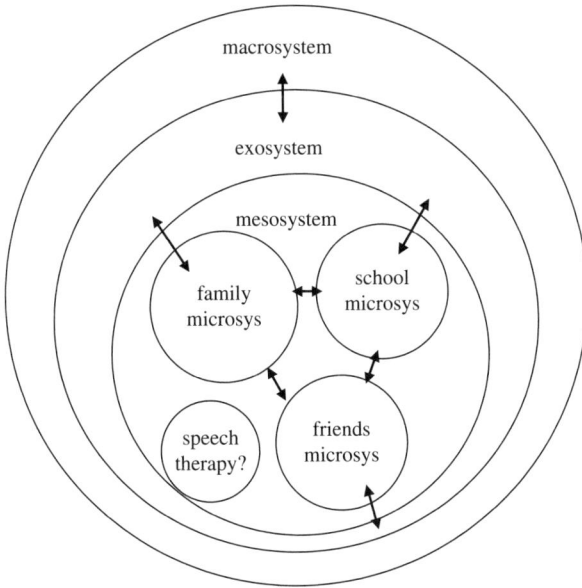

Figure 6.1 Bronfenbrenner's (1979) theory of ecological systems; illustration adapted by the author

interact with it. If they think the child's behaviour makes sense and is intelligible, they tune into his or her affectional state and attention focus, and they cause the action to be shared. If a child behaves in very untypical ways, it may be difficult for the parents and other communication partners to create interactive scaffolds, which the child would need to build up communicative competence. Therefore, the parents of children with high risks of developmental disabilities may need, or benefit from, early intervention procedures, which aim at preventing predictable problems in communication development before they appear.

Children with Down syndrome are known to have distinctive problems in their language development, and particularly in speech, which cannot be explained by their intellectual impairment only. In a Finnish long-term follow-up study, two groups of children with Down syndrome were compared (Launonen, 1996, 1998, 2003a). The research group ($n = 12$) consisted of children whose families took part in an early intervention program from the age of 6 months until the age of 3. Manual signs were taught to the families to augment the communication and language development of the children, and the active communicative role of the child was emphasised. The children of the comparison group ($n = 12$) did not participate in the programme. Other forms of early support were the same for the two groups. The development of the children was followed annually until the age of five, and an eight-year assessment was made five years after the intervention programme terminated. The results (Launonen, 1996, 1998) showed that the intervention had significant immediate and short-term benefits for the children of the research group. At the age of eight there were still significant differences in the interaction, communication, and language skills of the two groups (Launonen, 1998, 2003a). The results support the view that early language intervention is important for later achievements and adjustment of children with Down syndrome, and that a successful early interaction forms an important basis for later general development, social adjustment and quality of life.

Even though manual signing gives beneficial support to the early communication development of children with Down syndrome, generally, the findings of case studies indicate that there is large individual variation even within this diagnostic group (see Launonen, 2003a). Manual signing as an alternative communication form may have beneficial effects even if it is not started as early as the first year of life, but later in childhood. A family of a boy with Down syndrome adopted manual signs in its communication, when the boy was three years old and had not started to speak (Launonen & Grove, 2003). The boy quickly learned hundreds of manual signs and started to combine them and use his total communication, consisting of manual signs, gestures, lively mime and action, as a linguistic system. His vocal system was very dyspractic, and he was practically non-speaking until the age of 12, when he started gradually to attempt spoken words. At the age of 17, he was a fluent speaker but his speech was almost unintelligible to strangers, and he benefited greatly from manual signs as an augmentative system.

Another case study indicates that even though children may learn manual signs at a very early age, it does not guarantee that their communication will develop without problems (Launonen, 2005a, 2005b). A family of a boy with Down syndrome actively participated in an early intervention programme from when the boy was aged 6 months. The parents used manual signs with him, and he even learned to use them in signed songs and routine contact games. However, his reciprocal communication skills remained very poor, and he could not actively use manual signs nor any other communication means. Only after the focus of his communication intervention was shifted, at the age of 3, from learning more signs to reciprocal interaction by any means, did he gradually become aware of his own role in communication. This might easily have been regarded as a step backwards in intervention, because the attention was shifted from the demands of active sign use to shared activities, in practice even to early interpersonal attunement (e.g. Stern, 1985). However, when he learned, very slowly, to initiate shared activities intentionally, and to direct and control his own behaviour in them, he also could later actively use his manual sign vocabulary. At the age of 6, he started to attempt spoken words, which gradually displaced manual signs. However, his spoken expressions were, for a long time, formed by endings of the words he aimed at, which made most of his speech unintelligible, particularly when he was referring to something outside the immediate physical context. Therefore, this boy also continued to benefit from manual signs alongside his speech. The cognitive level of this boy was lower than in people with Down syndrome on average. Earlier studies on children with poor cognitive skills have also shown that shifting the attention to intensive interaction on the child's own terms may open up opportunities for the development of alternative communication for children with whom intervention has not seemed to make progress until then (Launonen, 2000a, 2001).

But children's development does not always make positive progress, new skills do not always build on the old ones. Sometimes children have progressive diseases, which lead to the loss of skills and, finally, even death. In these cases, parents may need support and alternative communication forms to maintain contact and interaction with their child. Reports of studies on the communication intervention with children with progressive diseases are practically nonexistent. In a small Finnish study, the families of three children with a progressive encephalopathy (infantile neuronal ceroid lipofuscinosis, INCL), took part in a one-year intervention programme aimed at creating opportunities for interaction between children with very few and limited skills and their parents (Pullola-Teeriaho, 2000; Pullola-Teeriaho & Launonen, 2002). The parents developed tangible signs (i.e. concrete objects) or sounds with a sign function (e.g. ringing of a bell before starting a singing session), in order for their child to anticipate shared activities. These activities were either nursing (e.g. taking a bath) or contact games, and mother and father found signs for different routines. The results showed that even though the children's development regressed during the follow-up year, the observations of their parents on their skills became more detailed and more accurate. It is, thus, presumable that the parents were also able to create more functional interaction with their child, when they could see not only regression but also a potential for sharing, in the child. Efforts like this intervention experiment show that it is possible to maintain or even increase the quality of life for people whose life is drawing to a close.

With the constantly increasing tendency to develop intervention practices that build on everyday communication and parents' alternative communication skills, it has also become topical to develop evaluation methods that would allow the involvement of parents in the evaluation process. Parents have been found to make reliable evaluations of their normally developing children's early language development (Dale, 1991; Lyytinen *et al.*, 1994), and the same seems to apply to many parents of children learning alternative communication forms. Parents can evaluate the number of manual signs used by their children very accurately when there are less than 100, and the accuracy seems to be reasonably good up to 200 signs, after which the parents often just say: 'it is impossible to give an estimation – hundreds' (Launonen, 1996, 1998). With small children or older individuals with very limited communication skills, it is often difficult for the speech and language therapist to ascertain what an individual really can do with his or her communication repertoire. Parents can give information and examples from everyday life, which may be invaluable for the speech and language therapist to be able to develop their child's communication and intervention together with them (Launonen 1998, 2003a, 2004). They may not know automatically what they should pay attention to and what to tell the professional, but with the help of well-directed questions and even ready-made evaluation forms – if they are detailed enough – parents may learn to pay attention even to very early and small steps in development (Launonen & Olkku, 2000; Olkku, 1997; Pullola-Teeriaho, 2000; Pullola-Teeriaho & Launonen, 2002; see also Pulli *et al.*, 2005). Sometimes these evaluations may be accurate enough for planning the intervention, so that, for example, video analysis gives no added value (see Launonen & Olkku, 2000; Olkku, 1997), but it is clear that the availability of video techniques has created invaluable, new opportunities for the evaluation of communication with alternative systems. New methods are being developed for the self-evaluation of staff working with people who need alternative communication (e.g. Burakoff, 2001; Martikainen, 2004), and these practices will eventually also help the development of communication in families who need alternative communication systems.

If children and their families take part in communication intervention, it is important that daycare personnel are also included, particularly if alternative communication forms are used (Launonen 1998; 2003a; Hildén *et al.*, 2001; Merikoski & Hildén 2000). There are, however, large differences between daycare personnel, individually and also between nurseries or preschools. This seems to depend partly on the education of the individual employees, both on their professional training, and on their education in augmentative and alternative communication (Launonen, 2002a, 2002b). Also the attitudes, general atmosphere, and work load experienced by the personnel, seem to determine whether and to what extent they are able and willing to take the trouble of implementing alternative communication in their daily routines (Launonen, 1998).

The significance of the knowledge and skills of professionals working with people who need alternative communication forms becomes accentuated because a great deal of the interaction of these individuals inevitably takes place in institutional settings. A number of recent Finnish studies have addressed the question of alternative communication skills of professionals. These studies have looked at the communication of daycare personnel (Hildén *et al.*, 2001; Hildén & Merikoski, 2002; Merikoski &

Hildén, 2000), as well as people working in schools (Hurmola, 2001), institutions (Markus, 2000), and in sheltered work units (Burakoff, 2001; Burakoff & Launonen, 2002). A large survey was carried out in the fall of 1999 in five Finnish districts (Launonen, 2002a, 2002b), aiming at ascertaining the knowledge, skills and attitudes in augmentative and alternative communication of staff working in different communities with people who use or are in need of these communication forms. Questionnaires were distributed in nurseries, schools, daycare centres, group homes and institutions. Most of the people in these communities had intellectual disabilities of differing severity, but there were also communities with people whose main diagnosis was autism or motor disability.

In the first of the three main sections of the questionnaire, the participants were asked to describe their probable behaviour in an imagined situation at work, as partners of a person using alternative communication. In the second section they evaluated how important 10 central functions of communication, given in the form, were for their imagined partner in his or her daily life. In the last section, the participants evaluated how well they knew different alternative communication matters, also given in the form. In the first and last sections, they evaluated both their own behaviour and knowledge, and that of their community in general.

According to the results, based on 635 returned questionnaires from 77 communities, members of the staff of different communities were well aware of good practices in their double role as partners and assistants in alternative communication. They evaluated that they behaved according to good practices most of the time, and so did their whole community, even if to a slightly lesser degree than themselves. They considered expressions of daily needs and emotions to be the most important communicative functions for their partner, while the use of communication to express imagination and controlling other people's behaviour were the least important. Even though manual signs were the most common communication form used in the communities, the staff evaluated that they did not know manual signs as well as they knew gestures, pictures and Pictograms. Blissymbols (Bliss, 1965) were neither used nor known very well. Neither were the participants very familiar with communication technology, but they estimated that other people in their community knew the field slightly better. According to the answers, the time spent daily in interaction seems to be very limited (a few times per day, 13.8 minutes each, on the average) for many people who use augmentative and alternative communication.

The results of the survey mainly confirmed the expectations of the speech and language therapists who participated in carrying out the survey. There were, however, also some unexpected findings. Based on observations in the communities, everyday interaction with people who use alternative forms of communication is rarely as ideal as the answers indicate. The staff's tendency to give an ideal picture, and an even more ideal picture of themselves than of other staff members, indicates, however, that they are aware of good practices. People with higher basic education (e.g. teachers) and more training in alternative communication seemed to be generally best aware of good communication practices and also seemed to be able to follow them best in their daily work. The findings of this survey highlighted, once again, that the education and other development projects of the future should aim at providing the staff of communities with people using alternative communication with both communicative tools and work conditions which would make ideal interaction possible.

It is not only the daily communication partners with whom people should be able to communicate, even if they are using alternative communication forms. For their empowerment, participation and integration, it is essential that they can manage their own business as independently as it is individually necessary, and have a shared language even with strangers. A Finnish project aimed at developing alternative communication skills of people working in professional services, such as libraries, social services or cabs (Huuhtanen, 2002a, 2004). It turned out, not surprisingly, that most of these professionals knew very little, if anything, about alternative communication. They were also nervous or afraid of the thought of having a client who would communicate using an alternative communication form. The very basic information given to these professionals during the project helped many of them overcome their nervousness, but the motivation to keep the alternative communication skills active is often low, because most of the professionals meet very few people who use them, particularly in small municipalities.

The main project in supporting individuals in independent communication presently in Finland is the *interpreter service model* (Pulli, 1994, 1996; Sundblad *et al.*, 2002). This model was created in the late 1980s, and was included in Finnish legislation in 1987. The act guarantees interpreter services, free of charge, a minimum of 120 hours per year, for people with speech disabilities (240 hours for deaf people using sign language). The service can be used, for example, in work, studies, business, social participation or leisure. Interpreter services connected to education are allowed as much as the person needs them individually to get through his or her studies.

Even if this legislation on interpreter services is important and even internationally exceptional, the implementation of it was not without problems. After the law became active, education of interpreters for people with communication disabilities was begun in numerous social studies schools, with no specified curriculum or defined criteria of professional skills for the interpreters, and for a while it seemed that almost anybody could claim to be an interpreter. Even after the educational criteria were officially defined, it has not always been easy to find interpreters whose skills would have met the needs of an individual requiring the service. The problem is accentuated with those individuals whose communication disabilities are the most severe. One of the biggest obstacles in the utilization of the interpreter services, up to now, has been that the general awareness of the law has increased very slowly.

It will be a challenge for future research to describe interaction in contexts where interpreters are used to transmit messages that are conveyed using alternative communication forms. This research, which has already been started in Finland, will be methodologically, as well as ethically, as challenging as is the interpreter activity itself.

The impact of *peers and friends* on the communication skills and language use of individuals has been little studied in general. It is known, however, that particularly in adolescence, the microsystems formed by peers are central for building up an individual's social identity, and that the micro-language community, shared by young people, plays an important role in this identification (Chambers, 2003: 186–194). However, children and adolescents who use alternative communication forms often lack genuine peer groups, the members of which they would call their friends. Even when the inclusion of children in the group of normally developing children seems otherwise to be successful, it may turn out that they and their peers do not have a genuinely shared language form, which they could use without adults as interpreters or supporters. In a case study by Herkman (2000) (see also Herkman & Launonen, 2002), a 7-year-old boy, who used a communication program in his computer, managed to convey messages to adults, particularly to those who were familiar with aided communication. However, when the communication partner was a peer, the boys needed an adult's help to be able to communicate with each other. It also happens that the vocabulary which is made available in communication aids is often chosen by adults. Thus, the vocabulary may not be ideal for communication between young people, who have their own interests, which adults may not even be aware of (see also Beukelman *et al.*, 1991; Murphy *et al.*, 1996; Sundblad, 2005).

Even if it may often be difficult to create natural communication situations with peers for young people who use alternative communication forms, sometimes artificially created interaction contexts, such as speech and language therapy in groups, may also add to the intervention beneficial factors, which only peers can offer each other. Different games and play, which are often used as therapy methods, gain new interest and challenges when there is a peer as a partner, and not always a therapist with her or his superior communication skills (Heikurainen, 2004; Heikurainen & Launonen, 2004). Acting in a group with equal partners makes children consider their own role and responsibility in interaction in a different way than with a therapist, who is always able to control the interaction with her or his professional sensitivity and skill (Widell *et al.*,

2002). In addition to the motivation factor, peers may also provide each other with communication models, if they have different strengths in their communication and different communication strategies in use (Heikurainen, 2004; Heikurainen & Launonen, 2004). Group projects have proved useful in creating opportunities for interaction and developing communication skills even in adults with severe learning disabilities, who use alternative communication (Grove & Park, 1996; Huuhtanen 2002b; Pulli *et al.*, 2002).

Augmentative and alternative communication has established its position worldwide mainly in the intervention with people with developmental disabilities. This was also the case for a long time in Finland. By the turn of the millennium however, the situation started to change, and alternative communication forms are now considered increasingly often with people who have lost their former ability to communicate by speech, for example, due to a stroke. As with the developmental disabilities, here too the focus is primarily on pragmatic aspects of language, and in ecological approaches, where the family members and friends of people with disabilities have been included both in intervention and evaluation (Rautakoski, 2002, 2005). Along with, or instead of, individual intervention, many people with aphasia take part in group speech therapy, often with their spouses or other relatives or friends. These group approaches enable them to practise genuine interaction using new strategies, not only alternative communication systems but also utilising non-verbal resources such as gestures, prosody of speech, laughter and drawing (Klippi, 1996).

Communication and Information Transmission Between Microsystems

A mesosystem is formed by the relationships between individual's microsystems. This could mean, for example, the interaction between children's home and daycare. It is essential for the development of communication skills of a child using alternative communication forms that this interaction is functional, and that the family and daycare personnel share their view on the communication needs and skills of the child (Hildén *et al.*, 2001). Later, when individuals are at school or work, the consistency of the views on their communicative opportunities and needs, of people in their microsystems, is, likewise, important. It seems, however, that this is not always the case (see Sundblad, 2005; Widell, 1999; Widell & Launonen, 2000). Along with the increasing emphasis on ecological and community-based approaches in intervention, it will be an increasing challenge for and responsibility of professionals to develop procedures and tools enabling the discussion and transmission of information between the microsystems of individuals who use alternative communication forms (e.g. Launonen, 2005c; Pulli *et al.*, 2005; see also Hildén *et al.*, 2001; von Tetzchner & Martinsen, 1999, 2000).

The knowledge and skills of the members of microsystems, as well as the interaction at the mesosystem level, is largely dependent on certain processes of the *exosystem* level. According to Bronfenbrenner's defini-tion, an exosystem is formed by connections in which the developing child has not necessarily a direct role, but which may have an indirect impact on him or her through the actions of other members of his or her microsystems. Talking about ecological and community-based approaches, the rehabilitation system can largely be seen as an exosystem (even if direct speech and language therapy, be it individual or group therapy, can be seen to form one of the microsystems of an individual with com-munication disability). In order for intervention with individuals with severe communication disorders to be efficacious, family members and friends need to communicate effectively with professionals and authori-ties to obtain all the information they need. For example, when an infant has a high risk of developing severe communication disorders, it is impor-tant that the professionals and the families recognise what sort of support and intervention the parents need, to be able to support their child in his or her zone of proximal development and to help their child learn (e.g. Brekke & von Tetzchner, 2003; Launonen, 1998; Pullola-Teeriaho, 2000; Smith, 2003).

The knowledge and skills of teachers, nurses, and other professionals working with people with communication disabilities are largely depen-dent on the quality and quantity of their education (Alant, 2003; Collier & Blackstien-Adler, 1998; Launonen, 2002a, 2002b; Ratcliff & Beukelman, 1995). Particularly for teachers, the question is not only that of supporting and developing children's daily interaction. Language, be it transmitted by speech or alternative communication forms, is always an important tool in teaching and learning. According to the observations of many pro-fessionals in communication intervention, the staff of the communities of people who use augmentative and alternative communication, do not, however, always sufficiently master the use of these communication forms, so that they would be consistently in use in all daily interactions. Hence, there seems to be a need for more effective education in the field, in professional training, updating training, and on-the-job training. Very many people will need these various sorts of education, and, because of the turnover of the staff, the need is also continuous. Planning education at different levels should be based on a careful analysis of the present knowledge and skills to guarantee that the future education will corre-spond to the needs and be cost-effective. A couple of recent or ongoing Finnish studies have addressed these questions, mainly at the levels of updating training and on-the-job training (Martikainen, 2004; see also Huuhtanen, 2002; Launonen, 2002a, 2002b).

Also different methods of distributing knowledge in augmentative and alternative communication should be tried and carefully analysed. Papunet, a comprehensive Finnish Internet site, has been created to serve people who have difficulty in producing and understanding speech, for users of plain language, for their proxies and professionals (Papunet, 2007). Papunet provides information to all these groups in written standard Finnish and Swedish, plain language Finnish and Swedish,[1] Bliss and other graphic communication forms. The site also includes games pages, designed particularly for people of different ages, using alternative communication forms. Some of the content is available with voice support or in a text version. Papunet has quickly become frequently visited by people with disabilities, their friends and families, and professionals, both in Finland and other Nordic countries. There is also ongoing logopedic research on its usability and application, from the point of view of the users.

Opportunities for a Shared Language at Societal Level

Macrosystem refers to different mechanisms of societies, having an influence on individuals' development. Each society has its historically and culturally determined practices, as well as structural and economical constituents, which direct their legislation and social-political solutions, also those that make different intervention practices possible (see also Launonen, 2002a, 2002b, 2003b). The attitudes of the general public and decision-makers towards minorities of a given society determine how people's human rights and equality are realised, how people with disabilities are included, integrated or segregated in relation to the rest of society. This includes questions, such as how the special needs of people with severe communication disabilities are taken into account in public environments and their planning. Policies concerning people with disabilities have been changing in many countries from segregation and diagnostic labels to integration, inclusion and empowerment, and to discussions on the opportunities of these people to participate as full members in their society. Language plays a decisive role in this participation. A minority language, also an alternative communication system, has to be acceptable as a symbol of authenticity; it must have credibility as an authentic language in the community of its users (Fasold, 1984).

The social policies of each individual country strongly affect the official status of different language groups in a given country. The Constitution of Finland can be used as an example. It states:

> The Sami, as an indigenous people, as well as the Roma and other groups, have the right to maintain and develop their own language and culture [...] The rights of persons using sign language and of

persons in need of interpretation or translation aid owing to disability shall be guaranteed by an Act. (Constitution of Finland, 1999: Chapter 2 – Basic Rights and Liberties; Section 17 – Right to one's language and culture)

Finland pursues this same policy also with immigrants; they are encouraged to keep their own language and culture along with their new Finnish language and culture. Political actions do not, however, define the status of given minority groups, as has been demonstrated by numerous examples in different countries. For example in Finland, of the two language groups mentioned in the Constitution, Sami has gained a positive status with public support, but Roma may be burdened by old prejudices against gypsies. Or, immigrants who speak English as their mother tongue may have a higher status than those who use, for example, Somali – even though Somali is the third most common language among preschool children in the capital area, right after the two official languages of the country, Finnish and Swedish.

The attitudes of the general public are not easily changed by political actions, but with great efforts they may have gradual effects, as has been demonstrated by the progress in the status of sign languages. In Finland, as in many other countries, television broadcasts the daily news in sign language, sign language interpreters get a first-class education, and sign language courses are often so popular that participants have to queue to get in. People who use sign language get proper basic education, they may study at universities and continue their studies up to the highest academic degrees.

Not only the shared language of deaf people but also their own culture has been emphasised. It has received positive attention, and hearing parents of deaf children have been advised to give their child an opportunity to join in the sign language community, in order to build a positive identity as a person using sign language. However, the situation has recently seen a drastic change in Finland and in many other countries, and the discussion on the status and rights of deaf people is returning to the old debate of oral and manual schools. This change has been caused by the new technology of cochlear implants (see also Lonka in this volume). Many parents of young children who will get an implant want to abandon sign language and give their child an opportunity to identify only with the hearing and speaking society. They are supported by many professionals – and so are the people who have learned sign language as their first language and who emphasise the importance of sign language, the identity of deaf people and their shared community. This return to the old debate, albeit with different reasons, reflects the strong role of language in the definition of people's rights and equality. It also demonstrates the complexity of the definition of the linguistic community of different minority language groups, which have a need to identify with the majority group of their society. The parents of children with developmental communication disabilities may seem to have a freedom of choice, as to their child's linguistic community, but actually they are highly dependent on the social and health care politics, as well as the attitudes to people with disabilities, in their own country (see also Alant, 1996).

The Finnish rehabilitation system is based mainly on public services and is enacted by law. The rehabilitation that people with severe disabilities need is paid for by the Social Insurance Institution of Finland. People who need alternative communication forms can practically always be defined as having a severe communication disability, which means that they would always be entitled to intervention funded by public money. However, this rehabilitation system builds strongly on traditional intervention practices, namely on individual approaches, and it is still not always easy to get authorities' approval of arguments which speak for more ecological approaches in intervention. Old practices are, however, changing. Recent logopedic research in Finland, which has had a strong emphasis on ecological approaches, has probably played a role in this positive progress.

People who need alternative communication will always form a small minority in their societies. Only very few of them will ever be able to take part in societal decision-making. Therefore, it will be the responsibility of their speaking partners to make their communication forms known and credible as language variants, which can be shared. Only this will make real participation possible for people who need these communication forms. The level and scope of ideal individual participation may vary considerably, but ethically sustainable solutions in arranging the living conditions of these people will always include considerations of how to make their communication not only possible but also genuinely shared (see also von Tetzchner & Jensen, 1999).

Note

1. Plain language writing is a technique of organising information in ways that most effectively present ideas to the reader. It uses straightforward, concrete, familiar words, and it aims at reaching people who cannot read well.

References

Alant, E. (1996) Augmentative and alternative communication in developing countries: Challenge of the future. *AAC Augmentative and Alternative Communication* 12, 1–12.

Alant, E. (2003) A developmental approach towards teacher training: A contradiction in terms? In S. von Tetzchner and N. Grove (eds) *Augmentative and Alternative Communication. Developmental Issues* (pp. 335–356). London: Whurr.

Beukelman, D.R., McGinnis, J. and Morrow, D. (1991) Vocabulary selection in augmentative and alternative communication. *AAC Augmentative and Alternative Communication* 7, 171–185.

Bliss, C. (1965) *Semantography (Blissymbolics)*. Sydney: Semantography Publications.

Brekke, K.M. and von Tetzchner, S. (2003) Co-construction in graphic language development. In S. von Tetzchner and N. Grove (eds) *Augmentative and Alternative Communication. Developmental Issues* (pp. 176–210). London: Whurr.

Bronfenbrenner, U. (1979) *The Ecology of Human Development. Experiments by Nature and Design* (3rd edn, 1980). Cambridge, Massachusetts: Harvard University Press.

Bronfenbrenner, U. (1995) Developmental ecology through space and time: A future perspective. In P. Moen, G.H. Elder and K. Lüscher (eds) *Examining Lives in Context. Perspectives on the Ecology of Human Development* (pp. 619–647). Washington, DC: American Psychological Association.

Bronfenbrenner, U. and Ceci, S.J. (1994) Nature-nurture reconceptualized in developmental perspective: A bioecological model. *Psychological Review* 101 (4), 568–586.

Bruner, J. (1983) *Child's Talk. Learning to Use Language*. New York: Norton.

Burakoff, K. (2001) Miten kukka viitotaan? Tapaustutkimus kolmen vuorovaikutusparin puhetta korvaavasta kommunikoinnista [How do you sign a flower? A case study on alternative communication of three interaction pairs]. Unpublished Master's thesis, University of Helsinki, Helsinki, Finland.

Burakoff, K. and Launonen, K. (2002) Conversation of three interaction pairs using alternative communication. Conference proceedings of the *10th Biennial Conference of the International Society for Augmentative and Alternative Communication*, August 2002, Odense, Denmark, 125–126.

Burkhart, L. (1994, October) Organizing vocabulary on dynamic display devices: Practical ideas and strategies. Paper presented at the *6th Biennial Conference of the International Society for Augmentative and Alternative Communication*, Maastricht, Netherlands.

Chambers, J.K. (2003) *Sociolinguistic Theory. Linguistic Variation and Its Social Significance* (2nd edn). Oxford: Blackwell Publishing.

Collier, B. and Blackstien-Adler, S. (1998) Building competencies in augmentative and alternative communication among professionals. *AAC Augmentative and Alternative Communication* 14, 250–260.

Constitution of Finland (1999) On WWW at http://www.finlex.fi/fi/laki/kaannokset/1999/en19990731.pdf. Accessed November 22, 2007.

Dale, P. (1991) The validity of a parent report measure of vocabulary and syntax at 24 months. *Journal of Speech and Hearing Research* 34, 565–571.

Fasold, R. (1984) *The Sociolinguistics of Society. Introduction to Sociolinguistics* (Vol. 1). Oxford: Blackwell.

Grove, N. and Park, K. (1996) *Odyssey Now*. London: Jessica Kingsley Publishers.

Heikurainen, I. (2004) "Mä haluun lainaa sun tota." Tapaustutkimus kahden lievästi kehitysvammaisen puhevammaisen nuoren kommunikoinnista ryhmäpuheterapiatilanteissa ["I want to borrow your that". A case study on the communication in group speech therapy situations of two adolescents with a mild learning disability and a speech disability]. Unpublished Master's thesis, University of Helsinki, Helsinki, Finland.

Heikurainen, I. and Launonen, K. (2004, October) "I want to borrow your that." Communication in a group. Poster session presented at the *11th Biennial Conference of the International Society for Augmentative and Alternative Communication*, Natal, Brazil.

Herkman, P. (2000) Arvaa mitä? Tapaustutkimus puhelaitetta käyttävän lapsen ja viiden keskustelukumppanin välisestä vuorovaikutuksesta [Guess what? A case study on the interaction between a child using VOCA, and his five conversation partners]. Unpublished Master's thesis, University of Helsinki, Helsinki, Finland.

Herkman, P. and Launonen, K. (2002) Guess what – computer-aided conversations of a six-year-old boy. Conference proceedings of the *10th Biennial Conference of the International Society for Augmentative and Alternative Communication*, August 2002, Odense, Denmark, 122–124.

Hildén, S. and Merikoski, H. (2002, August) The interaction between children and kindergarten personnel. Poster presentation at the *10th Biennial Conference of the International Society for Augmentative and Alternative Communication*, Odense, Denmark.

Hildén, S., Merikoski, H. and Launonen, K. (2001) Yhteisöpohjainen kuntoutus [Community-based rehabilitation]. In K. Launonen and M. Lehtihalmes (eds) *Lapsen kielen käytön kehitys ja sen ongelmat – pragmaattinen näkökulma* (pp. 113–119). Suomen logopedis-foniatrisen yhdistyksen julkaisuja 33.

Hurmola, S. (2001) "Tämä kuuluu tehtäviini" – Erityiskoulujen työntekijöiden arvioita omista kommunikointitiedoistaan ja -taidoistaan ["This belongs to my tasks". – Self-evaluations of the staff in special schools on their own communication knowledge and skills]. Unpublished Master's thesis, University of Helsinki, Helsinki, Finland.

Huuhtanen, K. (1992) *Puhetta tukevat ja korvaavat kommunikaatiomenetelmät Suomessa 1990-luvun taitteessa [Augmentative and alternative communication methods in Finland at the turn of the 1990s]*. Helsinki: Kehitysvammaliitto ry.

Huuhtanen, K. (ed.) (2001) *Puhetta tukevat ja korvaavat kommunikointimenetelmät Suomessa vuosituhannen taitteessa [Augmentative and alternative communication methods in Finland at the turn of the millennium]*. Helsinki: Kehitysvammaliitto ry.

Huuhtanen, K. (2002a, August) Let's be on speaking terms – or shall we? Poster presentation at the *10th Biennial Conference of the International Society for Augmentative and Alternative Communication*, Odense, Denmark.

Huuhtanen, K. (2002b, August) Odyssey in Finland. Video presentation at the *10th Biennial Conference of the International Society for Augmentative and Alternative Communication*, Odense, Denmark.

Huuhtanen, K. (2004, October) Let's be on speaking terms – or shall we? Part II. Poster presentation at the *11th Biennial Conference of the International Society for Augmentative and Alternative Communication*, Natal, Brazil.

Johnson, R. (1981) *The Picture Communication Symbols*. Solana Beach, CA: Mayer-Johnson.

Klippi, A. (1996) *Conversation as an Achievement in Aphasics*. Studia Fennica Linguistica 6. Helsinki: Finnish Literature Society.

Launonen, K. (1996) Enhancing communication skills of children with Down syndrome: Early use of manual signs. In S. von Tetzchner and M.H. Jensen (eds) *Augmentative and Alternative Communication. European Perspectives* (pp. 213–231). London: Whurr.

Launonen, K. (1998) *Eleistä sanoihin, viittomista kieleen. Varhaisviittomisohjelman kehittäminen, kokeilu ja pitkäaikaisvaikutukset Downin syndrooma -lapsilla [From gestures to words, from signs to language. Development, application, and long-term effects of an Early Signing Programme in the early intervention of children with Down syndrome]*. FAMR Research Publications, No.75. Helsinki: Kehitysvammaliitto ry.

Launonen, K. (2000a) Just for fun. Turn-taking and joint attention in alternative communication. Conference proceedings of the *9th Biennial Conference of the*

International Society for Augmentative and Alternative Communication, August 2000, Washington, DC, USA, 174–176.

Launonen, K. (2000b, July) Communication skills of four adolescents with Angelman syndrome. Paper presented at the *1st World Conference of the International Angelman Syndrome Organisation*, Tampere, Finland.

Launonen, K. (2001) Huvin vuoksi. Vuorottelu ja jaettu tarkkaavuus puhetta korvaavan kommunikoinnin kehityksen pohjana [Just for fun. Turn taking and joint attention as bases for alternative communcation development]. *Puhe ja kieli [Speech and Language]* 21, 25–36.

Launonen, K. (2002a) The use of augmentative and alternative communication in Finnish communities. Conference proceedings of the *10th Biennial Conference of the International Society for Augmentative and Alternative Communication*, August 2002, Odense, Denmark, 318–319.

Launonen, K. (2002b) Tunnen, tiedän ja toteutan. Puhetta tukevaa ja korvaavaa kommunikointia käyttävän yhteisön ja puheterapeutin yhteistyön edellytykset nyky-Suomessa [I know, I am aware of, and I carry out. Prerequisites of collaboration between speech therapists and communities using augmentative and alternative communication in Finland today]. *Puheterapeutti* 2/2002, 14–19.

Launonen, K. (2003a) Manual signing as a tool for communicative interaction and language: The development of children with Down syndrome and their parents. In S. von Tetzchner and N. Grove (eds) *Augmentative and Alternative Communication. Developmental Issues* (pp. 83–122). London: Whurr.

Launonen, K. (2003b) The feasibility of sociolinguistic theories in augmentative and alternative communication. In S. von Tetzchner and M.H. Jensen (eds) *Perspectives on Theory and Practice in Augmentative and Alternative Communication* (pp. 39–55). Toronto, Ontario: International Society for Augmentative and Alternative Communication.

Launonen, K. (2004, October) Parents' and teachers' evaluations of communications skills of children with Angelman syndrome. Paper presented at the *11th Biennial Conference of the International Society for Augmentative and Alternative Communication*, Natal, Brazil.

Launonen, K. (2005a, June) Manual signs and intensive interaction in building up the communicative competence of a child with Down syndrome. Paper presented at the *2nd Conference of the International Society for Gesture Studies, 'Interacting Bodies'*, Lyon, France.

Launonen, K. (2005b, July) Early grammatical development of a boy with Down syndrome using manual signs and spoken Finnish. Paper presented in the *X International Congress for the Study of Child Language*, Berlin, Germany.

Launonen, K. (2005c, August) Communication in communities with members who have autism. Invited paper at *'Who Cares?' Congress*, Lahti, Finland.

Launonen, K. and Grove, N. (2003) A longitudinal study of sign and speech development in a boy with Down syndrome. In S. von Tetzchner and N. Grove (eds) *Augmentative and Alternative Communication. Developmental Issues* (pp. 123–154). London: Whurr.

Launonen, K. and Olkku, S. (2000) Computer analysis and subjective evaluation of expressive means of communication. Conference proceedings of the *9th Biennial Conference of the International Society for Augmentative and Alternative Communication*, August 2000, Washington, DC, USA, 96–98.

Lyytinen, P., Lari, N., Lausvaara, A. and Poikkeus, A.-M. (1994) Lasten varhaisen sanaston ja kommunikoinnin arviointi [Evaluation of children's early vocabulary and communication]. *Psykologia* 29, 244–252.

Maharaj, S.C. (1980) *Pictogram Ideogram Communication*. Regina, Canada: The George Reed Foundation for the Handicapped.

Markus, M. (2000) Kehitysvammalaitoksissa työskentelevien tiedot ja taidot puhetta korvaavan kommunikoinnin mahdollistavista tekijöistä [The knowledge and skills of the staff in insitutions for people with intellectual impairments, on factors making alternative communication possible]. Unpublished Master's thesis, University of Oulu, Oulu, Finland.

Martikainen, K. (2004) *Tikoteekin ja Uudenmaan erityishuoltopiirin kommunikaatioprojekti 2002–2003*. [Final report of a communication project of Tikoteekki and Uudenmaan erityishuoltopiiri]. Tikoteekin raportteja 2/2004. Helsinki: Kehitysvammaliitto ry.

Martinsen, H. and von Tetzchner, S. (1996) Situating augmentative and alternative language intervention. In S. von Tetzchner and M.H. Jensen (eds) *Augmentative and Alternative Communication. European Perspectives* (pp. 37–48). London: Whurr.

Merikoski, H. and Hildén, S. (2000, August) Community based rehabilitation in special day care centres and AAC. Poster session presented at the *9th Biennial Conference of the International Society for Augmentative and Alternative Communication*, Washington DC, USA.

Murphy, J., Marková, I., Collins, S. and Moodie, E. (1996) AAC systems: Obstacles to effective use. *European Journal of Disorders of Communication* 31, 31–44.

Olkku, S. (1997) Tapaustutkimus vaikeasti monivammaisen nuorukaisen kommunikaatiokeinoista [A case study on communication means of a youth with severe multi-impairments]. Unpublished Master's thesis, University of Helsinki, Helsinki, Finland.

Papunet (2007) On WWW at http://www.papunet.net/english/info.en.php. Accessed November 22, 2007.

Porter, G. (2000) 'Low-tech dynamic displays': 'User friendly' multi-level communication books. Conference Proceedings of the *9th Biennial Conference of the International Society for Augmentative and Alternative Communication*, August 2000, Washington, DC, USA, 587–590.

Pulli, T. (1994, August) Interpreting services for persons with severe speech handicaps according to a Finnish law extention. Paper presented at the *6th Biennial Conference of the International Society for Augmentative and Alternative Communication*, Maastricht, The Netherlands.

Pulli, T. (1996, August) A training program for workers in AAC service delivery. Paper presented at the *7th Biennial Conference of the International Society for Augmentative and Alternative Communication*, Vancouver, Canada.

Pulli, T., Hildén, S., Puistolinna, H. and Hämäläinen, V. (2002, August) *Come on board! Pragmatic use of AAC in interactive exhibitions*. Workshop presented in the *10th Biennial Conference of the International Society for Augmentative and Alternative Communication*, Odense, Denmark.

Pulli, T., Launonen, K. and Saarela, M. (2005) *AURA yhteisön ja sen autistisen jäsenen vuorovaikutuksen ja viestinnän kehittämiseen [AURA for the development of interaction and communication of communities and their members with autism]*. Lahti: Avainsäätiö and Pääjärven kuntayhtymä.

Pullola-Teeriaho, R. (2000) INCL-perheiden vuorovaikutuksen tukeminen [Supporting interaction in INCL families]. Unpublished Master's thesis, University of Helsinki, Helsinki, Finland.

Pullola-Teeriaho, R. and Launonen, K. (2002) Supporting interaction within families with children who have INCL disease. Conference proceedings of the *10th Biennial Conference of the International Society for Augmentative and Alternative Communication*, August 2002, Odense, Denmark, 98–99.

Ratcliff, A. and Beukelman, D. (1995) Preprofessional preparation in augmentative and alternative communication: State-of-the-art report. *AAC Augmentative and Alternative Communication* 11, 61–73.

Rautakoski, P. (2002, August) AAC methods for aphasic persons and their significant others. Poster session presented at the *10th Biennial Conference of the International Society for Augmentative and Alternative Communication*, Odense, Denmark.

Rautakoski, P. (2005) *Vaikeasti afaattisten henkilöiden ja heidän läheistensä kommunikointitaitojen kuntoutuminen: seurantatutkimus [The change in communication abilities of people with severe aphasia and their significant others during a rehabilitation course: a follow-up study]*. Publications of the Department of Speech Sciences, 52. Helsinki: University of Helsinki.

Salminen, A-L. (2001) Daily life with computer augmented communication. Real life experiences from the lives of severely disabled speech impaired children. Research report 119. Helsinki: Stakes.

Smith, M.M. (2003) Environmental influences on aided language development: The role of partner adaptation. In S. von Tetzchner and N. Grove (eds) *Augmentative and Alternative Communication. Developmental Issues* (pp. 123–154). London: Whurr.

Stern, D.N. (1985) *The Interpersonal World of the Infant. A View from Psychoanalysis and Developmental Psychology*. New York: Basic Books.

Sundblad, I. (2005) Puhelaitteen käyttö ja sanaston valinta [The use of voice output communication aid and the selection of vocabulary]. Unpublished Master's thesis, University of Helsinki, Helsinki, Finland.

Sundblad, I., Ohtonen, M. and Johansson, S. (2002, August) Interpreter service model in Finland. Poster session presented at the *10th Biennial Conference of the International Society for Augmentative and Alternative Communication*, Odense, Denmark.

von Tetzchner, S. and Grove, N. (eds) (2003a) *Augmentative and Alternative Communication. Developmental Issues*. London: Whurr.

von Tetzchner, S. and Grove, N. (2003b) The development of alternative language forms. In S. von Tetzchner and N. Grove, N. (eds) *Augmentative and Alternative Communication. Developmental Issues* (pp. 1–27). London: Whurr.

von Tetzchner, S. and Jensen, K. (1999) Communicating with people who have severe communication impairment: Ethical considerations. *International Journal of Disability, Development and Education* 46, 453–462.

von Tetzchner, S. and Martinsen, H. (1999) *Johdatus puhetta tukevaan ja korvaavaan kommunikointiin*. [The Finnish translation of the Norwegian original of Introduction to Augmentative and Alternative Communication.] Helsinki: Kehitysvammaliitto ry.

von Tetzchner, S. and Martinsen, H. (2000) *Introduction to Augmentative and Alternative Communication* (2nd edn). London: Whurr.

Vygotsky, L.S. (1978) *Mind in Society. The Development of Higher Psychological Processes*. In M. Cole, V. John-Steiner, S. Scribner and E. Souberman (eds). Cambridge, Massachusetts/London, England: Harvard University Press.

Widell, A-L. (1999) CP-vammaisen ihmisen ja hänen vuorovaikutuskumppaninsa kommunikatiiviset taidot avusteisen vuorovaikutuksen toimivuuden edellytyksenä [The communicative skills of a person with cerebral palsy and her interaction partners, as prerequisites of functional aided communication]. Unpublished Master's thesis, University of Helsinki, Helsinki, Finland.

Widell, A-L. and Launonen, K. (2000) Increasing communicative skills in children with severe communication impairments. Conference proceedings of the *9th Biennial Conference of the International Society for Augmentative and Alternative Communication*, August 2000, Washington, DC, USA, 236–238.

Widell, A-L., Vuokila, L. and Honkanen, T. (2002, August) Look at us playing! Taking turns and sharing social closeness. Paper presented at the *10th Biennial Conference of the International Society for Augmentative and Alternative Communication*, Odense, Denmark.

World Health Organization (2005) *International Classification of Functioning, Disability and Health (ICF)*. On WWW at http://www3.who.int/icf/. Accessed November 22, 2007.

Part 3

Characteristics of Finnish and the Study of Adult Speech and Language Disorders

Chapter 7

Text Production of Finnish Speakers with Aphasia

ANNA-MAIJA KORPIJAAKKO-HUUHKA

Introduction

Orientation to studies of discourse

Neurolinguistic studies of discourse (term adopted from Stemmer, 1999) have followed research within linguistics and psychology with a delay of approximately one decade (cf. Dressler & Pléh, 1988; Joanette & Brownell, 1990). In Europe, text linguistics of the 1970s questioned the generative tradition, and in the United States the new approach was called discourse analysis (de Beaugrande, 1997; van Dijk, 1981). Simultaneously in psychology, the study of memory and text comprehension developed (cf. Kintsch, 1994). The contribution of these disciplines to the development of neurolinguistic studies of discourse in the 1980s has been significant (Joanette & Brownell, 1990; Patry & Nespoulous, 1990), and resulted in a paradigmatic conception that discourse problems of people with aphasia are due to disorders at the micro level (word search and syntactic problems) rather than the macro level (problems in text production or in pragmatic skills).

According to Stemmer (1999), different current and future orientations within neurolinguistics can be classified as follows:

(1) Traditional aphasia research has aimed at describing the spared and disordered skills at the level of both linguistic structures and interaction. Studies focusing on the production and comprehension of words and sentences, as well as text linguistic approaches and sociolinguistic research, conversation analysis included, belong to this category of research, according to Stemmer.
(2) Theories of how the human brain processes discourse have also been developed. The pivotal method has been to correlate the disorders in micro level and macro level processes with the location of the lesion in the brain.

(3) More knowledge about the contribution of specific cognitive domains, such as working memory, attention and executive functions, to discourse processing is needed.

(4) In addition to traditional behavioural methods, new neuroimaging technologies are expected to increase our understanding of the biological basis and neurophysiological mechanisms contributing to discourse processing.

Neurolinguistic studies of discourse in Finland have followed the international developments belonging mostly to the first of Stemmer's categories; text linguistic and sociolinguistic orientations to aphasia started to strengthen in the late 1980s. As discourse is a relatively new topic in Finnish neurolinguistics, international publications are few (see below). As examples of the emergent study of text production, one can mention the work by this author (Korpijaakko-Huuhka & Aulanko, 1994) concerning the relevance of prosody in the evaluation of narrative speech, and the work by Laine *et al.* (1998), which focused on the role of semantic breakdown and attentional or memory disorders in discourse processing of people with vascular dementia or probable Alzheimer's disease; the last mentioned study belongs to the third of Stemmer's categories.

In logopedics, and more specifically in aphasia research, orientation to functional communication, along with the adoption of pragmatic theories of the 1970s and 1980s, resulted in Finnish versions of functional or pragmatic evaluation methods, such as the Edinburgh Functional Communication Profile for elderly people and people with aphasia (Skinner *et al.*, 1984; Terva-Heinonen, 1985), the Communicative Abilities of Daily Living for persons with aphasia (Holland, 1980; Malkamäki, 1995), and the Pragmatic Protocol for people with traumatic brain injury (Prutting & Kirchner, 1987; Tykkyläinen, 1992). On the other hand, some studies from the late 1980s and early 1990s focused on the communicative efficiency of the narrative speech of people with aphasia (Korpijaakko-Huuhka, 1987, 1989, 1991a, 1991b, 1992) and their conversational discourse (Klippi, 1989). Simultaneously, the influence of sociolinguistics, especially conversation analytic orientation, was growing in Finland (for a review see Klippi, 1996). For this author, however, the interaction of interlocutors in conversation, and especially the impact of context in construing meaning in discourse became relevant through another route, namely via the Systemic Functional Linguistic (SFL) framework by Michael Halliday and his co-workers. The SFL approach to aphasia research and rehabilitation has been developed mainly in Australia (see Togher & Ferguson, 2005). In Europe, the SFL framework seems relatively unknown amongst aphasia researchers, and in Finland, it has been the privilege of this author to promote the neurolinguistic study of text production by being the first speech therapist to apply SFL approach to larger clinical data (cf. Korpijaakko-Huuhka, 2003). Finnish linguists, however, have acknowledged SFL theory since the 1980s (e.g. Iivonen, 1988; Kalliokoski 1989; Shore, 1991, 1992; Ventola, 1987).

In SFL theory, language is seen as a means of making many meanings simultaneously (Eggins, 1994; Halliday, 1994; Matthiessen & Halliday, 1997). That is, language has several metafunctions. When studying the interpersonal metafunction, a clause is seen as an exchange of information (or goods and services). Interpersonal meanings include information about the roles of the speakers, and about their attitudes towards the situation and their own performance in it. We also use language for relating experience, and ideational meanings refer to representations of the world around (also inside) us. This chapter will focus on the textual metafunction, that is, the ways language is used for organising information into larger or smaller chunks so that the message is coherent. Textual meanings are realised, for example, in thematic and schematic structures of the discourse, and in the use of cohesive means of language in organising a text into a coherent whole.

The textual metafunction is the enabling function of language. According to Matthiessen and Halliday (1997: 13) it 'serves to enable the presentation of ideational and interpersonal meanings as information that can be shared: it provides the speaker with strategies for guiding the listener in his/her interpretation of the text'. In this chapter, the usage of linguistic options to realise textual meanings by Finnish-speaking people with and without aphasia will be descibed, as well as some problems speakers with aphasia have in organising what they say into a coherent story (see also Armstrong, 2005).

Role of aphasic language in text production

The afore-mentioned view, that discourse problems of people with aphasia are based on deficits in microprocessing (i.e. linguistic processes) while macroprocessing (i.e. cognitive processes, e.g. memory, inference) is spared, was based on studies showing that people with aphasia, at least those with mild-to-moderate disorder, comprehend and produce stories basically in the same way as people without aphasia; for example, their retelling and self-generated texts include the most relevant content units and structures of a story (Berko-Gleason *et al.*, 1980; Brookshire & Nicholas, 1993; Ernest-Baron *et al.*, 1987; Huber, 1990; Ulatowska *et al.*, 1981, 1983, 1990, 1993). In addition, people with fluent aphasia have been reported to produce thematically coherent narratives about their life, although the words and clauses they use may be deviant and cohesive ties missing or insufficient (Glosser & Deser, 1990). In Glosser and Deser's study (1990: 73–74), the subjects were interviewed about their family and work, and listeners rated coherence of the texts based on their 'impressions of the meaning of a speaker's whole verbalization with respect to meaning in the adjoining discourse, regardless of lexical or syntactic errors'.

New findings have shown, however, that the picture of discourse skills and problems of people with aphasia is not at all as clear-cut as was earlier thought (for a critical review see Chantraine *et al.*, 1998). In recent years, the question has been raised about the role of aphasic difficulties in using the lexicogrammatical resources of language to construct coherent discourse (Armstrong, 2005; Korpijaakko-Huuhka, 2004; Ulatowska & Streit Ollnes, 2000). For example, Bond Chapman *et al.* (1998: 65) noticed that 'individuals with aphasia exhibited marked difficulty in lexicalizing their ideas as manifested by increased hesitations, revisions, circumlocutions, paraphasic errors, and ambiguous pronouns as compared with normal control subjects. This formulation difficulty disrupted the coherence of the various texts'.

The notion that the frequent and multifaceted word-finding problems in aphasia reflect directly on the syntactic level and the cohesion of the text is not new (e.g. Glosser & Deser, 1990; Huber, 1990). When a speaker with aphasia is unable to access the words he or she is searching for, a clause may remain incomplete (Bird & Franklin, 1996), and relevant information may be missing from the intended message (Christiansen, 1995). The speaker may also start a complicated repair sequence or a new search with, for example, a circumlocution. This may break down the clause structures (Helasvuo *et al.*, 2001), and disrupt the thematic continuity of the text (Korpijaakko-Huuhka, 2003).

Other forms of word-finding problems, such as the use of neologisms, semantic substitutions and nonspecific terms (e.g. thing, guy, do, happen) may result in lexical ambiguity and thus loosen the lexical cohesion of the text (Glosser, 1993; Glosser & Deser, 1990). In addition, speakers with aphasia have been observed to refer to earlier mentioned participants and things more often with pronouns than proper nouns (Ulatowska *et al.*, 1983). They also use pronouns without any referents in the preceding text more often than speakers without aphasia (Armstrong, 1991; Berko-Gleason *et al.*, 1980; Ulatowska *et al.*, 1983). This imprecision of pronominal reference affects the grammatical cohesion of the text. As the cohesive means of language are 'building blocks' of textual coherence (Armstrong, 1991: 41; see also Bond Chapman *et al.*, 1998; Ulatowska & Streit Ollnes, 2000), the ways in which people with aphasia use words and clauses (micro level means) to generate a coherent text (macro level result) need more attention (for a review see Armstrong, 2000). In this chapter, the role of aphasic language will be examined in the generation of a story based on cartoon frames.

Coherence and cohesion

As the concepts 'coherence' and 'cohesion' are used in various meanings in various studies, and as they are essential for the purposes of this chapter, some definitions need to be given. Various researchers make a distinction between local and global coherence. In some studies (e.g. Coelho, 1995; Glosser & Deser, 1990; Laine *et al.*, 1998), *local coherence* is defined as a thematic relationship between two consecutive utterances. In other studies (e.g. Patry & Nespoulous, 1990), it refers to the ways clauses are locally linked with lexical and grammatical ties. This definition of local coherence corresponds to what Halliday and Hasan (1976) call *cohesion*, as will be discussed below (see also Dressler & Pléh, 1988). *Global coherence*, in all these studies, is defined as the relatedness of the content of utterances with the overall topic of the discourse.

According to Halliday and Hasan (1976: 4), cohesive links are semantic relations: 'cohesion occurs where the interpretation of some element in the discourse is dependent on that of another'. The use of (local) lexical and grammatical links, such as reiteration or hyponyms and anaphoric reference or conjunction, is one way to increase the unity of the text. A text is also tied together by its thematic patterning and thematic continuity (Halliday & Hasan, 1976: 324–326, 1985: 84). Here, the above-mentioned definition of local coherence as a thematic relationship between verbalisations seems to meet an equivalent. In addition, the text's macrostructure is also significant in keeping it together. The schematic structure of a story realises the *generic coherence* of a narrative (Eggins & Martin, 1997).

Thus, in order to make a coherent interpretation of a text, the participants in a discourse may rely on the afore-mentioned linguistic features. However, a text lacking these explicit links can be considered coherent when it is relevant and understandable in the context in which language is used, that is, 'coherent with respect to the context of situation' (Halliday & Hasan, 1976: 23). In this chapter, coherence is considered as emerging from the thematic progression, the generic (episodic) structure and the cohesive relations in the texts.

Materials and Methods

Speakers

The participants with aphasia were selected from an age-cohort (55–85 years) of 482 stroke patients (see Pohjasvaara *et al.*, 1998). In this cohort, 65 patients were diagnosed as having an aphasic disorder at the mean of four months after the stroke, and 15 of these had a cortical/subcortical lesion in the left hemisphere. These 15 speakers participated in this study. Their aphasic disorders varied from very severe, global aphasia to relatively mild, anomic aphasia (Table 7.1). Most of the aphasias were classified as fluent; only two speakers had non-fluent aphasia.

Seven age-matched individuals without aphasia out of a larger pool of normal speakers served as controls. They all suffered from voice problems and produced the stories during their voice assessment (Table 7.2). Although most of them had moderate-to-severe dysphonia in terms of

Table 7.1 Background data of the speakers with aphasia

Type of aphasia	n	AQ range	Age range	Sex
Fluent aphasias				
• Anomic	7	82.5–93.5	68–85 years	4 F 3 M
• Wernicke's	4	25.1–49.0	63–82 years	2 F 2 M
• Transcortical sensory	1	65.9	73 years	M
• Conduction	1	50.7	74 years	F
Non-fluent aphasias				
• Global	1	10.8	60 years	M
• Transcortical motor	1	68.7	80 years	F
Total	15	10.8–93.5	60–85 years	8 F 7 M

AQ = Aphasia Quotient from The Western Aphasia Battery; F = female, M = male.

deteriorated voice quality, they could produce as long and as detailed stories as speakers with milder disorders (Korpijaakko-Huuhka, 1995).

Elicitation and prosodic notation of the texts

The speakers were shown a nine-frame cartoon by Henning Dahl Mikkelsen – a little man, *Ferd'nand* attempting to keep away the crows that came to peck at the seeds he planted in his garden (see Korpijaakko-Huuhka & Aulanko, 1994: 93). The speakers were instructed to follow the order of the picture frames and generate a narrative based on the pictures. They were expected to proceed in monologue, and the therapist was supposed to give minimal feedback only. The stories were recorded on audiotape and then transcribed for linguistic analysis.

Table 7.2 Background data of the control speakers

Aetiology of the voice disorder	n	Age	Sex
Vocal cord paralysis	3	61–76 years	2 F 1 M
Vocal cord surgery	1	82 years	M
Vocal cord atrophy	1	75 years	M
Spasmodic dysphonia	1	79 years	F
Functional dysphonia	1	60 years	M
Total	7	60–82 years	4 F 3 M

The prosodic notation loosely followed examples from Finnish researchers using conversation analysis (e.g. Seppänen, 1997; see Example 1). The numbered lines are, however, intonation units, that is, information units that are perceived as complete tonal contours, and that are typically separated by pauses (cf. Chafe, 1980, 1998; cf. tone groups in Halliday & Hasan, 1976: 325). Intonation units may be clauses or clause complexes that construe one thematic entity (Example 1).

Example 1: Intonation units in control speaker P45's text. A comma refers to slightly and a full stop to prominently falling intonation. Phrasal stress is indicated by capital letters. The durations of pauses ≥0.5 seconds are given in parentheses; shorter pauses are marked with (.). A rough English translation is given in the line under the original Finnish transcription.

(1) *no nyt tässäk (.)* *kertoa pitäis SEMmosta* *että (1.1)* *tämä (0.7)* *kaveri* *istuttaa SIEmeniä*
     well now here   one should tell such   that   this   guy   plants seeds
     MAAhan   *ja,*
     in the ground   and
(2) *(1.2)* *kuvittelee sitte että*   *minkäm*   *miten ison SAdon hän ((rykäisy)) saa*   *näistä (0.8) siemenistään.*
            imagines then that   what   how big a harvest he ((cough)) will get   from these seeds of his
(3) *(1.5)* *mutta yhtä äkkiä*   *hä HUOmaa että (0.7)*   *varikset nokkii hänen*   *siemenet maasta.*
            but suddenly   he notices that   crows are pecking at his   seeds in the ground

Analysis of textual meanings

In this study, as mentioned earlier, textual meanings are seen to be realised in the thematic and schematic (episodic) structures of the texts, and in ways the speakers use the cohesive means of language for organising the message into a coherent whole. In order to find out the structures of the texts, the ways the speakers marked both the discontinuities of the story line, and the connectedness of the events they were describing, were examined. First, the study focussed on thematic progression by looking at the topical participants of each clause, that is, whom the speaker is telling about in consecutive clauses (cf. Downing, 1991; Shore, 1992: 322). Simultaneously, the 'oral punctuation marks' (Armstrong, 1992) were examined, for example, pauses, intonation and connectors, which indicate the structural units of a text. In addition to the boundaries of the units, the study also investigated the speakers' ways of indicating the connectedness of the clauses with cohesive means (lexical and grammatical ties). Finally, the aim was to see if thematic shifts matched changes in the type of cohesive ties, and how together these structured the text into episodes.

The many-faceted analysis is illustrated by Example 2 below. This detailed description of the text from a non-aphasic speaker is meant to give an example of how the Finnish language is used in construing textual meanings and to help the reader understand the less detailed examples that follow. The *thematic progression* can be followed by looking at whom the speaker is talking about (topical participant theme) in each of the clauses.

Example 2: The thematic units (indicated with → ←) of control speaker P45's story. Øx refers to each presupposed theme, and the index to its lexical correlate (indicated by [ ]x) earlier in the text. Rising intonation is marked with ? Cohesive ties are underlined.

(1) *no nyt tässäk (.)   kertoa pitäis SEMmosta   että → (1.1) [tämä (0.7)   kaveri]1   istuttaa SIEmeniä MAAhan ja,*
     well now here   one should tell such   that → (1.1) [this   guy]1   plants seeds in the ground and,

(2) *(1.2) Ø1 kuvittelee sitte että minkäm   miten ison SAdon hän ((rykäisy)) saa   näistä (0.8) siemenistään .←*
     (1.2.) Ø1 imagines then that what   how big a harvest he ((cough)) will get   from these seeds of his .←

(3) *→(1.5) mutta   yhtä äkkiä   hä HUOmaa   että (0.7)   varikset nokkii hänen siemenet   maasta .←*
     →(1.5.) but   suddenly   he notices   that   crows are pecking at his seeds   in the ground .←

(4) *→(1.4) ja sittemh (.)   [tämäh (0.7)   mies]2 KEKsii että tehdäänpäs siinä   variksempelätij ja,*
     →(1.4) and then   [this   man]2 thinks that let's make there   a scarecrow and,

(5) *(0.8) Ø2 [pistää]3   pystyym   semmosen PUUristikon?*
     (0.8) Ø2 [sets]3   up   that kind of a wooden framework?

(6) *(0.9) ja:: ja Ø2 Ø3 takin   siiher ristikkooj+ja   hatum päähän,*
     (0.9) and and Ø2 Ø3 a coat   on the framework and   a hat on its head,

(7) *ja näin on (0.9)   valmis tämä (0.7)   VAriksempelätin .←*
     and so is   completed this   scarecrow . ←

(8) *→(1.1) mut ei siitä ollu paljon Apua   [nää varikset]4 (1.0)   menit ym   siihen (.)*
     →(1.1) but it was not of much help   [these crows]4   went hmm   there
     hänen PElättimem päälle   istumaaj   ja nauramaaj+ja   Ø4 syövät Edelleen   siemeniä ja .←
     on his scarecrow   to sit   and to laugh and   Ø4 keep on eating   the seeds and .←

(9) *→(1.3) no nyt tämä SUUttuu [tämä mies]5   ja Ø5 menee ja (1.1)   Ø5 ottaa*
     →(1.3) well now this gets angry [this man]5   and Ø5 goes and   Ø5 takes
     kokom (.)PElättimen käteensä ja,
     the whole scarecrow in his hand and,

(10) *(0.6) Ø5 hätistää VAriksia sitten (1.5)   sittem   POis hänen kasvimaaltaan .←*
     (0.6) Ø5 chases the crows then   then   away from his garden . ←

(11) *(4.1) että sem PItuinen se .*
     (4.1) so that that was it [in length] .

In line 1, the speaker starts the story talking about *tämä kaveri* ('this guy'), referring to the main character. This theme continues in the following clause (line 2): the speaker presupposes the previous theme, that is, does not mention the guy again, indicating that the theme is common to the two consecutive clauses (cf. Halliday & Hasan, 1976: 143). The speaker continues to talk about the main character in the following clause, but now, when describing the main character's cognition, he uses the pronoun *hän* ('he' or 'she'). In line 3, we see that the speaker repeats the pronominal reference, a colloquial form *hä* of the pronoun *hän*.

A new theme is started with the noun *varikset* ('crows'), in line 3. However, the speaker has clearly chosen to talk about the main character, and turns back to that theme (line 5) by referring to him with *tämä mies* ('this man'). The themes of the two following clauses are presupposed, that is, the speaker continues to talk about the same man.

Then, a thematic shift is seen. In line 7, the speaker introduces a new participant *variksenpelätin* ('scarecrow'). This becomes a new theme and is indicated with the pronoun *siitä* (elative form of *se*; 'it') in line 8. After that, the speaker talks again about the crows mentioned earlier (*nää varikset*; 'these crows'), and uses ellipsis as an indicator of the continuing theme.

In line 9, the speaker returns to the main character. He repeats the previously used phrase *tämä mies* ('this man'), and presupposes this theme in the next to last clause. Thus, this text is mainly about the main character (main theme), but the two other themes, the crows and the scarecrow, have an important role in the making of the event structure (schematic structure), as we will see below.

Simultaneously with the previously presented analysis, the study looked at the ways in which the speakers marked the thematic units with *prosodic, lexical and grammatical ties*. As is seen in the analysis above, the speaker uses a consistent pattern of referential chains: a new participant theme is realised with a noun (or noun group), and later in the same unit the noun is substituted with a pronoun or an ellipsis (i.e. it is presupposed). These chains realise lexical cohesion of the text, as do the other types of substitutions, such as repeated phrases ('this man') and hypo/hyperonymous expressions ('this guy – this man') (see Halliday & Hasan, 1985: 80–85).

In addition to lexical means, the speaker P45 indicates the thematic units prosodically, and by using different kinds of connectors and conjunctions. In line 1 we see that the first thematic unit starts with a pause of 1.1 seconds. The first clause ends with slightly falling intonation and the connector *ja* ('and'). The next clause also starts after a pause and the speaker uses an elliptic tie (Ø) to indicate that these two clauses hang together. The next clause about the main character dreaming of crops completes the thematic unit with clearly falling intonation. This pattern of an extended falling intonation contour covering several clauses that are tied together with 'and' and ellipsis is typical of the thematic structure of this text. This same pattern, consecutive clauses sharing the same theme being connected with coordinate 'and' and the elliptic tie, was also found in the Pear Stories of Finnish-speaking people by Kalliokoski (1989) (see also Chafe, 1980). In addition, the perceptually defined intonation patterns of this text match well with acoustic measurements by Korpijaakko-Huuhka and Aulanko (1994); Finnish speakers tend to use greater intonational shifts at thematic borders than within thematic units.

The next clause (line 3) starts with a pause and the grammatical conjunction *mutta* ('but') indicating a contrast, a change in the event flow. The following clause starting a new theme ('crows') is completed with falling intonation. After this short shift from one theme to another, the speaker indicates the return to the main theme (line 4) with *ja sitten* ('and then') that can be interpreted as a temporal connector indicating the flowing of time in the story world, as well as the speaker's shift from one thematic unit (or from one picture frame and event) to another (see Kalliokoski, 1989: 172). Again, typically, the speaker uses 'and' with ellipsis and slightly falling intonation (and also rising intonation in line 5) to indicate thematic continuity. In this example, the shifts from one theme to another are clearly marked by changing the type of cohesive tie and, most often, by using longer pauses at the borders than within the thematic units. This difference in the durations of pauses depending on their location in the text has also been acoustically verified by Korpijaakko-Huuhka and Aulanko (1994).

As the thematic structure was explicit in P45's text, the *schematic structure* of the story (cf. Eggins, 1994: 89; Joanette & Goulet, 1990: 133; Labov, 1977: 363) was easy to interpret. The first two lines, the first thematic unit about the main character, include information about the setting, that is, the necessary background information needed to understand the events to follow (orientation). A problem (complication) is expressed in line 3; the crows are coming to the garden. The main theme continues in the next unit telling about the man's attempts to scare away the birds (resolution). These lines form the first of the two episodes of the story; the motivation for what followed and the result of that action are clearly expressed. That the scarecrow was of no help starts the second episode: the reason for the little man's further efforts is that the birds flew back to the garden (complication). The last thematic unit (lines 9 and 10) is again about the main character as he furiously attacks the crows (resolution). The story ends with a coda (line 10). The schematic structure of this text is realised in a prototypical way, the prototype of the *Ferd'nand* story being based on texts by 45 non-aphasic Finnish speakers (see Korpijaakko-Huuhka, 1995). When putting all these three facets of the analysis together, we can see that the text by the speaker P45 represents a well-formed story, which is coherent with respect to the context of situation (the speaker having been asked to generate a story based on cartoon frames in a clinical evaluation) and with respect to itself (cohesion).

Results

Before going to the results of the textual analysis, a brief comment on the speakers' orientation to the task and attitudes towards their own performance in it is in order. It is important to be sure that the speakers had understood the instruction given to them; if not, the results would be invalid.

Comprehension of the demands of the task

According to the analysis of the interpersonal metafunction (in Korpijaakko-Huuhka, 2003), all speakers, perhaps with the exception of one aphasic speaker with global aphasia, understood what they had been asked to do. For example, they started, as is expected when telling a story, by identifying or by trying to identify the main character (e.g. 'this little guy'; 'this farmer here'; 'it's bad that I don't know the name is it Osmo or Alto'). In addition, many of them expressed the obligation to talk in a specific way ('I ought to tell a story'; 'I should talk vividly'). This means that the speakers were aware of the demands of the narrative genre and that the difficulties found in completing the task did not result from difficulties in understanding the instruction or from a broader cognitive deficit.

The speakers also expressed their attitudes and feelings, that is, they talked about their cognition concerning their own performance during the task. In making interpersonal meanings, the speakers with aphasia did not differ much from control speakers without aphasia, except that they appealed to their word-finding difficulties and memory problems more often than the control speakers did (cf. Korpijaakko-Huuhka, 2003). This word-finding problem is probably also the reason why the speakers with aphasia were clearly less confident in their ability to tell the story, and used modal and hedging expressions more often than the control speakers. It also explains why only half of the speakers with aphasia could proceed by themselves (as expected) while the rest of them needed help and prompting from the therapist to complete the task. Eight of the texts can thus be considered dialogues, but in two cases it was the speech therapist who mostly contributed to the completion of the story; this will be discussed later.

Well-formed stories despite word-finding problems

Of the 22 speakers with and without aphasia participating in this study, nine produced a unitary story telling about the main character's (main theme) attempts in his garden to scare away the birds that came to peck at the seeds. Five of these were control speakers, and four were speakers with aphasia. They all indicated the thematic structure of the story with explicit prosodic and lexicogrammatical means (cohesion), and it was easy for the listener to follow the logical flow of events (schematic structure) during the narration. These texts can be considered coherent with respect to the narrative genre, and with respect to the context of situation as the speakers were asked to generate a story in monologue. This group of speakers completed the task in monologue, except for the one person with conduction aphasia who was about to break off the narration because of her enormous difficulties in finding the correct phonological forms for the words she used. With the therapist's support, she could complete the task and produce a coherent story.

The other three people with aphasia producing coherent stories had anomic disorders and typical problems in accessing words. This did not, however, prevent them from fulfilling the demands of the task (Example 3).

Example 3: Thematic continuity over a word-search sequence in speaker A312's (anomic aphasia, AQ = 82.4) text. Themes are bolded and search sequence is indicated with slashes (// \\). Øx refers to each presupposed theme, and the index to its lexical correlate. *A* refers to the speaker with aphasia, and *T* to the therapist.

(5) *(4.5) A: ja sitten (.)* **isäntä** *(0.9)* *vähä niinku* *SUUttuu siinä ja,*
         A: and then   **the farmer**   a bit like   gets angry there and
(6) *(.) A: sitte [hän]1 (0.7)* *me- (.)*   *menee ha- (1.0)* *hakemaan tuolta //(1.9)*   *niin+kun*
         A: then [**he**]1   go-   goes to fe-   fetch from there //   like
      (1.3) kuinkas **mä** *nyt sanoisin (2.4)* *niin+kun (1.0)* *että (.)* *jo (2.1)*   *kuinka* **mä** *nyt*
         how   *I*   now should say like   that   already how   *I*   now
      SAnoisin tän,
      should say this
(7) *(3.5) A: kyl* **mä** *sen (.)* *niin+ku (1.0)* *ymmär::* **se** *on* *niinku* *näyttää (.)* \\ *PElottimen .*
         A: surely I that   like   underst- **it** is like   seems   \\ a scarecrow
(8) *T: yhm.*
      T: hmm
(9) *(1.3) A: ja sitten* **Ø1** *pistää (.)* *NArut ja?,*
         A: and then **Ø1** puts   ropes and
(10) *(0.8) A:* **hänel** *on jo (.) ja* **Ø1** *pistää (.)*   *kato (2.0)* *niin+ku* *sem* *PYstyyn .*
         A: **he**'s already got and **Ø1** puts see   like   it   up

Speaker A312 interrupts the storyline for word-search in line 6. This sequence has two themes of its own (*mä*, 'I' and *se*, 'it'), but the speaker mainly talks about his difficulty to get access to the target word (*kuinka mä nyt sanoisin tän*; 'how should I say this now'). After he remembers the word *pelottimen* (genitive form of *pelotin*, a dialectal form of *linnunpelätin*; 'scarecrow') he continues the story-telling as if there was no interruption in the thematic flow: the theme of the next clause (line 9) is presupposed and its correlate *hän* ('he') is found earlier in the text (in line 6), just before the word search started. Thus, despite anomic difficulty some people with mild aphasia may succeed in generating coherent stories.

Omission of relevant information

It was, however, more typical for the people with aphasia in this study to be unable to produce coherent stories. Of the 22 texts, 13 were more or less incoherent, and 11 of these were produced by people with aphasia (some together with the therapist; see below). Two texts by speakers without aphasia lacked generic coherence because the speakers mainly produced a list of guesses and non-related descriptions about the events depicted in the cartoon frames. In two cases with aphasia, the speakers' text production problems were realised with frequent questions. In addition, although both of these speakers could maintain the main theme, some information was left out or ambiguous. This made it hard for the listener to follow the logical sequence of the events (Example 4).

Example 4: Structures of speaker A161's (anomic aphasia, AQ = 93,5) text. Linguistic elements of special interest in this example are set in courier font.

ORIENTATION

(7)   *(5.2) A: siellä on   niinku se (.)   niinku se jotain* IStut IStuttais *tossa sitte toi toi*
      A: there is   like it/he   like it/he something plant- plants here then that that
      on ainaki tossa noi ja,
      is at least here and
(8)   *(0.9) A: ja tää* onko tääh *(0.5)* onko tää sitte *.hh JUU siin on LApio tommonen se on*
      A: and this is this   is this then   yeah there is a spade that kind it is
(9)   *(2.1) A: KAI se jotain on* IStuttamassa *jotain tossa,*
      A: probably it/he something is planting something here
(10) *(0.8) A:* mutta mitä se sitten KUvittelleeko se *.h joo   se kuvittellee tietysti*
      A: but what it/he then does it/he imagine yes   it/he imagines of course
      että hänel hän saa tommosia hedelmiä   sitten niin kovasti (1.0)   kovasti sitte sitte
      that he's g- he'll get that kind of fruit   then   so lots of   lots of then then
(11) *(1.2) A: tuo sa:: sadosta (1.6)   s::adosta   ja sitten?,*
      A: from that cro- crops   crops   and then
(12) *(5.9) A: juu ja sielä on ne ?,*
      A: yes and there they are
(13) *(0.6) A: seuraa niiden kos KASvua ?*
      A: follows their gra growth

COMPLICATION?

(14) *(1.2) A:* mitäs sielä LINtujakin *sielä hätyyttelee*
      A: what there birds too there chases

RESOLUTION?

(15) *(1.0) A: ((rykii)) (3.3) joo:: ja* mitä se tos *tossa se vie (5.5)*   viekö se
      A: ((coughs)) yeah and what it/he her- here it/he takes   does it/he take
      tossai jotain *(1.4)   JOO se vie jotain (.)   PElotinta niille linnuille sitte*
      here something   yes it/he takes some   scarecrow for the birds then
(16) *(1.0) A: tässä näi jah   tuos tuola onkin sitte jo   tommone variksenpeläti .*
      A: here and   ther there is then already   that kind of a scarecrow
(17) *(1.2) A: jah sitte täälä* onh-ö *(1.6)   TÄÄla on sitten   KA:NSsa.,*
      A: and then here is   here is then   also

COMPLICATION & RESOLUTION

(18) *(2.5) A:* mutta mitä se *(1.2)*   miten se TUOSsa sitten tekee
      A: but what it/he   how does it/he here then do
(19) *(17.2) A:* siin+on *(.) ((rykii))* siin+on *(0.5)   niitten   lintuja   takasin   mut se hä (0.5)*
      A: there is ((cough)) there is   their   birds   back   but it/he he
      HÄtyyttelee niitä pois kyllä .,
      does chase them away

CODA

(20) *A: em+mä EM+mä osaa   muuta siihe sanookkaa (2.4)   että se (1.6)   että mitäh*
      A: I cannot I cannot   anything else say to it   so that it   that what
(21) *(5.7)T: no HYvä .*
      T: OK fine

The main theme of speaker A161's text is the personal pronoun *se* ('it/he/she') referring to the main character; in spoken Finnish, the pronoun *se* is used to refer to both human and non-human referents (cf. 'they' in English). In line 10 the speaker substitutes *se* with *hän* ('he/she'), which is used in reported and quoted speech in spoken Finnish (Seppänen, 1998: 35–38, 82–92). Here it is used when describing the inner world of the main character: *se* ('it/he') imagines that *hän* ('he') will get a lot of fruit. The thematic progression is quite easy to follow since there are no other themes in the text, except for *tää* and *se* ('this'; 'it') in line 8 referring to *lapio* ('spade'; 'and this is this yeah there is a spade'...'it is of that kind'). There are, however, some difficulties in interpreting the schematic structure of speaker A161's text. The elliptic tie in line 13 is in accordance with the notion that themes may be presupposed in clauses belonging to the same larger thematic unit (Halliday & Hasan, 1976: 143). In this example, all that the speaker has said up to this point can be interpreted as construing the orientation to the events to follow.

Then, in line 14, the speaker uses presupposition again ('birds [it] chases') as if she were indicating that the next clause is also part of the orientation. In addition, the previous clause was completed with rising intonation, supporting the interpretation that the speaker is going to add something to the orientation of the story. If this is the case, there is no motivation for the events to follow, that is, that the main character takes a scarecrow to the garden. The speaker mentions, however, that the birds returned (line19), but the first episode of the story, because the birds flew to the garden to peck at the seeds the man built a scarecrow, but it did not help, is not realised in a logical way. If, however, we look at the way the speaker uses the many questions and prosody in this text, it might be interpreted that she does indicate a major move (complication) in the storyline in line 14. She starts with a question, answers with putting the word 'birds' in a topical position, and maintains a flat intonation as far as line 16, where she tells that the scarecrow has been finished, and brings the clause to an end with prominently falling intonation. A similar pattern is seen in lines 18 and 19: the second episode starts with a question, and the speaker produces the rest of the narrative content in one intonation unit. Despite these speculations, one can positively find only one explicit episode in this text: in line 15 the speaker tells that the main character is taking the scarecrow to the garden, and in line 19 that the birds have returned, and that the man chases the birds away himself.

In addition to what is presented above, there are some other features of language use that make the text of speaker A161 somewhat ambiguous. It is typical that she frequently refers to the human and non-human participants with pronouns *se* ('he/it') or *ne* ('they'; human/non-human) and with a non-specific term *jotain* ('something'); their referents can be understood only in relation to the context, that is, the pictures in front of the speaker.

For example, in line 9 the speaker is assuming that 'he/it' (the main charac-ter) is planting 'something' (*KAI se jotain on IStuttamassa jotain tossa*). It appears, in lines 12 and 13, that she refers again to this 'something' with the pronouns *ne* ('they') and *niiden* ('their') (*juu ja sielä on ne; seuraa niiden kos KASvua*). The 'something' and the pronouns used most probably refer to seeds the man was planting, but this can be interpreted only by a partner with shared knowledge about the picture frames in front of the speaker.

The use of questions, non-specific terms, and especially ambiguous pronominal reference loosens the cohesion of the text, as has been reported in many studies on text production of people with aphasia (e.g. Armstrong, 1991; Glosser, 1993; Glosser & Deser, 1990). Still, these are not necessarily aphasic symptoms, since these features were also found in three texts of the eldest control speakers of this study (see also Stover & Haynes, 1989). Questioning may also indicate that the speaker has difficulties either in visual perception or in reading the cartoon genre, as explicitly stated by control speaker P1 (*mie oon niin huono (.) sarjakuvien TULkit(h)sija e(h)ttä he he*; 'I am such a poor interpreter of cartoons'). However, when a speaker is asking questions and answering them him- or herself, as was the case with speaker A161, the text may turn to a list of consecutive but non-related guesses. This kind of a texture does not make a coherent narrative (cf. Halliday & Hasan, 1976: 326–327).

Substitutions and reiterations

When the aphasic problem is more serious than in the cases presented above, the thematic progression is not as easy to follow as it is in milder disorders. This is clearly seen in the texts of three speakers with Wernicke's aphasia. In order to understand the meanings of the typically frequent substitutions (semantic and phonological paraphasias) and reiterated expressions (traditionally referred as perseveration), it is necessary to rely on contextual cues. In this study, the pictures in front of the speaker (known to this author) and the on-line interpretations of the therapist made it possible to estimate the intended meanings (Example 5).

Example 5: Substitutions and reiterations in speaker A128's (Wernicke's aphasia, AQ = 25,1) text. Linguistic elements of special interest in this example are set in `courier` font.

(19) *(.) A: .hh no .hh ja* `PIkku`*poika katselaa ja katseloo ihan KOtona ja.*
     A: well   and `little` `boy` is watching and watching right at home and
(20) *(.) A: .hh ja HUOmaa,*
     A: and notices
(21) *A: .hh on* `PIkku`*poikat vie Edussa,*
     A: are `little` `boys` still in front
(22) *(.) A: .hh .hh ja .h* `Iso poika` *katselee ja katselee.*
     A: and   `big boy`   is watching and watching

(23) *(0.6) A: .HH [Ö HE ovat POis,*
      A: they are away

(24) *T: [yhm ?*
      T: hmm

(25) *A: kukaan ei oo VIEty ?*
      A: no one has been taken

(26) *(0.5) A: [.hh ja TÄÄLLäki* PIkkukoisa *.hh katselee koko ju::ttua,*
      A: and here also [pikkukoisa] is watching the whole thing

(27) *T: [yhm .*
      T: hmm

(28) *(0.5) A: .hh ja lähetää vielä TÄÄllä on se ku VIEdää .*
      A: and [they] leave again here is the one that is taken

(29) *T: yhm*
      T: hmm

(30) *A: jap ja* pik- Iso pikkupoika *nau-nauraa et*
      A: and and lit- big little boy is laughing that
        koko ju::ttua et NOIha se kävi tietet .hh
        the whole thing that that of course was the way it happened

Without any knowledge about the contents of the picture frames, the listener would have a major problem in understanding about whom the speaker A128 is talking – for many reasons. First, many themes are realised with reiterated (perseverated) substitutes, some with phonological distortions. In line 19 the speaker seems to refer to the main character (a little man) with *pikkupoika* ('little boy') who is looking at something at home. This theme is presupposed by ellipsis in the following clause, and – surprisingly – *pikkupoikat* (a morphologically deviant form of plural *pikku-pojat*; 'little boys') are introduced in line 21; 'the little boy notices that little boys are still there'. It is obvious that instead of introducing new boys, the speaker has referred to the birds pecking at the seeds there in front of the house. This sequence might, thus, be interpreted as the complication (birds coming to the field), which leads to the main character's (a phonologically distorted form *pikkukoisa*; line 26) action of taking something somewhere, that is, the resolution. Thus, when all the contextual information is taken into account, this example may be interpreted as a coherent episode. However, if we were to evaluate this text purely based on the words used, we presumably would not come to the same conclusion.

The second difficulty for the listener is that the speaker does not include any theme in some clauses (lines 25 and 28). These clauses are realised with the Finnish passive verb forms *ei ole viety* ('has not been taken') and *lähetää(n)* (leave-passive), which can correspond either to the English passive or to a generalised verb form 'one/they/we/people in general leave(s)' (see Shore, 1988). With the Finnish passive, the speaker does not indicate who the actor is, the one who is leaving and taking something, and thus the topical participant themes are missing. In addition, in line 25 the speaker does not indicate explicitly who or what the 'no-one' (*kukaan*) who has not been taken, is. Third, referential ambiguity is also noticed in line 23 where the theme is realised with the pronoun *he* ('they'; used only for human referents). The speaker has just been talking about 'little boys' and a 'big boy', so *he* seems to be an appropriate pronoun. However, we can assume that these phrases are substitutes for the word 'birds'. Thus, *he* would not be the appropriate pronoun, as it is not used to refer to animals. To conclude, the linguistic choices available for this speaker make the interpretation of the thematic and schematic structures of this text very difficult. It would be almost impossible unless the contextual cues were utilised.

The repetition of same or similar words, that is, recurrent perseveration, described above, is considered typical of people with fluent aphasia (e.g. Albert & Sandson, 1986; Vilkki, 1989). In addition, some speakers with fluent aphasia repeat whole constructions, that is, they seem to be unable to move from one idea to the next (stuck-in-set perseveration; cf. Kaczmarek, 1987: 234) (Example 6).

Example 6: Poverty of new ideas in speaker A361's (Wernicke's aphasia, AQ = 59,7) text. Linguistic elements of special interest in this example are set in `courier` font.

(23) (*6.2 ot .hhh hhh.*) *A: en+en Osaa .*
        ((breathing in-out)) A: I can not

(24) (*3.1*) *T: ihan HYvin se meni tähän asti   sanoitte että että nuo tuli SYÖmään   niitä SIE[meniä*
        T: it went pretty well this far   you said that those came to eat   the seeds

(25) *A: [kyllä ne syö ja sitten ne syö TÄmä:kin tästä ?,*
        A: yes they eat and then they eat this also from here

(26) (*1.4*) *A: ja sitte tästä* `se tekee UUdestaas UUden kuopan,`
        A: and then from `this it makes again a new hole`

(27) (*1.7*) *A: ja TAAS* `takii tekee kuopan,`
        A: and again `((makes)) makes a hole`

(28) (*1.6*) *A:* `tekee niinku UUden` (*1.8*) `työn?,`
        A: `makes like a new`   `job`

(29) (*0.8*) *A: ja SITte vasta tulee tää* (*3.6 ot mt*)   `sit se tulee UUdestaan` *toi ?,*
        A: and after that comes this   `then it comes again` that

(30) (*2.4*) *A: noh* `se on tulee` *tä* (*4.6 ot .hh hh.*)   *tule-tulee se on sano* (*2.0*)   *no MIStä ne*
        A: well `it is comes` th-   come-comes it is say   well from where they
        nyt TUlee tuol[ta,
        now come from there

(31) *T: [yhm ?*
        T: hmm

(32) *A: joo.*
        A: yeah

(33) (*0.7*) *A: ja:: (.) ja sitte sehä::* `tekee tästä se tekee` (*2.5*) `laittaa sinne` (*1.7*)
        A: and   and then it   `makes from this it makes puts there`
        `sen UUdestaan,`
        `it again`

(34) (*2.4*) *A: ja sit* `se TUlee taas,`
        A: and then `it comes again`

(35) (*2.5*) *A: mistä se OTtaa tuolta .*
        A: from where it takes from there

In this example, the speaker A361 first mentions that he is not able to talk. This is due to his enormous difficulties in remembering the words he wants to use, explicit in the text preceeding this example (cf. Korpijaakko-Huuhka, 2003). In line 24, the therapist refers to the speaker's former utterances and interprets their meaning. After this (from line 26 on) the speaker continues to tell the story. The events he describes do not, however, bring much new information to the storyline: after the birds arrived in the garden, *se* ('he/it'; assumed to be the main character) makes something new over and over again, and someone (either the man or the birds) come again and again from somewhere. The speaker seems to be able to use only a very limited vocabulary for both nouns and verbs, and with these very common verbs ('make, come, put, take') and stuck-in-set constructions he is unable to provide the listener with content that would make the interpretation of the schematic structure of the story possible. Thus, it is not possible for the listener to interpret the text as a generically coherent story.

Coherence through co-authorship

As is obvious from Example 6 above, people with severe aphasia recognise their difficulty of talking (for data from conversational contexts, see Laakso, 1997). In this story-telling condition, many of them were about to interrupt the task because of their evident word-finding problems. However, with the therapist's help, the speakers with severe aphasia could also maintain their role as active participants in construing the story (Example 7).

Example 7: Therapist's contribution to story-generation with speaker A275 (Wernicke's aphasia, AQ = 49.0)

(46)   A: *EI sitä saa*
       A: not get it
(47)   T: *yhm . (0.5)   se on se VArik[senPElätin .*
       T: hmm   it is the scarecrow
(48)   A: *[(–) joo-o sä tiiät TÄÄ+on tää .*
       A: yes yes you know this is this
(49)   T: *PElätin .*
       T: scare((crow))
(50)   A: *tässä tää m[m (--) jo MEni .*
       A: here this ((unintell)) already went
(51)   T: *[yhm . (.) yhm . yhm .*
       T: hmm hmm hmm
(52)   A: *.hhh nii*
       A: ((inhalation)) yeah
(53)   *(1.0) T: Yhm .*
       T: hmm
(54)   *(0.5) A: j::o (0.9) tässä sitte se::   i- (0.5)   no se i-ISk-k   mikä se o-on .*
              A: ((yes?)) here then it   hi-   well it hi-hit   what it is
(55)   *(3.5) A: ((naputtaa kuvaa)) #y tota:: (1.1)   ((naputtaa kuvaa)) TOta:: tota::*
              A: ((taps on the picture)) that   ((taps on the picture)) that that

(56) *(0.5) T: no NII ? JUstiinsa .*
      T: well yes that's it
(57) *A: tota (--) [tota*
      A: that   that
(58) *T: [Yhm .*
      T: hmm
(59) *(3.3) A: SItä:: .*
      A: that
(60) *(1.3) T: elikä ne LINnut*
      T: that is the birds
(61) *A: j::oo [sit LINnut LINnut joo et ta taa tampe(--)   JAA-a JAAha .*
      A: yeah then birds birds yeah that ((syllables)) oh yeah oh yeah
(62) *T: [LINnut TAAs (.) TUlee (.) yhm .*
      T: birds again   arrive   hmm
(63) *(1.2) A: j::a (3.6) ja täällä (1.7) täällä kans (1.9) on nuo (1.0) ((naputtaa kuvaa)) j::a (0.5) yhm .*
      A: and   and here   here also   are those   ((taps on the picture)) and hmm
(64) *(2.3) A: EI VOi ? (0.5) ei voi . (.) [he he*
      A: can not   can not ha ha
(65) *T: [yhm . ei VOI s(h)anoa [he he*
      T: hmm   cannot say   ha ha
(66) *A: [e(h)ei [(.) ja joo ja TÄss+o[n (1.3) pa (--)*
      A: no   and yeah and here's ((syllable))
(67) *T: [NII [yhm .*
      T: yes   hmm
      hmm hmm
      yhm . yhm .
(68) *(0.7) T: nii elikä siinä se HÄÄtää niitä pois .*
      T: yes that is there it chases them away

This example is the latter part of a very long text, and it starts with the speaker A275's comment on his inability to get access to a specific word. The therapist has followed the speaker's attempts, and offers the most probable target word *variksempelätin* ('scarecrow'). The speaker, then, confirms this target, and continues to tell the story in line 50. The theme of the clause is *tää* ('this') referring obviously to the main character (*tässä tää m[m (--) jo MEni*; 'here <u>this</u> already went'). In line 56, the speaker is trying to describe that the main character (referred to with *se*; 'it') then hits something. He does not, however remember the targeted word, and the therapist offers *linnut* ('birds') for the speaker (line 60). Then again, the speaker tries to continue, but now, the therapist takes the initiative and leads the construction of the complication: the birds have returned to the field. The speaker's next contribution is the notion that there are birds in other pictures, too. But this attempt also breaks down, due to the inability to remember the words needed. This is clearly expressed in lines 64 and 65, where the interlocutors seem to share a face-saving laugh (cf. Haakana, 1999). Once again, the speaker attempts to continue, but the therapist completes the story by expressing that the main character is chasing the birds away. Thus, this second of the two episodes of the Ferd'nand story was co-authored (cf. Goodwin, 1979, 1995).

Discussion

The aim of this study was to describe how Finnish speakers with aphasia used their micro level means (words and clauses) to gain a macro level result (a well-formed story). The main result is that people with aphasia have many and various kinds of problems in text production. Although a few of them could generate a well-formed story in spite of their anomic disorder, most of the texts produced by speakers with aphasia could not be considered coherent stories. In this study, coherence was seen to emerge from the speakers' ways of using their linguistic options in order to provide the listener/reader with information that guides the interpretation of the text into thematic entities and episodes (cf. Matthiessen & Halliday, 1997). The lexicogrammar, including prosody, available to the speakers was examined to find out how they marked the connectedness, as well as the discontinuities, of the events they were describing. As was expected, according to earlier findings based on the English language (e.g. Armstrong, 1991; Bond Chapman *et al.*, 1998; Ulatowska & Streit Ollnes, 2000), most of the speakers with aphasia had problems in accessing target words, used deviant word forms and non-specific terms, and substituted proper nouns with ambiguous pronouns. These hindered or at least complicated the interpretation of the thematic structure and loosened the cohesion of the texts. In some cases, iteration of same words and ideas (perseveration) resulted in a shortage of information necessary for the interpretation of the event structure (episodes). In other cases, some relevant content was missing, or at least not explicitly expressed. Thus, the logical links between the events were hard to find.

In spite of the obvious problems described above, it is evident that speakers with aphasia have not totally lost their text production skills. They recognise the narrative genre and struggle for the completion of the story. Although their texts might not be well-formed stories, one can find fragments of narrative structures or individual coherent episodes in them. Often, however, the listener has to use all the contextual cues available in order to be able to understand the message of the speaker with aphasia. On the other hand, speakers with aphasia seem to rely on their partner's ability to interpret their utterances with the aid of contextual information. The more severe the aphasic disorder, the more frequent the use of contextual (exophoric) reference as a compensatory strategy seems to be. In the most severe cases, help and prompting from the partner serve as resources for the speakers with aphasia, supporting them to complete the task and to save face in a difficult situation.

It can be concluded, then, that according to this study, the role of aphasic language in text production is fundamental. There is no coherent text if the listener is unable to understand what the speaker is talking about and how the events he or she is describing are related to each other and to the context of the situation. Metaphorically: if the (enabling) tool (language) is broken, it does not serve its (textual) function. The 'building blocks' of textual coherence in the Finnish language, and the realisations of text production problems in Finnish-speaking people with and without aphasia seem similar to those reported in the English language and in English-speaking persons. Based on this study, it is impossible to say if there are some fundamental differences in lexicogrammatical patterns and patterns of deteriorations in text production of Finnish speakers compared with speakers of other languages. Thus, systematic comparative neuro-linguistic research on language usage in discourse is needed.

The Systemic Functional Linguistic framework applied in this study has proved valuable in the understanding of the nature of text production problems due to aphasia, and in the near future, it is expected to influence aphasia research and rehabilitation in Finland in many ways. Traditional clinical assessments, like psycholinguistic tests, focus on some basic levels of linguistic processing, but they do not reveal the ways the linguistic options available for people with aphasia are used in various discourses (Armstrong, 1995; Holland, 1982; Klippi, 1996: 15). Through a detailed linguistic analysis focusing on the meanings construed in the text and on the various possible reasons for difficulties in meaning-making, it is also possible to define the aims of logopedic intervention more precisely and make its results more transparent and measurable (for detailed examples, see Armstrong, 2005). In addition to using tradi-tional methods for processing words and clauses, the therapists might strive to open up opportunities for the client with aphasia to use his or her linguistic options in discourse tasks, like story generation as used in this study, retelling film clips (cf. Ramsberger & Rende, 2002) and conver-sational story-telling (cf. Aaltonen & Laakso, 2000). In these contexts, it is possible to consciously focus on the crucial textual elements, for example, how to enhance thematic progression, and how to increase logical connections between the events, to strengthen the client's ability to pro-duce understandable messages. The most natural situations for relating experiences, thoughts and feelings are, of course, every-day conversa-tions with family members or significant others. Thus, it is necessary to have them involved in the intervention, as it is evident that people with (severe) aphasia can maintain an active speaker role, for example the storyteller's role, only when their partners operate as co-authors.

Acknowledgement

This chapter has benefited from valuable comments by Susanna Shore, PhD, University of Helsinki.

References

Aaltonen, T. and Laakso, M. (2000) Aphasia and conversational story telling. *Journal of Neurolinguistics* 13, 265–266.

Albert, M.L. and Sandson, J. (1986) Perseveration in aphasia. *Cortex* 22, 103–115.

Armstrong, E. (1991) The potential of cohesion analysis in the analysis and treatment of aphasic discourse. *Clinical Linguistics & Phonetics* 5 (1), 39–51.

Armstrong, E. (1992) Clause complex relations in aphasic discourse: A longitudinal case study. *Journal of Neurolinguistics* 7 (44), 261–275.

Armstrong, E. (1995) A linguistic approach to the functional skills of aphasic speakers. In C. Code and D. MŸller (eds) *The Treatment of Aphasia: From Theory to Practice* (pp. 70–89). London: Whurr.

Armstrong, E. (2000) Aphasic discourse analysis: The story so far. *Aphasiology* 14 (9), 875–892.

Armstrong, E. (2005) Language disorder: A functional linguistic perspective. *Clinical Linguistics & Phonetics* 19 (3), 137–153.

de Beaugrande, R. (1997) The story of discourse analysis. In T.A. van Dijk (ed.) *Discourse as Structure and Process. A Multidisciplinary Introduction 1* (pp. 35–62). London: SAGE.

Berko-Gleason, J., Goodglass, H., Obler, L., Green, E., Hyde, M.R. and Weintraub, S. (1980) Narrative strategies of aphasic and normal-speaking subjects. *Journal of Speech and Hearing Research* 23 (2), 370–382.

Bird, H. and Franklin, S. (1996) Cinderella revisited: A comparison of fluent and non-fluent aphasic speech. *Journal of Neurolinguistics* 9 (3), 187–206.

Brookshire, R.H. and Nicholas, L.E. (1993) Comprehension of narrative discourse by aphasic listeners. In H.H. Brownell and Y. Joanette (eds) *Narrative Discourse in Neurologically Impaired and Normal Aging Adults* (pp. 151–170). San Diego: Singular.

Bond Chapman, S., Peterson Highley, A. and Thompson J.L. (1998) Discourse in fluent aphasia and Alzheimer's disease: Linguistic and cognitive considerations. In M. Paradis (ed.) *Pragmatics in Neurogenic Communication Disorders* (pp. 55–78). Oxford: Elsevier Science.

Chafe, W.L. (1980) The deployment of consciousness in the production of a narrative. In W.L. Chafe (ed.) *The Pear Stories. Cognitive, Cultural, and Linguistic Aspects of Narrative Production* (pp. 9–50). Norwood: Ablex.

Chafe, W. (1998) Language and the flow of thought. In M. Tomasello (ed.) *The New Psychology of Language. Cognitive and Functional Approaches to Language Structure* (pp. 93–111). London: LEA.

Chantraine, Y., Joanette, Y. and Cardebat, D. (1998) Impairments in discourse-level representations and processes. In B. Stemmer and H.A. Whitaker (eds) *Handbook of Neurolinguistics* (pp. 261–274). San Diego: Academic Press.

Christiansen, J.A. (1995) Coherence violations and propositional usage in the narratives of fluent aphasics. *Brain and Language* 51, 291–317.

Coelho, C.A. (1995) Discourse production deficits following traumatic brain injury: A critical review of the recent literature. *Aphasiology* 9 (5), 409–429.

Downing, A. (1991) An alternative approach to theme: A systemic-functional perspective. *Word* 42, 119–143.

Dressler, W.U. and Pléh, C. (1988) On text disturbances in aphasia. In W.U. Dressler and J.A. Stark (eds) *Linguistic Analyses of Aphasic Language* (pp. 151–178). New York: Springer Verlag.

Eggins, S. (1994) *An Introduction to Systemic Functional Linguistics.* London: Pinter.

Eggins, S. and Martin, J.R. (1997) Genres and registers of discourse. In T.A. Van Dijk (ed.) *Discourse as Structure and Process. Discourse Studies: A Multidisciplinary Introduction* (Vol. 1) (pp. 230–256). London: SAGE.

Ernest-Baron, C.R., Brookshire, R.H. and Nicholas, L.E. (1987) Story structure and retelling of narratives by aphasic and non-brain-damaged adults. *Journal of Speech and Hearing Research* 30, 44–49.

Glosser, G. (1993) Discourse production patterns in neurologically impaired and aged populations. In H.H. Brownell and Y. Joanette (eds) *Narrative Discourse in Neurologically Impaired and Normal Aging* (pp. 191–212). San Diego: Singular.

Glosser, G. and Deser, T. (1990) Patterns of discourse production among neurological patients with fluent language disorders. *Brain and Language* 40, 67–88.

Goodwin, C. (1979) The interactive construction of a sentence in natural conversation. In G. Psathas (ed.) *Everyday Language: Studies in Ethnometodology* (pp. 97–121). New York: Erlbaum.

Goodwin, C. (1995) Co-constructing meaning in conversations with an aphasic man. *Research on Language and Social Interaction* 28 (3), 233–260.

Haakana, M. (1999) Laughing matters. A conversation analytical study of laughter in doctor–patient interaction. Unpublished doctoral thesis. University of Helsinki, Helsinki, Finland.

Halliday, M.A.K. (1994) *An Introduction to Functional Grammar* (2nd edn). London: Edward Arnold.

Halliday, M.A.K. and Hasan, R. (1976) *Cohesion in English*. London: Longman.

Halliday, M.A.K. and Hasan, R. (1985) *Language, Context, and Text: Aspects of Language as a Social-Semiotic Perspective*. Victoria: Deakin University Press.

Helasvuo, M-L., Klippi, A. and Laakso, M. (2001) Grammatical structuring in Brocas's and Wernicke's aphasia in Finnish. *Journal of Neurolinguistics* 14, 231–254.

Holland, A.L. (1980) *Communicative Abilities of Daily Living. Manual*. Baltimore: University Park Press.

Holland, A.L. (1982) Observing functional communication of aphasic adults. *Journal of Speech and Hearing Disorders* 47, 50–56.

Huber, W. (1990) Text comprehension and production in aphasia: Analysis in terms of micro-and macrostructure. In Y. Joanette and H.H. Brownell (eds) *Discourse Ability and Brain Damage. Theoretical and Empirical Perspectives* (pp. 154–179). New York: Springer-Verlag.

Iivonen, A. (1988) Functional interpretation of prosody within the linguistic system. *The 1988 Yearbook of the Linguistic Association of Finland* (pp. 69–91). Helsinki: The Linguistic Association of Finland.

Joanette, Y. and Brownell H.H. (1990) Introduction. In Y. Joanette and H.H. Brownell (eds) *Discourse Ability and Brain Damage. Theoretical and Empirical Perspectives* (pp. xiii–xvi). New York: Springer-Verlag.

Joanette, Y. and Goulet, P. (1990) Narrative discourse in right-brain-damaged right-handers. In Y. Joanette and H.H. Brownell (eds) *Discourse Ability and Brain Damage. Theoretical and Empirical Perspectives* (pp. 131–153). New York: Springer-Verlag.

Kaczmarek, B.L.J. (1987) Regulatory function of the frontal lobes. A neurolinguistic perspective. In E. Perecman (ed.) *The Frontal Lobes Revisited* (pp. 225–240). New York: The IRBN Press.

Kalliokoski, J. (1989) *Ja. Rinnastus ja rinnastuskonjunktion käyttö [Ja. Coordination and the Use of the Coordinating Conjunction in Finnish]*. Helsinki: Finnish Literature Society.

Kintsch, W. (1994) The psychology of discourse processing. In M.A. Gernsbacher (ed.) *Handbook of Psycholinguistics* (pp. 721–740). New York: Academic Press.

Klippi, A. (1989) The communicative effectiveness of aphasic patients in discourse. *Proceeding of the XXIst Congress of the International Association of Logopedics and Phoniatrics*, vol. 1, August 1989, Prague, Czechoslovakia, 73–75.

Klippi, A. (1996) *Conversation as an Achievement in Aphasics*. Studia Fennica Linguistica 6. Helsinki: Finnish Literature Society.

Korpijaakko-Huuhka, A-M. (1987) Kertovan puheen tehokkuuden mittaaminen. Tapaustutkimus nimeämisvaikeuden aiheuttaman kommunikaatiohaitan arvioimisesta [Measuring the efficiency of narrative speech. The evaluation of communication handicap caused by word-finding difficulty: a case study]. *Suomen logopedis-foniatrinen aikakauslehti* (1), 2–18.
Korpijaakko-Huuhka, A-M. (1989) Clinical measurement of communicative efficiency: A case study and plans for further research. *Proceeding of the XXIst Congress of the International Association of Logopedics and Phoniatrics*, vol. 1, August 1989, Prague, Czechoslovakia, 76–79.
Korpijaakko-Huuhka, A-M. (1991a) Narrative speech in aphasia: Experiments in communicative efficiency. In R. Aulanko and M. Leiwo (eds) *Studies in Logopedics and Phonetics* (pp. 57–70). Publications of the Department of Phonetics, University of Helsinki, Series B: Phonetics, Logopedics and Speech Communication 3.
Korpijaakko-Huuhka, A-M. (1991b) Narrative speech styles in non-brain-damaged subjects. In M. Laine and J. Niemi and P. Koivuselkä – Sallinen (eds) *Proceedings of the 4th Finnish Conference of Neurolinguistics, Turku 1991* (pp. 61–74), University of Joensuu, Faculty of Arts, 23.
Korpijaakko-Huuhka, A-M. (1992) Communicative efficiency in narrative speech. *Proceedings of the XXII IALP Congress*, August 1992, Hannover, Germany, 386–392.
Korpijaakko-Huuhka, A-M. (1995) Kertomuksen koherenssi: Sarjakuvak-ertomuksen normaalivariaation piirteitä ja kuuden afaatikon kertomuksen analyysi [Coherence of a story: Features of normal variation in a cartoon-story task, and analysis of stories of six aphasic speakers]. Unpublished Licentiate thesis, University of Helsinki, Helsinki, Finland.
Korpijaakko-Huuhka, A-M. (2003) *Kyllä se lintupelotintaulujuttu siinä nyt on käsittelyssä Afaattisten puhujien kielellisiä valintoja sarjakuvatehtävässä [Aphasic Speakers' Linguistic Choices in a Cartoon-Story Task]*. Helsinki: Publications of the Department of Phonetics, University of Helsinki 46.
Korpijaakko-Huuhka, A-M. (2004, August–September) Aphasic speakers' linguistic choices in a cartoon-story task. Paper presented at the *26th World Congress of the International Association of Logopedics and Phoniatrics*, Brisbane, Australia.
Korpijaakko-Huuhka, A-M. and Aulanko, R. (1994) Auditory and acoustic analyses of prosody in clinical evaluation of narrative speech. In R. Aulanko and A-M. Korpijaakko-Huuhka (eds) *Proceedings of the Third Congress of the International Clinical Phonetics and Linguistics Association*. Helsinki 1993 (pp. 91–98). Publications of the Department of Phonetics, University of Helsinki 39.
Laakso, M. (1997) *Self-Initiated Repair by Fluent Aphasic Speakers in Conversation*. Helsinki: Finnish Literature Society.
Labov, W. (1977) *Language in the Inner City. Studies in the Black English Vernacular*. Oxford: Basil Blackwell.
Laine, M., Laakso, M., Vuorinen, E. and Rinne, J. (1998) Coherence and informativeness of discourse in two dementia types. *Journal of Neurolinguistics* 11 (1), 79–87.
Malkamäki, A. (1995) Afasiapotilaiden kommunikaatiotaitojen arviointi Communicative Abilities of Daily Living –tutkimusmenetelmällä (CADL) [The evaluation of communication skills of aphasic patients with the Communicative Abilities of Daily Living assessment (CADL)]. Unpublished Master's thesis, University of Helsinki, Helsinki, Finland.
Matthiessen, C. and Halliday, M.A.K. (1997) *Systemic Functional Grammar: A First Step into the Theory*. Australia: Macquarie University, Department of Linguistics.

Patry, R. and Nespoulous, J-L. (1990) Discourse analysis in linguistics: Historical and theoretical background. In Y. Joanette and H.H. Brownell (eds) *Discourse Ability and Brain Damage. Theoretical and Empirical Perspectives* (pp. 3–27). New York: Springer-Verlag.

Pohjasvaara, T., Erkinjuntti, T., Vataja, R. and Kaste, M. (1998) Correlates of dependent living 3 months after ischemic stroke. *Journal of Cerebrovascular Diseases* 8, 259–266.

Prutting, C.A. and Kirchner, D.M. (1987) A clinical appraisal of the pragmatic aspect of language. *Journal of Speech and Hearing Disorders* 52, 105–119.

Ramsberger, G. and Rende, B. (2002) Measuring transactional success in the conversation of people with aphasia. *Aphasiology* 16 (3), 337–353.

Seppänen, E-L. (1997) Vuorovaikutus paperilla [Interaction on paper]. In L. Tainio (ed.) *Keskustelunanalyysin perusteet [Basics in Conversation Analysis]* (pp. 18–31). Tampere: Vastapaino.

Seppänen, E-L. (1998) *Läsnäolon pronominit. Tämä, tuo, se ja hän viittaamassa keskustelun osallistujiin [Pronouons of participation. The Finnish pronouns tämä, tuo, se and hän as deviced for referring to co-participants in conversation].* Helsinki: Finnish Literature Society.

Shore, S. (1988) On the so-called Finnish passive. *Word* 39, 151–176.

Shore, S. (1991) A systemic-functional perspective on mood. In J. Niemi (ed.) *Papers from the Eighteenth Finnish Conference of Linguistics* (pp. 235–255). Studies in Linguistics 24, University of Joensuu.

Shore, S. (1992) Aspects of a systemic-functional grammar of Finnish. Doctoral thesis, School of English and Linguistics, Macquarie University, Sydney, Australia.

Skinner, C., Wirtz, S., Thompson, I. and Davidson, J. (1984) Edinburgh Functional Communication Profile. An observation procedure for the evaluation of disordered communication in elderly patients, Buckingham.

Stemmer, B. (1999) Discourse studies in neurologically impaired populations: A quest for action. *Brain and Language* 68, 402–418.

Stover, S.E. and Haynes, W.O. (1989) Topic manipulation and cohesive adequacy in conversations of normal adults between the ages 30 and 90. *Clinical Linguistics & Phonetics* 3 (2), 137–149.

Terva-Heinonen, K. (1985) 'The Edinburgh Functional Communication Profile' suomalaisten afaatikkojen ja laitosvanhusten funktionaalisen kommunikaation kuvaajana [The Edinburgh Functional Communication Profile as an indicator of functional communication of Finnish elderly people and people with aphasia]. Unpublished Master's thesis, University of Helsinki, Helsinki, Finland.

Togher, L. and Ferguson, A. (eds) (2005) Special Issue: Systemic Functional Linguistics and the Study of Language Disorders. *Clinical Linguistics & Phonetics* 19, 3.

Tykkyläinen, T. (1992) Tuotteliaisuus ja sisällön informatiivisuus aivoruhjevammapotilaiden keskustelussa [Productiveness and informativeness in conversation of people with traumatic brain injury]. Unpublished Master's thesis, University of Helsinki, Helsinki, Finland.

Ulatowska, H.K., Allard, L. and Bond Chapman, S. (1990) Narrative and procedural discourse in aphasia. In Y. Joanette and H.H. Brownell (eds) *Discourse Ability and Brain Damage. Theoretical and Empirical Perspectives* (pp. 180–198). New York: Springer-Verlag.

Ulatowska, H.K., Freedman-Stern, R., Weiss Doyel, A., Macaluso-Haynes, S. and North, A.J. (1983) Production of narrative discourse in aphasia. *Brain and Language* 19, 317–334.

Ulatowska, H.K., North, A.J. and Malacuso-Haynes, S. (1981) Production of narrative and procedural discourse in aphasia. *Brain and Language* 13, 345–371.

Ulatowska, H.K., Sadowska, M., Kordys, J. and Kadzielawa, D. (1993) Selected aspects of narratives in Polish-speaking aphasics as illustrated by Aesop's fables. In H.H. Brownell and Y. Joanette (eds) *Narrative Discourse in Neurologically Impaired and Normal Aging Adults* (pp. 171–190). San Diego: Singular.

Ulatowska, H.K. and Streit Ollnes, G. (2000) Discourse revisited: Contributions of lexico-syntactic devices. *Brain & Language* 71, 249–251.

van Dijk, T.A. (1981) *Studies in the Pragmatics of Discourse*. The Hague: Mouton.

Ventola, E. (1987) *The Structure of Social Interaction. A Systemic Approach to the Semiotics of Service Encounters*. London: Frances Printer.

Vilkki, J. (1989) Differential perseverations in verbal retrieval related to anterior and posterior left hemisphere lesions. *Brain and Language* 36, 543–554.

Chapter 8

Semantic Impairment in Finnish-Speaking People with Alzheimer's Disease: A Review

SEIJA PEKKALA

Introduction

Alzheimer's disease (AD) is characterised by a progressive semantic memory impairment, which is manifested as an inability to process semantically related information. The semantic impairment causes difficulties in communication and language processing skills at an early phase of the disease (Appell *et al.*, 1982; Bayles & Tomoeda, 1983; Chan *et al.*, 1993; Chertkow & Bub, 1990; Hodges *et al.*, 1990). These problems can be demonstrated as impaired speech production and comprehension, deteriorated reading and writing abilities and poor conversational skills (Appell *et al.*, 1982; Fromm & Holland, 1989; Kempler, 1995; Luzzatti *et al.*, 2003; Ripich & Ziol, 1998). Despite the semantic deficit, phonological (Croot *et al.*, 2000; Kempler, 1995) and morpho-syntactic (Bayles, 1982; Kempler *et al.*, 1987) abilities are relatively well preserved even in the moderate and late stages.

There seem to be four main accounts to explain the cause of the semantic impairment in AD. First, the semantic impairment may be caused by a visuoperceptual deficit (Bayles & Tomoeda, 1983; Hodges *et al.*, 1999; Lukatela *et al.*, 1998; Rochford, 1971). Second, a breakdown or loss of information in the representations in the semantic system may underlie the deficit (i.e. a storage deficit) (Chertkow & Bub, 1990; Hodges *et al.*, 1992; Hodges & Patterson, 1995; Huff *et al.*, 1986; Mickanin *et al.*, 1994). Third, the deficit may follow from a failure in the processes called upon to retrieve and exploit the relatively well preserved semantic representations (i.e. an access deficit) (Cronin-Golomb *et al.*, 1992; Johnson *et al.*, 1995; Nebes, 1989; Nebes *et al.*, 1984; Nebes & Halligan, 1996). Fourth, a multifactor deficit may underlie the disturbed semantic processing, in which both the degradation of semantic structure and the impaired retrieval of information are involved (Carew *et al.*, 1997; Crowe, 1998; Hagoort, 1998).

In Finland, as in other Western societies, the number of people with dementia increases as the population ages, which makes varying demands on the society in terms of providing services for those in need. In northern Europe, the prevalence of dementia among people older than 65 years is 5–9%, whereas the incidence among people aged 60–65 years is 0.1% and among people with 85–89 years, 5% (Fratiglioni *et al.*, 2000; Viramo & Sulkava, 2001). It was estimated that in 2000, approximately 30,000 people of the population of 5 million inhabitants suffered from mild dementia and 80,000 from moderate to severe dementia in Finland, and that in 2030 the number of people with moderate to severe dementia would increase to 130,000 (Viramo & Sulkava, 2001). Therefore, increasing the knowledge of communication and language difficulties in dementia, such as AD, helps speech pathologists to assess the nature and severity of the communication problems and meet the increasing communicative needs of individuals with dementia and their family members. Thus, knowing the structure and functioning of semantic memory and the ways it can be impaired in dementia is necessary for clinicians.

Nature and Structure of Semantic Information

According to the view broadly accepted in cognitive (neuro)psychology, semantic memory, a part of the long-term memory system, is responsible for the permanent storage of meaning-related knowledge. In modern theories of memory (e.g. connectionism), semantic knowledge is represented as a dynamic and interconnected network of semantic features that make up different constellations of meaning (Pulvermüller, 1999; Schwartz & Reisberg, 1991: 5–7, 406–427). These semantic features involve physical information about the shape, size, colour, taste, smell etc. of objects (Persson, 1995: 73–76; Tyler *et al.*, 2000) and functional features about the manner and the rules by which objects move or interact with the environment or how one moves one's body when manipulating objects (Bird *et al.*, 2000, 2001; Marshall *et al.*, 1996; Persson, 1995: 77–79; Tyler *et al.*, 2000; see also Labov, 1973; Rosch *et al.*, 1976; Tversky & Hemenway, 1984). Thematic features imply information concerning spatial locations and causal and interactional relationships between objects and actions, as well as cultural information (Barsalou, 1982, 1983, 1987; Lucariello & Rifkin, 1986; Nelson, 1996: 234). So called encyclopaedic knowledge, such as facts learned from books (e.g. penguins live in Antarctica), are also part of the semantic representation (Tyler *et al.*, 2000).

Some of the semantic features are shared features that are common to many semantically related words denoting objects, whereas distinctive features may be shared only by one or a few members in a category. Therefore, they are crucial for differentiating between co-ordinates (Devlin *et al.*, 1998; Gonnerman *et al.*, 1997; McRae *et al.*, 1997; Persson, 1995: 1, 18–124;

Tyler & Moss, 2001; Vinson *et al.*, 2003). For example, lions and tigers share such features as 'have-4-legs', 'have-fur' and 'have-a-tail', but only tigers have the feature 'have-stripes', by which they can be differentiated from lions (Gonnerman *et al.*, 1997). The features that co-occur in a systematic fashion are called correlated features. For example, things that have legs typically also have ears and eyes and are able to move (Bird *et al.*, 2000, 2001; Caramazza, 2000; Gonnerman *et al.*, 1997; McRae *et al.*, 1997; Persson, 1995: 1, 18–124; Pulvermüller, 1999; Pulvermüller *et al.*, 2001; Rosch, 1978; Rosch *et al.*, 1976; Tyler *et al.*, 2000; Tyler & Moss, 2001; Vandenberghe *et al.*, 1996; Vinson *et al.*, 2003). Because of their shared and correlated properties, semantically close items have strong and rapid connections to each other in the semantic network and they can be thought to form different semantic categories. These categories can be divided into living and non-living categories and further into different subcategories (e.g. birds and fruit vs. vehicles and tools) on the basis of their unique set of semantic features, which are not shared by other subcategories (Farah & McClelland, 1991; Garrard *et al.*, 2001; Gonnerman *et al.*, 1997; McRae & Cree, 2002; Moss *et al.*, 2002; Small, 1997; Vinson *et al.*, 2003).

Categories of objects are believed to form hierarchies of different levels of specificity, which are tightly interconnected (Collins & Quillian, 1969; Persson, 1995: 92–94; Warrington, 1975; Warrington & McCarthy, 1983). Categories can be vertically divided into the super-superordinate (e.g. 'thing', 'stuff'), the superordinate (e.g. 'animals', 'furniture'), basic ('cat', 'table') and the subordinate (e.g. 'Persian', 'dinner table') levels (Persson, 1995: 93–94; Rosch *et al.*, 1976; Smith *et al.*, 1974; Tversky & Hemenway, 1984). Horizontally the internal structure of categories can be considered graded, meaning that categories tend to have more central or more proto-typical and more marginal members (e.g. 'robin' vs. 'ostrich') (Rosch, 1975, 1978; Rosch & Mervis, 1975). The more typical of a category a member is the more features it shares with other members of the category, and the faster it can be identified as a member of a particular category. Conversely, the marginal, 'poor' members have only a few attributes in common with other members of the category.

The semantic structure of concrete verbs is different from that of concrete nouns in the sense that they are conceptually-semantically depen-dent on different entities that compose the meaning of verbs, whereas concrete nouns tend to stand semantically on their own (Huttenlocher & Lui, 1979; Levelt, 1989: 90–94; Persson, 1995: 96–104; Pinker, 1989: 165–246; Reyna, 1987). For example, the verb 'give' involves three components: a giving part, a transferred entity and a receiving part. Similar to nouns, rich and systematic correlational features can also underlie the semantic representation of specific verbs (Bird *et al.*, 2000; Kersten & Billman, 1997; Marshall *et al.*, 1996; McClelland & Kawamoto, 1986; Persson, 1995: 100; Pulvermüller, 1999; Pulvermüller *et al.*, 2001; Vinson & Vigliocco, 2002).

For example, the verbs 'hammer' and 'saw' specify the use of particular tools and motions associated with the actions, as well as the result of the actions. However, relative to nouns, very little is known about the principles of how actions are classified but assumptions have been made that correlated features account also for their classification process (Kersten & Billman, 1997; Persson, 1995: 99; Vinson & Vigliocco, 2002). Some verbs can form hierarchical structures with different levels of specificity (e.g. 'communicate', 'talk', 'babble' for the speech act verbs) (Fellbaum, 1998: 80; Miller & Fellbaum, 1991; Pulman, 1983: 111–112) and have a graded structure with some verbs being more prototypical than others (Pulman, 1983: 110–133; see also Ungerer & Schmid, 1996: 100, 191). For example, 'murder' can be a better example of killing than 'execute'.

Damage to semantic features and/or their connections, noise in the system and changes in the rate at which activated information decays in the semantic network may interfere with performance on semantic tasks (Dell, 1986; Devlin *et al.*, 1998; Farah & McClelland, 1991; Gonnerman *et al.*, 1997; Harley, 1998; Hinton *et al.*, 1986; Hinton & Sejnowski, 1986; Martin *et al.*, 1994; Smolensky, 1986). Damage to semantic features may lead to many types of degradation in performance in AD, including naming, matching and feature decisions (Harley, 1998; Moss *et al.*, 2002). In word production, damaged or lost features may affect the functioning of the semantic, the lemma (lexical) and the phonological levels, due to the interconnectivity between the levels (Harley, 1998).

Besides a number of studies conducted with English- and German-speaking individuals with AD, strong evidence of semantic impairment has also been obtained from studies in which the performance of Finnish-speaking people with AD was investigated. The three studies described below involved people with mild and moderate AD scoring between 15.9 and 23.5 on the Mini Mental State Examination Test (MMSE) (Folstein *et al.*, 1975). They were asked to perform different tasks requiring conscious processing of various semantic features, naming, as well as generating words belonging to various semantic categories and grammatical classes.

Impaired Conscious Understanding of Semantic Relations

Laatu *et al.* (1997) and Laatu (1999, 2003) indicated that people with mild and moderate AD ($n = 14$, MMSE score $M = 21.9$, SD $= 3.1$) had difficulty defining concepts for both concrete and abstract words (e.g. *majava* 'beaver', *sandaali* 'sandal', *miniä* 'daughter-in-law' and *pessimisti* 'pessimist'). In the definition task, the people with AD generated significantly fewer features for the superordinate categories and fewer physical and functional features for the concepts than healthy elderly control subjects (see also Abeysinghe *et al.*, 1990; Garrard *et al.*, 2005; Grober *et al.*, 1985; Hodges *et al.*, 1996; Moss *et al.*, 2002). When the spontaneous description lacked some of the essential features expected in the answer, the task was eased first with cueing questions given by the experimenter (e.g. *Minkälainen häntä ja minkälaiset hampaat majavalla on?* 'What is the tail and what are the teeth of a beaver like?'). Later, forced-choice questions were provided if the cueing questions were unhelpful (e.g. *Onko majavalla iso litteä häntä vai ohut kippura häntä?* 'Does a beaver have a big and flat or a thin and curled tail?'). The results indicated that the individuals with AD needed significantly more questions than the control subjects in order to find the correct information about concrete and abstract concepts from their semantic memory. They also made significantly more incorrect responses to the forced-choice level questions.

Laatu *et al.* (1997) and Laatu (1999) also indicated that individuals with AD were poorer than normal control subjects at mastering precise knowledge of the nature and strength of the semantic connection between the object and its different features. The subjects were given a concept with four attributes. The concept was embedded in four different written sentences that were in the form 'X is always ...', 'X is often ...', 'X is seldom ...' and 'X is never ...'. The attributes were given in a random order below the sentences. The subjects were told that one attribute fit only one sentence and were asked to complete the sentence with the given features so that the sentences made sense. For example, for the concept *timantti* 'diamond', the following meaningful combinations were possible: *Timantti on aina kova; timantti on usein koru; timantti on harvoin halpa; timantti ei ole koskaan metalli* 'A diamond is always hard; a diamond is often a jewel; a diamond is seldom inexpensive; a diamond is never metal.' Findings of diminished connections between objects and their attributes in AD have been reported also by Garrard *et al.* (2005), Grober *et al.* (1985), as well as Hodges *et al.* (1996).

Finally, the study of Laatu *et al.* (1997) showed that people with AD performed significantly worse than healthy adults in understanding hierarchies with both very concrete and more abstract concepts (see also Grossman *et al.*, 1996a). Laatu *et al.* (1997) asked the subjects to recognise errors in wrongly arranged conceptual hierarchies with superordinate concept at the top (e.g. *ruoka* 'food'), followed by three subcategories, each having two instances at the bottom (*hedelmät: sitruuna, päärynä* 'fruit': 'lemon', 'pear', *juurekset: porkkana, lanttu* 'rootcrop': 'carrot', 'turnip' and *vihannekset: tomaatti, kurkku* 'vegetables': 'tomato', 'cucumber'). The people with AD showed poor performance in pointing out the misplaced cards and in correcting the hierarchies. They were also impaired in their ability to assemble the whole hierarchy from 10 written cards. It was as difficult for them to correct some of the misplaced concepts as it was to construct a whole hierarchy by themselves. However, they tended to be as good as the control subjects at recognising the errors in the incorrect hierarchies. Thus, the people with AD obviously understood that something was wrong in these hierarchies and were able to point out the misplaced concept but they could not correct the hierarchy.

On the basis of their findings, Laatu *et al.* (1997) concluded that the performance of the individuals with AD reflected a deficit in the conscious understanding of semantic relationships, rather than defective visuo-constructive functions, which appeared not to have a significant effect on the results [controlled by the WAIS Block Design (Wechsler, 1955)]. Laatu *et al.* (1997) suggested that the semantic deficit could be caused both by insufficient conscious access to, and a degradation of, conceptual-semantic representations. The breakdown of semantic information involved both concrete and abstract concepts, the relationships between concepts and their attributes, and sub- and superordinate category knowledge. These findings are in line with many other studies conducted with speakers of English (Garrard *et al.*, 2005; Grober *et al.*, 1985; Grossman *et al.*, 1996a; Martin & Fedio, 1983; Nebes, 1989, 1992). The finding indicating a remarkable difficulty in maintaining the superordinate category information early in the disease, however, challenged the notion of its robustness and contrasted with earlier reports (Chertkow & Bub, 1990; Chertkow *et al.*, 1989; Cronin-Golomb *et al.*, 1992; Hodges *et al.*, 1992; Huff *et al.*, 1986; Martin & Fedio, 1983; Tippett *et al.*, 1995; cf. Grossman *et al.*, 1996a). Laatu *et al.* (1997) interpreted the finding that people with AD needed external guidance in order to consciously access meanings and that they tended to recognise, though not correct, errors in the hierarchy task as a sign of the access deficit. However, in their later study, Laatu *et al.* (2003) indicated that semantic memory impairment contributed also to deficits in visual object recognition in early AD. Consequently, semantic memory deficit may be manifested in several ways in the difficulties that people with AD experience in everyday life.

Anomia as a Reflection of the Semantic Impairment

The study of Laine *et al.* (1997) indicated that individuals with mild and moderate AD ($n = 13$, MMSE score $M = 18.2$, SD $= 3.5$) suffered from a substantial semantic deficit, which could be manifested as anomia, that is, the inability to find words for naming, and a tendency to make semantically related errors when producing words (see also Appell *et al.*, 1982; Nicholas *et al.*, 1996; Shuttleworth & Huber, 1988; Williamson *et al.*, 1998). Laine *et al.* (1997) measured semantic performance and, in particular, the naming ability of the subjects with an extensive battery of tests.

Laine *et al.* (1997) first modified the Finnish version of the Boston Naming Test (BNT) (Laine *et al.*, 1994) for the purposes of their study so that half of the test items were selected to match the frequency range of the Finnish BNT version and to fall into eight semantic categories (furniture, building, plant, animal, vehicle, tool, musical instrument and game accessory). Forty-five seconds was allowed for spontaneous naming, after which multiple-choice tasks measuring meaning-related and word form-related information followed. In the first multiple-choice task for measuring the preservation of meaning-related information, the subjects had to choose the specific semantic feature related to the target picture from four alternatives (e.g. for *helikopteri*: *se liikkuu vedessä, sillä lennetään, se liikkuu kiskoilla, se liikkuu lumessa* 'helicopter': 'one moves with it in the water', 'one flies with it', 'it moves on tracks', 'it moves in the snow'). In the second semantic multiple-choice task, the subjects had to find the correct superordinate out of eight written category names. The individuals with AD made significantly more errors on the semantic feature choice than did the healthy controls. Also, when choosing the superordinate, the control group performed significantly better than the AD group. Unlike the controls, the people with AD made significantly more errors when choosing semantic features rather than superordinate categories. Thus, the findings of this study add to the reports stating that superordinate information can also be affected in AD (see also Grossman *et al.*, 1996a; Laatu *et al.*, 1997).

In their first multiple-choice task measuring word form-related information (i.e. whether at least partial lexical retrieval had taken place), Laine *et al.* (1997) asked the subjects to choose the initial syllable of the target from four alternatives. The task design was based on the notion that semantic foils could be mistakenly chosen if the target was not well differentiated at the semantic level. Thus, two of the alternatives represented words that were semantically close to the target whereas one of them was unrelated (e.g. for *helikopteri* 'helicopter': *he, ra* (*raketti* 'rocket'), *len* (*lentokone* 'airplane'), and *ruo* (unrelated)). In the second task requiring word form-related information, the subjects were asked to point to the target word that was presented in written form together with four alternatives. Two of them were semantically related and one was phonologically related to the target (i.e. sharing the initial consonant-vowel with the target; e.g. for *helikopteri* 'helicopter': *helikopteri* 'helicopter', *raketti* 'rocket', *lentokone* 'airplane', *helistin* 'rattle'). The individuals with AD differed significantly from the control subjects in both the syllable choice task and the word choice task (cf. Hodges *et al.*, 1999). On the syllable choice task, 84% of the errors were semantically related foils and the rest were omissions. On the word choice task, 97% of the errors were semantically related to the target.

Second, Laine *et al.*'s (1997) study indicated that the naming performance of people with AD on the 60-item BNT was significantly poorer than that of normal controls. Phonological cueing appeared to help the people with AD to produce the correct target in a significant manner. However, the division of responses into different error types (i.e. perseverations, visual errors, semantic-associative, superordinate, functional/featural, semantic-visual, lexical-phonological, egocentric, segmental-phonological, unrelated, non-response and unclassifiable) indicated that the relative naming error distributions did not vary between the groups. The finding is in accordance with that of Lukatela *et al.* (1998) and Nicholas *et al.* (1996) but does not fully coincide with the finding of Bayles and Tomoeda (1983), Cuetos *et al.* (2005), Hodges *et al.* (1991) and Martin and Fedio (1983).

Third, Laine *et al.* (1997) used an odd-man-out task as a non-verbal test of semantic abilities. The subjects were presented with five pictures representing semantically related items, four of which were semantically very close to each other and one which did not go with the others (e.g. desk, chair, sofa, rocking chair and stool). The results indicated that the individuals with AD were significantly poorer than the healthy adults at doing a fine-grained semantic analysis between semantically related items, a finding in accordance with the study of Grossman *et al.* (1996a).

Fourth, Laine *et al.* (1997) utilised the word repetition and the word reading sections from the Finnish version of the Boston Diagnostic Aphasia Examination (BDAE) (Laine *et al.*, 1994), in which the people with AD performed as well as the control subjects, indicating normal functioning of the phonological output lexicon and the phoneme assembly for motor output. The finding is in contrast with that of Pekkala (2006), who indicated that difficulties in phonological processing emerged in the speech production of a Finnish-speaking male with mild AD (MMSE score 25) when he repeated pseudowords and words of foreign origin rather than stimuli from common clinical tests such as BDAE. Impaired phonological processing has also been found in different repetition tasks among English-speaking people with mild and moderate AD (Biassou *et al.*, 1995; Croot *et al.*, 2000; Glosser *et al.*, 1997, 1998).

Finally, the study of Laine *et al.* (1997) involved the Heinonen visual pattern matching task (Portin & Rinne, 1980), in which 40 geometric designs were to be matched with their identical counterparts, each from four alternatives. The people with AD made significantly more errors than the healthy controls, indicating a visuoperceptual deficit, a finding in accordance with many other studies (Bayles & Tomoeda, 1983; Cronin-Golomb *et al.*, 1991; Hodges *et al.*, 1999; Lukatela *et al.*, 1998; Rochford, 1971; but see Grossman *et al.*, 1998; Laatu *et al.*, 2003).

According to Laine *et al.* (1997), the poor overall performance and the semantic errors of the individuals with AD in the different verbal and non-verbal semantic tasks indicated that the mechanism underlying anomia in AD was likely to result from a semantic deficit (i.e. a difficulty in accessing information about specific semantic attributes or other subordinate categories) rather than a phonological or a lexical component (i.e. inability to retrieve the name of an object although it has been identified successfully). However, they also suggested that a combination of deficits may have caused the impairment, that is, a semantic disorder combined with impaired lexical retrieval. The visuoperceptual disorder may only have had latent effects on the naming ability of the people with AD. Similar conclusions have been drawn on the basis of several other studies, in which English-speaking participants with AD were examined (Chenery *et al.*, 1996; Hodges *et al.*, 1991).

Impaired Semantic Fluency Performance

Pekkala (2004) demonstrated that people with both mild AD ($n = 20$, MMSE score $M = 23.5$, SD $= 2.0$) and moderate AD ($n = 20$, MMSE score $M = 15.9$, SD $= 2.4$) had difficulty in producing concrete nouns and verbs in a semantic fluency task, in which participants were asked to list as many members of a semantic category as possible within 60 seconds. The semantic categories employed in the study involved clothes, vegetables, vehicles and animals as the noun categories, and preparing food, playing sports, constructing and cleaning as the verb categories. The task is performed as a cycle of clustering and switching (Troyer *et al.*, 1997) so that listing the most prototypical words of a very common subcategory takes place first (e.g. farm animals: *lehmä, hevonen, lammas* 'cow', 'horse', 'sheep'), after which switches to other subcategories (e.g. exotic animals) follow, and clusters of semantically related items are generated from these subcategories (e.g. *tiikeri, leijona, kirahvi* 'tiger', 'lion', 'giraffe') until the time allocated has passed. Words can also be clustered according to their phonemic similarity (e.g. *porkkana, peruna, palsternakka* 'carrot', 'potato', 'parsnip'). This task is employed to investigate not only spoken word production but also the organisation and function of, as well as the access to the lexical-semantic systems (Hodges & Patterson, 1995; Huff, 1988; Joanette & Goulet, 1986; Lafosse *et al.*, 1997). The semantic fluency task has thus far been limited to assess noun production but Pekkala (2004) demonstrated that it can also be applied to cover and analyse the production of different types of verbs (see also Östberg *et al.*, 2005; Piatt *et al.*, 1999a, 1999b).

Pekkala (2004: 97–154, 162–164, 186) showed that the ability of people with AD to flexibly process semantic information corresponding to a semantic category, to integrate related information as clusters of semantically or phonologically similar words, and to switch between different semantic dimensions was reduced compared to healthy elderly adults. For the noun category fluency tasks, similar results have been reported earlier (e.g. Beatty *et al.*, 1997, 2000; Binetti *et al.*, 1995; Carew *et al.*, 1997; Martin & Fedio, 1983; Ober *et al.*, 1986; Troyer *et al.*, 1998; Tröster *et al.*, 1989, 1998). Pekkala (2004: 97–154) indicated that individuals with mild AD were significantly poorer than control subjects, but better than those with moderate AD at processing the semantic-lexical information and producing words, clusters and switches for both types of tasks. The finding is consistent with the studies by Bayles *et al.* (1993), Crossley *et al.* (1997), Hodges and Patterson (1995) and Mickanin *et al.* (1994).

Pekkala (2004: 114–118, 125–127, 140–144, 150–151) also revealed that the AD groups showed a significantly reduced range of semantic subcategories for both noun and verb production. In the noun categories, the most relevant semantic features for the cluster formation consisted mainly of thematic and functional features that denote contextual, spatial and temporal information of the items, as well as their functional purpose. Physical features denoting the appearance (e.g. parts, colour or size) of objects or strictly taxonomic relations between words (e.g. birds, fish) emerged relatively rarely, mainly in the group of normal controls and the mild AD group. Thematic and functional features seemed to allow a cross-classification of different lexical items over the semantic subcategories, which may explain their high occurrence among the subject groups (e.g. Barsalou, 1982, 1983; Lucariello *et al.*, 1992; Lucariello & Rifkin, 1986; Nelson, 1996: 232–248). For example, vehicles were clustered as items used on water, in the air, on the roads, in the snow or by the public in an urban environment.

As far as the verb fluency task was concerned, Pekkala (2004: 150–151, 164) demonstrated that the semantic features that were mostly used to activate semantic dimensions involved mostly agent-initiated and goal-directed actions denoting tools or instruments with which the action was carried out (e.g. *sahata, vasaroida* 'to saw', 'to hammer'), the outcome or the result of the action (e.g. *keittää, paistaa* 'to boil', 'to fry') and spatial configurations of the action (e.g. *kattaa, valaa perusta* 'to build a roof', 'to pour foundation'). In the category of playing sports, form-functional features denoting the specific body parts in charge of the action (e.g. hands for *heittää, työntää* 'to throw', 'to push') played an important role in the selection of verbs for production. Sports verbs were also clustered based on thematic features that specified seasonal information implied by the verb (*hiihtää, luistella* 'to do cross-country skiing', 'to skate'). Verbs were also produced by applying the temporal-causal, sequential order (i.e. scripts) in which actions are likely to take place in the real world. Yet another way to form clusters of verbs was to combine the semantic information according to the manner in which actions are carried out (e.g. *tampata, puistella* 'to beat', 'to shake' [carpets]; see Fellbaum, 1998: 79; Marshall *et al.*, 1996; Miller & Fellbaum, 1991).

Pekkala's (2004: 109–112, 136–140) study also indicated that people with mild and moderate AD produced significantly more errors in the semantic fluency task than the control subjects, with the people with mild AD exhibiting a more accurate performance than those with moderate AD. In general, the error analysis appeared insufficiently sensitive to differentiate the AD groups from each other at the level of individual noun and verb categories. Nevertheless, the errors consisted mainly of semantically related intrusions (e.g. fruit, such as *omena* 'apple', were listed as vegetables) and perseverations (repetitions of earlier responses). The number of intrusions in the noun categories remained relatively low, which is in accordance with earlier studies with Dutch- and English-speaking subjects (Beatty *et al.*, 2000; Diesfeldt, 1985; Ober *et al.*, 1986; Tröster *et al.*, 1989). Pekkala (2004: 135–139, 146–150, 164) showed that intrusions produced for the verb categories consisted mainly of concrete nouns referring to tools and instruments needed for different actions (e.g. *rätti* 'rag' for the category of cleaning and *hella* 'stove' for the category of preparing food). One reason for the occurrence of intrusions during semantic fluency performance may be an unsuccessful semantic feature integration in semantic memory and/or at the lemma and phonological levels (Dell, 1986; Dell *et al.*, 1997b; Foygel & Dell, 2000; Pekkala, 2004: 120–123, 148–150, 165–171; Persson, 1995: 35–39, 125–135, 177–182).

Pekkala's (2004: 109–112, 124–125, 138–140, 150) error analysis revealed that very many perseverations were produced by people with both mild AD and moderate AD for both types of fluency tasks. Perseverations may hinder production of words, cluster formation and shifting between subcategories which interferes with activation of new words for the output (Dell, 1986; Dell *et al.*, 1997a; Laine, 1989: 75–80; Martin *et al.*, 1994; Pekkala, 2004: 165–169; Persson, 1995: 66). As a consequence of an insufficient spread and decay of activation in the lexicon, previously produced words may remain active because they are not 'turned off' properly by the self-inhibition system, and new items do not receive enough activation to compete successfully (Dell, 1986; Dell *et al.*, 1997a). Perseverations may also indicate an impoverished active vocabulary in AD, which is why subjects tend to activate and produce the same words and clusters over and over again. Repetitions may also be an attempt to activate new semantic dimensions to facilitate the retrieval of new words (Gruenewald & Lockhead, 1980; Pekkala, 2004: 166; Persson, 1995: 33–35).

Concluding Remarks

The three Finnish studies discussed in this chapter have provided evidence that people with mild and moderate AD have difficulty retaining the semantic knowledge of concrete and abstract nouns as well as concrete verbs. The semantic deficit appeared as a difficulty defining concepts for words, grasping relations between concepts, naming words and producing responses for the semantic fluency tasks. Clinically, the studies provided guidelines for the quantitative and qualitative performance of healthy elderly control subjects and people with AD in different types of semantic tasks, which can be used as the basis for comparing and assessing the performance of other subjects. The discussion of semantic features and their ability to flexibly activate and create different combinations with each other, forming varying semantic representations, gives an insight into their crucial role in both normal and deviant language processing. Furthermore, the error analyses can help clinicians analyse the loci or level of impaired speech processing in AD.

All studies, pointing out that Finnish-speaking people with AD had problems using the semantic features of words and the relations between semantically related words, contribute to similar findings recently reported on English-speaking people with AD (e.g. Garrard *et al.*, 2005; Gonnerman *et al.*, 1997; Hodges *et al.*, 1996; Moss *et al.*, 2002; Whatmough & Chertkow, 2002). Laatu *et al.* (1997) found that physical and functional features denoting an object were difficult to match, and that incorrect, although semantically related features, were introduced for some of the definitions. Laine *et al.* (1997) indicated that choosing appropriate semantic features for the target items was difficult and that there was a very strong tendency for semantically related errors in the word choice task. Pekkala (2004: 114–118, 125–127, 163–164), on the other hand, showed that physical features were seldom used as the basis for cluster formation in AD. Instead, the functional and thematic features served as the most strongly weighted connection between the items produced for the task. Consequently, the studies indicated that a deficit in semantic feature integration is likely to be present in AD.

The findings confirm the notion that different types of semantic features and their correlations may be sensitive to damage in the semantic network in AD (Devlin *et al.*, 1998; Garrard *et al.*, 2001; Gonnerman *et al.*, 1997; McRae & Cree, 2002; Moss *et al.*, 2002; Tyler *et al.*, 2000; Tyler & Moss, 2001; Vinson *et al.*, 2003; Whatmough *et al.*, 2003). According to current assumptions, strongly correlated sets of features tend to be heavily weighted and thus are more resistant to damage than features with weaker correlations. Consequently, distinctive features that are weakly correlated, in particular for living things, are likely to be more vulnerable to damage than the highly correlated shared features. As a result of damage to the vulnerable distinctive features of living things, naming pictures and matching words to pictures may cause confusion within a semantic category, whereas sorting items into semantic categories is preserved due to shared semantic features. Man-made objects tend to be more robust against damage than living entities because they have a strong correlation between the distinctive physical form and the specific function of the object (e.g. 'has-blade' and 'cuts' for 'knife') which make them mutually discriminative (Devlin *et al.*, 2002; Moss *et al.*, 2002; Persson, 1995: 80–81; Tyler *et al.*, 2000; Tyler & Moss, 2001; but see Vinson *et al.*, 2003). Thus, relating object concepts based on their physical features, which tends to require fine-grained differentiation between the feature patterns, may be more difficult for people with AD than relating items according to common thematic and functional features. However, to some extent, the findings of Laatu *et al.* (1997) Laatu (2003) and Laine *et al.* (1997) challenge this notion and some earlier empirical studies by indicating that problems in comprehending semantic information was not only restricted to the specific features of the items, but that people with AD also displayed difficulties in grasping more general, common information concerning superordinate knowledge that is shared by many items (cf. Chertkow & Bub, 1990; Chertkow *et al.*, 1989; Cronin-Golomb *et al.*, 1992; Hodges *et al.*, 1992; Huff *et al.*, 1986; Martin *et al.*, 1985; Martin & Fedio, 1983; Schwartz *et al.*, 1979; Shuttleworth & Huber, 1988; Tippett *et al.*, 1995; Warrington, 1975).

Despite methodological differences, the outcomes of the three studies summarised above shared the common finding of an impaired semantic processing in AD. On the basis of these studies it is difficult to point out whether the semantic deficit is caused by impaired conscious access to semantic memory or by a breakdown of its semantic representations. However, Laine *et al.* (1997) and Pekkala (2004: 167–171) speculated that not only the semantic level, but also other levels of speech processing, such as the lemma and phonological levels, were likely to contribute to the performance of their participants with AD on the word production tasks (see Dell, 1986; Dell *et al.*, 1997a, 1997b; Laine & Martin, 1996; Martin *et al.*, 1994). Furthermore, Pekkala (2004) clearly indicated that not only processing concrete nouns, but also concrete verbs can be affected in AD, a finding consistent with the study of Grossman *et al.* (1996b), Kim and Thompson (2001) and White-Devine *et al.* (1996). Consequently, people with AD may suffer from a multi-level deficit in which semantic disorder and impaired lexical retrieval of both nouns and verbs are involved.

It has been stressed that deterioration of other cognitive functions may be yet another plausible factor explaining the poor performance of people with AD on semantic tasks relative to normal control subjects. For example, failure in metalinguistic skills (Astell & Harley, 2002), impaired working memory and executive functions affecting planning, initiating and monitoring one's performance, cognitive flexibility to shift mental sets and so on, are likely to have a negative impact on the performance of the people with AD (Bayles, 2003; Chertkow & Bub, 1990; Diesfeldt, 1985; Kopelman, 1994; Morris, 1994; Rosen & Engle, 1997; Troyer *et al.*, 1998).

References

Abeysinghe, S.C., Bayles, K.A. and Trosset, M.W. (1990) Semantic memory deterioration in Alzheimer's subjects: Evidence from word association, definition, and associate ranking tasks. *Journal of Speech and Hearing Research* 33 (3), 574–582.

Appell, J., Kertesz, A. and Fisman, M. (1982) A study of language functioning in Alzheimer patients. *Brain and Language* 17 (1), 73–91.

Astell, A.J. and Harley, T.A. (2002) Accessing semantic knowledge in dementia: Evidence from a word definition task. *Brain and Language* 82 (3), 312–326.

Barsalou, L.W. (1982) Context-independent and context-dependent information in concepts. *Memory and Cognition* 10 (1), 82–93.

Barsalou, L.W. (1983) Ad hoc categories. *Memory and Cognition* 11 (3), 211–227.

Barsalou, L.W. (1987) The instability of graded structure: Implications for the nature of concepts. In U. Neisser (ed.) *Concepts and Conceptual Development: Ecological and Intellectual Factors in Categorization* (pp. 101–140). Cambridge: Cambridge University Press.

Bayles, K.A. (1982) Language function in senile dementia. *Brain and Language* 16 (2), 265–280.

Bayles, K.A. (2003) Effects of working memory deficits on the communicative functioning of Alzheimer's dementia patients. *Journal of Communication Disorders* 36 (3), 209–219.

Bayles, K.A. and Tomoeda, C.K. (1983) Confrontation naming impairment in dementia. *Brain and Language* 19 (1), 98–114.

Bayles, K.A., Trosset, M.W., Tomoeda, C.K., Montgomery, E.B. Jr and Wilson, J. (1993) Generative naming in Parkinson disease patients. *Journal of Clinical and Experimental Neuropsychology* 15 (4), 547–562.

Beatty, W.W., Testa, J.A., English, S. and Winn, P. (1997) Influences of clustering and switching on the verbal fluency performance of patients with Alzheimer's disease. *Aging, Neuropsychology, and Cognition* 4 (4), 273–279.

Beatty, W.W., Salmon, D.P., Testa, J.A., Hanisch, C. and Tröster, A.I. (2000) Monitoring the changing status of semantic memory in Alzheimer's disease: An evaluation of several process measures. *Aging, Neuropsychology, and Cognition* 7 (2), 94–111.

Biassou, N., Grossman, M., Onishi, K., Mickanin, J., Robinson, K.M. and D'Esposito, M. (1995) Phonologic processing deficits in Alzheimer's disease. *Neurology* 45 (12), 2165–2169.

Binetti, G., Magni, E., Cappa, S.F., Padovani, A., Bianchetti, A. and Trabucchi, M. (1995) Semantic memory in Alzheimer's disease: An analysis of category fluency. *Journal of Clinical and Experimental Neuropsychology* 17 (1), 82–89.

Bird, H., Howard, D. and Franklin, S. (2000) Why is a verb like an inanimate object? Grammatical category and semantic category deficits. *Brain and Language* 72 (3), 246–309.

Bird, H., Howard, D. and Franklin, S. (2001) Noun-verb differences? A question of semantics: A response to Shapiro and Caramazza. *Brain and Language* 76 (2), 213–222.

Caramazza, A. (2000), The organization of conceptual knowledge in the brain. In M.S. Gazzaniga (ed.) *The New Cognitive Neuroscience* (2nd edn) (pp. 1037–1046). Cambridge, MA: MIT Press.

Carew, T.G., Lamar, M., Cloud, B.S., Grossman, M. and Libon, D.J. (1997) Impairment in category fluency in ischemic vascular dementia. *Neuropsychology* 11 (3), 400–412.

Chan, A.S., Butters, N., Paulsen, J.S., Salmon, D.P., Swenson, M.R. and Maloney, L.T. (1993) An assessment of the semantic network in patients with Alzheimer's disease. *Journal of Cognitive Neuroscience* 5 (2), 254–261.

Chenery, H.J., Murdoch, B.E. and Ingram, J.C.L. (1996) An investigation of confrontation naming performance in Alzheimer's dementia as a function of disease severity. *Aphasiology* 10 (5), 423–441.

Chertkow, H. and Bub, D. (1990) Semantic memory loss in dementia of Alzheimer's type. What do various measures measure? *Brain* 113 (2), 397–417.

Chertkow, H., Bub, D. and Seidenberg, M. (1989) Priming and semantic memory loss in Alzheimer's disease. *Brain and Language* 36 (3), 420–446.

Collins, A.M. and Quillian, M.R. (1969) Retrieval time from semantic memory. *Journal of Verbal Learning and Verbal Behavior* 8 (2), 240–247.

Cronin-Golomb, A., Keane, M.M., Kokodis, A., Corkin, S. and Growdon, J.H. (1992) Category knowledge in Alzheimer's disease: Normal organization and a general retrieval deficit. *Psychology and Aging* 7 (3), 359–366.

Croot, K., Hodges, J.R., Xuereb, J. and Patterson, K. (2000) Phonological and articulatory impairment in Alzheimer's disease: A case series. *Brain and Language* 75 (2), 277–309.

Crossley, M., D'Arcy, C. and Rawson, N.S.B. (1997) Letter and category fluency in community-dwelling Canadian seniors: A comparison of normal participants to those with dementia of the Alzheimer or vascular type. *Journal of Clinical and Experimental Neuropsychology* 19 (1), 52–62.

Crowe, S.F. (1998) Decrease in performance on the verbal fluency test as a function of time: Evaluation in a young healthy sample. *Journal of Clinical and Experimental Neuropsychology* 20 (3), 391–401.

Cuetos, F., Gonzales-Nosti, M. and Martinez, C. (2005) The picture-naming task in the analysis of cognitive deterioration in Alzheimer's disease. *Aphasiology* 19 (6), 545–557.

Dell, G.S. (1986) A spreading-activation theory of retrieval in sentence production. *Psychological Review* 93 (2), 283–321.

Dell, G.S., Burger, L.K. and Svec, W.R. (1997a) Language production and serial order: A functional analysis and a model. *Psychological Review* 104 (1), 123–147.

Dell, G.S., Schwartz, M.F., Martin, N., Saffran, E.M. and Gagnon, D.A. (1997b) Lexical access in aphasic and nonaphasic subjects. *Psychological Review* 104 (4), 801–838.

Devlin, J.T., Gonnerman, L.M., Andersen, E.S. and Seidenberg, M.S. (1998) Category-specific semantic deficits in focal and widespread brain damage: A computational account. *Journal of Cognitive Neuroscience* 10 (1), 77–94.

Devlin, J.T., Russell, R.P., Davis, M.H., Price, C.J., Moss, H.E., Fadili, M.J. and Tyler, L.K. (2002) Is there an anatomical basis for category-specificity? Semantic memory studies in PET and fMRI. *Neuropsychologia* 40 (1), 54–75.

Diesfeldt, H.F.A. (1985) Verbal fluency in senile dementia: An analysis of search and knowledge. *Archives of Gerontology and Geriatrics* 4 (3), 231–239.

Farah, M.J. and McClelland, J.L. (1991) A computational model of semantic memory impairment: Modality specificity and emergent category specificity. *Journal of Experimental Psychology: General* 120 (4), 339–357.

Fellbaum, C. (1998) A semantic network of English verbs. In C. Fellbaum (ed.) *Wordnet. An Electronic Lexical Database* (pp. 69–104). Cambridge, MA: MIT Press.

Folstein, M.F., Folstein, S.E. and McHugh, P.R. (1975) 'Mini-mental state'. A practical method for grading the cognitive state of patients for the clinician. *Journal of Psychiatric Research* 12 (3), 189–198.

Foygel, D. and Dell, G.S. (2000) Models of impaired lexical access in speech production. *Journal of Memory and Language* 43 (2), 182–216.

Fratiglioni, L., Launer, L.J., Andersen, K., Breteler, M.M., Copeland, J.R., Dartigues, J.F., Lobo, A., Martinez-Lage, J., Soininen, H. and Hofman, A. (2000) Incidence of dementia and major subtypes in Europe: A collaborative study of population-based cohorts. *Neurology* 54 (Suppl. 5), S10–15.

Fromm, D. and Holland, A.L. (1989) Functional communication in Alzheimer's disease. *Journal of Speech and Hearing Disorders* 54 (3), 535–540.

Garrard, P., Lambon Ralph, M.A., Hodges, J.R. and Patterson, A. (2001) Prototypicality, distinctiveness, and intercorrelations: Analysis of the semantic attributes of living and nonliving concepts. *Cognitive Neuropsychology* 18 (2), 125–174.

Garrard, P., Lambon Ralph, M.A., Patterson, K., Pratt, K.H. and Hodges, J.R. (2005) Semantic feature knowledge and picture naming in dementia of Alzheimer's type: A new approach. *Brain and Language* 93 (1), 79–94.

Glosser, G., Kohn, S.E., Friedman, R.B., Sands, L. and Grugan, P. (1997) Repetition of single words and nonwords in Alzheimer's disease. *Cortex* 33 (4), 653–666.

Glosser, G., Friedman, R.B., Kohn, S.E., Sands, L. and Grugan, P. (1998) Cognitive mechanisms for processing nonwords: Evidence from Alzheimer's disease. *Brain and Language* 63 (1), 32–49.

Gonnerman, L.M., Andersen, E.S., Devlin, J.T., Kempler, D. and Seidenberg, M.S. (1997) Double dissociation of semantic categories in Alzheimer's disease. *Brain and Language* 57 (2), 254–279.

Grober, E., Buschke, H., Kawas, C. and Fuld, P. (1985) Impaired ranking of semantic attributes in dementia. *Brain and Language* 26 (2), 276–286.

Grossman, M., D'Esposito, M., Hughes, E., Onishi, K., Biassou, N., White-Devine, T. and Robinson, K.M. (1996a) Language comprehension profiles in Alzheimer's disease, multi-infarct dementia, and frontotemporal degeneration. *Neurology* 47 (1), 183–189.

Grossman, M., Mickanin, J., Onishi, K. and Hughes, E. (1996b) Verb comprehension deficits in probable Alzheimer's disease. *Brain and Language* 53 (3), 369–389.

Grossman, M., Robinson, K., Biassou, N., White-Devine, T. and D'Esposito, M. (1998) Semantic memory in Alzheimer's disease: Representativeness, ontologic category, and material. *Neuropsychology* 12 (1), 34–42.

Gruenewald, P.J. and Lockhead, G.R. (1980) The free recall of category examples. *Journal of Experimental Psychology: Human Learning and Memory* 6 (3), 225–240.

Hagoort, P. (1998) The shadows of lexical meaning in patients with semantic impairments. In B. Stemmer and H.A. Whitaker (eds) *Handbook of Neurolinguistics* (pp. 235–248). San Diego: Academic Press.

Harley, T.A. (1998) The semantic deficit in dementia: Connectionist approaches to what goes wrong in picture naming. *Aphasiology* 12 (4/5), 299–318.

Hinton, G.E., McClelland, J.L. and Rumelhart, D.E. (1986) Distributed representations. In D.E. Rumelhart, J.L. McClelland and the PDP Research Group (eds) *Parallel Distributed Processing. Explorations in the Microstructure of Cognition: Vol. 1. Foundations* (pp. 77–109). Cambridge, MA: MIT Press.

Hinton, G.E. and Sejnowski, T.J. (1986) Learning and relearning in Bolzmann machines. In D.E. Rumelhart, J.L. McClelland and the PDP Research Group (eds) *Parallel Distributed Processing. Explorations in the Microstructure of Cognition: Vol. 1. Foundations* (pp. 282–317). Cambridge, MA: MIT Press.

Hodges, J.R. and Patterson, K. (1995) Is semantic memory consistently impaired early in the course of Alzheimer's disease? Neuroanatomical and diagnostic implications. *Neuropsychologia* 33 (4), 441–459.

Hodges, J.R., Salmon, D.P. and Butters, N. (1990) Differential impairment of semantic and episodic memory in Alzheimer's and Huntington's disease: A controlled prospective study. *Journal of Neurology, Neurosurgery, and Psychiatry* 53 (12), 1089–1095.

Hodges, J.R., Salmon, D.P. and Butters, N. (1991) The nature of the naming deficit in Alzheimer's disease and Huntington's disease. *Brain* 14 (4), 1547–1558.

Hodges, J.R., Salmon, D.P. and Butters, N. (1992) Semantic impairment in Alzheimer's disease: Failure of access or degraded knowledge. *Neuropsychologia* 30 (4), 301–314.

Hodges, J.R., Patterson, K., Graham, N. and Dawson, K. (1996) Naming and knowing in dementia of Alzheimer's type. *Brain and Language* 54 (2), 302–325.

Hodges, J.R., Garrard, P., Perry, R., Patterson, K., Ward, R., Bak, T. and Gregory, C. (1999) The differentiation of semantic dementia and frontal lobe dementia (temporal and frontal variants of frontotemporal dementia) from early Alzheimer's disease: A comparative neuropsychological study. *Neuropsychology* 13 (1), 31–40.

Huff, F.J. (1988) The disorder of naming in Alzheimer's disease. In L.L. Light and D.M. Burke (eds) *Language, Memory, and Aging* (pp. 209–220). New York: Cambridge University Press.

Huff, F.J., Corkin, S. and Growdon, J.H. (1986) Semantic impairment and anomia in Alzheimer's disease. *Brain and Language* 28 (2), 235–249.

Huttenlocher, J. and Lui, F. (1979) The semantic organization of some simple nouns and verbs. *Journal of Verbal Learning and Verbal Behavior* 18 (2), 141–162.

Joanette, Y. and Goulét, P. (1986) Criterion-specific reduction of verbal fluency in right brain-damaged right-handers. *Neuropsychologia* 24 (6), 875–879.

Johnson, M.K., Hermann, A.M. and Bonilla, J.L. (1995) Semantic relations and Alzheimer's disease: Typicality and direction of testing. *Neuropsychology* 9 (4), 529–536.

Kempler, D. (1995) Language changes in dementia of the Alzheimer type. In R. Lubinski (ed.) *Dementia and Communication* (pp. 98–114). San Diego: Singular Publishing Group.

Kempler, D., Curtiss, S. and Jackson, C. (1987) Syntactic preservation in Alzheimer's disease. *Journal of Speech and Hearing Research* 30 (3), 343–350.

Kersten, A.W. and Billman, D. (1997) Event category learning. *Journal of Experimental Psychology: Learning, Memory, and Cognition* 23 (3), 638–658.

Kim, M. and Thompson, C.K. (2001) Verb deficits in Alzheimer's disease and agrammatism: Semantic versus syntactic impairments. *Brain and Language* 79 (1), 125–127.

Kopelman, M.D. (1994) Working memory in the amnesic syndrome and degenerative dementia. *Neuropsychology* 8 (4), 555–562.

Laatu, S. (1999) Käsitteiden ymmärtämisen vaikeuksia Alzheimerin taudissa, Parkinsonin taudissa sekä MS-taudissa [Difficulties in understanding concepts in Alzheimer's disease, Parkinson's disease and Multiple Sclerosis]. *Suomen logopedis-foniatrinen aikakauslehti* 19 (2), 72–85.

Laatu, S. (2003) *Semantic Memory Deficits in Alzheimer's Disease, Parkinson's Disease and Multiple Sclerosis. Impairments in Conscious Understanding of Concept Meanings and Visual Object Recognition.* Annales Universitatis Turkuensis, Ser. B., 259. Turku: University of Turku.

Laatu, S., Portin, R., Revonsuo, A., Tuisku, S. and Rinne, J. (1997) Knowledge of concept meanings in Alzheimer's disease. *Cortex* 33 (1), 27–45.

Laatu, S., Revonsuo, A., Jäykkä, H., Portin, R. and Rinne, J.O. (2003) Visual object recognition in early Alzheimer's disease: Deficits in semantic processing. *Acta Neurologica Scandinavica* 10 (2), 82–89.

Labov, W. (1973) The boundaries of words and their meaning. In C-J.N. Bailey and R.W. Shuy (eds) *New Ways of Analyzing Variation in English* (pp. 340–373). Washington, DC: Georgetown University Press.

Lafosse, J.M., Reed, B.R., Mungas, D., Sterling, S.B., Wahbeh, H. and Jagust, W.J. (1997) Fluency and memory differences between ischemic vascular dementia and Alzheimer's disease. *Neuropsychology* 11 (4), 514–522.

Laine, M. (1989) *On the Mechanisms of Verbal Adynamia. A Neuropsychological Study.* Annales Universitatis Turkuensis. Series B, Pt. 185. Turku: University of Turku.

Laine, M., Goodglass, H., Niemi, J., Koivuselkä-Sallinen, P., Tuomainen, J. and Marttila, R. (1994) Adaptation of the Boston Diagnostic Aphasia Examination and Boston Naming Test into Finnish. *Scandinavian Journal of Logopedics and Phoniatrics* 18, 83–92.

Laine, M. and Martin, N. (1996) Lexical retrieval deficit in picture naming: Implications for word production models. *Brain and Language* 53 (3), 283–314.

Laine, M., Vuorinen, E. and Rinne, J.O. (1997) Picture naming deficits in vascular dementia and Alzheimer's disease. *Journal of Clinical and Experimental Neuropsychology* 19 (1), 126–140.

Levelt, W.J.M. (1989) *Speaking: From Intention to Articulation.* Cambridge, MA: MIT Press.

Lucariello, J., Kyratzis, A. and Nelson, K. (1992) Taxonomic knowledge: What kind and when. *Child Development* 63 (2), 978–998.

Lucariello, J. and Rifkin, A. (1986) Event representations as the basis for categorical knowledge. In K. Nelson (ed.) *Event Knowledge: Structure and Function in Development* (pp. 189–203). Hillsdale, NJ: Lawrence Erlbaum.

Lukatela, K., Malloy, P., Jenkins, M. and Cohen, R. (1998) The naming in early Alzheimer's and vascular dementia. *Neuropsychology* 12 (4), 565–572.

Luzzatti, C., Laiacona, M. and Agazzi, D. (2003) Multiple patterns of writing disorders in dementia of the Alzheimer type and their evolution. *Neuropsychologia* 41 (7), 759–772.

Marshall, J., Chiat, S., Robson, J. and Pring, T. (1996) Calling a salad a federation: An investigation of semantic jargon. Part 2 – verbs. *Journal of Neurolinguistics* 9 (4), 251–260.

Martin, A., Browers, P., Cox, C. and Fedio, P. (1985) On the nature of the verbal memory deficit in Alzheimer's disease. *Brain and Language* 25 (2), 323–341.

Martin, A. and Fedio, P. (1983) Word production and comprehension in Alzheimer's disease: The breakdown of semantic knowledge. *Brain and Language* 19 (1), 124–141.

Martin, N., Dell, G.S., Saffran, E.M. and Schwartz, M.F. (1994) Origins of paraphasias in deep dysphasia: Testing the consequences of a decay impairment to an interactive spreading activation model of lexical retrieval. *Brain and Language* 47 (4), 609–660.

McClelland, J.L. and Kawamoto, A.H. (1986) Mechanisms of sentence processing: Assigning roles to constituents of sentences. In J.L. McClelland, D.E. Rumelhart and the PDP Research Group (eds) *Parallel Distributed Processing. Explorations in the Microstructure of Cognition. Vol. 2: Psychological and Biological Models* (pp. 272–325). Cambridge, MA: MIT Press.

McRae, K. and Cree G.S. (2002) Factors underlying category-specific semantic impairments. In E.M.E. Forde and G.W. Humphreys (eds) *Category Specificity in Brain and Mind* (pp. 211–249). Hove: Psychology Press.

McRae, K., de Sa, V.R. and Seidenberg, M.S. (1997) On the nature and scope of featural representations of word meaning. *Journal of Experimental Psychology: General* 126 (2), 99–130.

Mickanin, J., Grossman, M., Onishi, K., Auriacombe, S. and Clark, C. (1994) Verbal and nonverbal fluency in patients with probable Alzheimer's disease. *Neuropsychology* 8 (3), 385–394.

Miller, G.A. and Fellbaum, C. (1991) Semantic networks of English. *Cognition* 41 (1–3), 197–229.

Morris, R.G. (1994) Working memory in Alzheimer-type dementia. *Neuropsychology* 8 (4), 544–554.

Moss, H.E., Tyler, L.K. and Devlin, J.T. (2002) The emergence of category-specific deficits in a distributed semantic system. In E.M.F. Forde and G.W. Humphreys (eds) *Category Specificity in Brain and Mind* (pp. 115–147). Hove: Psychology Press.

Nebes, R.D. (1989) Semantic memory in Alzheimer's disease. *Psychological Bulletin* 106 (3), 377–394.

Nebes, R.D. and Halligan, E.M. (1996) Sentence context influences the interpretation of word meaning by Alzheimer patients. *Brain and Language* 54 (2), 233–245.

Nelson, K. (1996) *Language in Cognitive Development: The Emergence of the Mediated Mind.* Cambridge: Cambridge University Press.

Nicholas, M., Obler, L.K., Au, R. and Albert, M.L. (1996) On the nature of naming errors in aging and dementia: A study of semantic relatedness. *Brain and Language* 54 (2), 184–195.

Ober, B.A., Dronkers, N.F., Koss, E., Delis, D.C. and Friedland, R.P. (1986) Retrieval from semantic memory in Alzheimer-type dementia. *Journal of Clinical and Experimental Neuropsychology* 8 (1), 75–92.

Östberg, P., Fernaeus, S.-E., Hellström, Å., Bogdanović, N. and Wahlund, L.-O. (2005) Impaired verb fluency: A sign of mild cognitive impairment. *Brain and Language* 95 (2), 273–279.

Pekkala, S. (2004) *Semantic Fluency in Mild and Moderate Alzheimer's Disease.* Publications of the Department of Phonetics, 47. Helsinki: University of Helsinki. On WWW at http://ethesis.helsinki.fi/.

Pekkala, S. (2006) Impaired repetition of pseudowords and words of foreign origin as an indication of phonological difficulties in mild Alzheimer's disease. *Conference Proceedings of the 34th Annual Meeting of the International Neuropsychological Society*, February 2006, Boston, MA, 245 pp.

Persson, I.-B. (1995) *Connectionism, Language Production and Adult Aphasia. Elaboration of a Connectionist Framework for Lexical Processing and a Hypothesis of Agrammatic Aphasia.* Commentationes Humanarum Litterarum, 106. Helsinki: The Finnish Society of Sciences and Letters.

Piatt, A.L., Fields, J.A., Paolo, A.M., Koller, W.C. and Tröster, A.I. (1999a) Lexical semantic and action verbal fluency in Parkinson's disease with and without dementia. *Journal of Clinical and Experimental Neuropsychology* 21 (4), 435–443.

Piatt, A.L., Fields, J.A., Paolo, A.M. and Tröster, A.I. (1999b) Action (verb naming) fluency as an executive function measure: Convergent and divergent evidence of validity. *Neuropsychologia* 37 (13), 1499–1503.

Pinker, S. (1989) *Learnability and Cognition. The Acquisition of Argument Structure.* Cambridge, MA: MIT Press.

Portin, R. and Rinne, U.K. (1980) Neuropsychological responses of parkinsonian patients to long-term levodopa treatment. In U.K. Rinne, M. Klinger and G. Stamm (eds) *Parkinson's Disease: Current Progress, Problems and Management* (pp. 271–304). New York: Elsevier Science.

Pulman, S.G. (1983) *Word Meaning and Belief.* London: Croom Helm.

Pulvermüller, F. (1999) Words in the brain's language. *Behavioral and Brain Sciences* 22 (2), 253–336.

Pulvermüller, F., Härle, M. and Hummel, F. (2001) Walking or talking?: Behavioral and neurophysiological correlates of action verb processing. *Brain and Language* 78 (2), 143–168.

Reyna, V.F. (1987) Understanding verbs: Easy extension, hard comprehension. In A.W. Ellis (ed.) *Process in the Psychology of Language* (Vol. 3) (pp. 301–315). London: Lawrence Erlbaum.

Ripich, D.N. and Ziol, E. (1998) Dementia: A review for the speech-language pathologist. In A.F. Johnson and B.H. Jacobson (eds) *Medical Speech-Language Pathology: A Practitioner's Guide* (pp. 467–494). New York: Thieme Medical.

Rochford, G. (1971) A study of naming errors in dysphasic and in demented patients. *Neuropsychologia* 9 (4), 437–443.

Rosch, E. (1975) Cognitive representations of semantic categories. *Journal of Experimental Psychology: General* 104 (3), 192–233.

Rosch, E. (1978) Principles of categorization. In E. Rosch and B.B. Lloyd (eds) *Cognition and Categorization* (pp. 27–48). Hillsdale, NJ: Lawrence Erlbaum.

Rosch E. and Mervis, C.B. (1975) Family resemblance: Studies in the internal structure of categories. *Cognitive Psychology* 7 (4), 573–605.

Rosch, E., Mervis, C.B., Gray, W.D., Johnson, D.M. and Boyes-Bream, P. (1976) Basic objects in natural categories. *Cognitive Psychology* 8 (4), 382–439.

Rosen, V.M. and Engle, R.W. (1997) The role of working memory capacity in retrieval. *Journal of Experimental Psychology: General* 126 (3), 211–222.

Schwartz, B. and Reisberg, D. (1991) *Learning and Memory*. New York: W. W. Norton.

Schwartz, M.F., Marin, O.S.M. and Saffran, E.M. (1979) Dissociations of language function in dementia: A case study. *Brain and Language* 7 (3), 277–306.

Shuttleworth, E.C. and Huber, S.J. (1988) The naming disorder of dementia of Alzheimer type. *Brain and Language* 34 (2), 222–234.

Small, S.L. (1997) Semantic category imprecision: A connectionist study of the boundaries of word meanings. *Brain and Language* 57 (2), 181–194.

Smith, E.E., Shoben, E.J. and Ribs, L.J. (1974) Structure and process in semantic memory: A featural model for semantic decisions. *Psychological Review* 81 (3), 214–241.

Smolensky, P. (1986) Information processing in dynamical systems: Foundations of harmony theory. In D.E. Rumelhart, J.L. McClelland and the PDP Research Group (eds) *Parallel Distributed Processing: Explorations in the Microstructure of Cognition. Volume 1: Foundations* (pp. 194–281). Cambridge, MA: MIT Press.

Tippett, L.S., McAuliffe, S. and Farah, M.J. (1995) Preservation of categorical knowledge in Alzheimer's disease: A computational account. *Memory* 3 (3/4), 519–533.

Tröster, A.I., Salmon, D.P., McCullough, D. and Butters, N. (1989) A comparison of the category fluency deficits associated with Alzheimer's and Huntington's disease. *Brain and Language* 37 (4), 500–513.

Tröster, A.I., Fields, J.A., Testa, J.A., Paul, R.H., Blanco, C.R., Hames, K.A., Salmon, D.P. and Beatty, W.W. (1998) Cortical and subcortical influences on clustering and switching in the performance of verbal fluency task. *Neuropsychologia* 36 (4), 295–304.

Troyer, A.K., Moscovitch, M. and Winocur, G. (1997) Clustering and switching as two components of verbal fluency: Evidence from younger and older healthy adults. *Neuropsychology* 11 (1), 138–146.

Troyer, A.K., Moscovitch, M., Winocur, G., Leach, L. and Freedman, M. (1998) Clustering and switching on verbal fluency tests in Alzheimer's and Parkinson's disease. *Journal of the International Neuropsychological Society* 4 (2), 137–143.

Tversky, B. and Hemenway, K. (1984) Objects, parts, and categories. *Journal of Experimental Psychology: General* 113 (2), 169–193.

Tyler, L.K. and Moss, H.E. (2001) Towards a distributed account of conceptual knowledge. *Trends in Cognitive Sciences* 5 (6), 244–252.

Tyler, L.K., Moss, H.E., Durrant-Peatfield, M.R. and Levy, J.P. (2000) Conceptual structure and the structure of concepts: A distributed account of category-specific deficits. *Brain and Language* 75 (2), 195–231.

Ungerer, F. and Schmid, H.-J. (1996) *An Introduction to Cognitive Linguistics*. London: Longman.

Vandenberghe, R., Price, C., Wise, R., Josephs, O. and Frackowiak, R.S.J. (1996) Functional anatomy of a common semantic system for words and pictures. *Nature* 383 (6597), 254–256.

Vinson, D.P. and Vigliocco, G. (2002) A semantic analysis of grammatical class impairments: Semantic representations of object nouns, action nouns and action verbs. *Journal of Neurolinguistics* 15 (3–5), 317–351.

Vinson, D.P., Vigliocco, G., Cappa, S. and Siri, S. (2003) The breakdown of semantic knowledge: Insights from a statistical model of meaning representation. *Brain and Language* 86 (3), 347–365.

Viramo, P. and Sulkava, R. (2001) Muistihäiriöiden ja dementian epidemiologiaa [Epidemiology of memory disorders and dementia]. In T. Erkinjuntti, J. Rinne, K. Alhainen and H. Soininen (eds) *Muistihäiriöt ja Dementia* (pp. 20–36). Helsinki: Duodecim.

Warrington, E.K. (1975) The selective impairment of semantic memory. *Quarterly Journal of Experimental Psychology* 27 (4), 635–657.

Warrington, E.K. and McCarthy, R. (1983) Category specific access dysphasia. *Brain* 106 (4), 859–878.

Wechsler, D. (1955) *Manual for the Wechsler Adult Intelligence Scale.* New York: Psychological Corporation.

Whatmough, C. and Chertkow, H. (2002) Category-specific recognition impairments in Alzheimer's disease. In E.M.E. Forde and G.W. Humphreys (eds) *Category Specificity in Brain and Mind* (pp. 181–210). Hove: Psychology Press.

Whatmough, C., Chertkow, H., Murtha, S., Templeman, D., Babins, L. and Kelner, N. (2003) The semantic category effect increases with worsening anomia in Alzheimer's type dementia. *Brain and Language* 84 (3), 134–147.

White-Devine, T., Grossman, M., Robinson, K.M., Onishi, K., Biassou, N. and D'Esposito, M. (1996) Verb confrontation naming and word-picture matching in Alzheimer's disease. *Neuropsychology* 10 (4), 495–503.

Williamson, D.J.G., Adair, J.C., Raymer, A.M. and Heilman, K.M. (1998) Object and action naming in Alzheimer's disease. *Cortex* 34 (4), 601–610.

Chapter 9

The Interplay Between Verbal and Non-verbal Behaviour in Aphasic Word Search in Conversation

ANU KLIPPI and LIISA AHOPALO

Introduction

The linguistic processes during spoken language, especially in word production, are broadly studied within psycho- and neurolinguistics, and several models related to word production have been developed (see e.g. Nickels, 2002). In addition, the interplay between verbal and non-verbal behaviour during speaking has been studied to some extent (see e.g. McNeill, 2000). However, up to this point, few researchers have studied how non-verbal behaviour is related to language problems, for example the process of word search and disordered language production in general.

One typical and persistent behaviour characterising aphasic conversational interactions is word searching (Whitehouse *et al.*, 1978). Different types of fluent and non-fluent aphasic persons experience word-finding problems and these problems have been broadly studied in experimental contexts, mostly in confrontation naming experiments (e.g. Nickels, 2002). Yet these studies have been more interested in the end result of the word search, not in the process of the search as such. However, it is often observed that persons with aphasia take longer in searching for words than do normal speakers, and it is possible to observe the different stages in the aphasic word searching activity (e.g. Laakso & Klippi, 1999). By carefully analysing these stages, we can examine how the speaker approaches the target word.

Goodwin and Goodwin (1986) have studied the interactive structure of word searching in everyday conversation. They support the view that searching for a word is a visible and an auditory activity that others not only recognise, but can participate in, too. Speakers signal their word search activity by emitting speech perturbations such as pauses, cut-offs, vocal hesitations such as sound stretches, repetitions and 'uh's. These features can be regarded as self-repair initiations (Schegloff *et al.*, 1977).

According to Goodwin and Goodwin (1986), recipients typically gaze towards speakers during their word searches, and thus increase their attention towards the speaker. If the self-repair initiations do not lead to word finding, speakers often withdraw their gaze away from recipients during word searches, and at the same time they may produce a characteristic thinking face. In addition, other non-verbal behaviour may indicate the ongoing word search. For example, sometimes the speaker may turn his/her gaze back to the recipient and start to produce expressions such as 'what is it?' or 'what do you call it?' When the word has been found, the search can then be treated as being closed and the talk moves forward to other matters.

Hayashi (2003) has used the concept of *prospective indexical* when examining word searches in Japanese. This concept was first introduced by Goodwin (1996: 384–385) and he describes it as follows: 'The occurrence of a prospective indexical ... invokes a distributed, multiparty process. The cognitive operations relevant to the ongoing constitution of the event in process are by no means confined to speakers alone. Hearers must engage in an active, somewhat problematic process of interpretation in order to uncover the specification of the indexical that will enable them to build appropriate subsequent action at a particular place.' In Hayashi's (2003) study, the speaker who engaged in a word search deployed multiple practices in different semiotic modalities (linguistic and gestural) simultaneously. The analysis showed that these different practices work together and they mutually reinforce one another. Thus, they narrow down the domain of words to which the searched-for item belongs.

It is often observed that when speakers search for words, they begin moving their hands or bodies during that word search. It is argued that these gestural accompaniments to spontaneous speech can facilitate access to the mental lexicon (Rauscher *et al.*, 1996). Some researchers have suggested that gestures reflect an effort to facilitate impaired verbal processing (e.g. Fex & Månsson, 1998; Hadar, 1991; Hadar & Yadlin-Gedassy, 1994; Hanlon *et al.*, 1990; Rose *et al.*, 2002) Especially the role of iconic gestures has been at the focus of increased attention in the study of speech-related behaviour (e.g. Hadar & Butterworth, 1997; Laakso, 2003; Rose *et al.*, 2002).

Several studies maintain that people with aphasia use more non-verbal behaviours than do people with unimpaired language (Ahlsén, 1985; Feyereisen, 1983; Hadar, 1991; Herrmann *et al.*, 1989; Larkins & Webster, 1981; Le May *et al.*, 1988; Smith, 1987). In these studies, non-verbal behaviour includes the movements of the speaker's hands, head (including gaze), face, body and sometimes even the movements of his or her feet. Furthermore, many of these studies argue that aphasic speakers compensate for their verbal deficit by increasing the frequency of their non-verbal behaviour (see e.g. Ahlsén, 1991; Fex & Månsson, 1998; Feyereisen *et al.*,

1988; Hadar, 1991; Herrmann *et al.*, 1989; Le May *et al.*, 1988; Smith, 1987). In addition, Ahlsén (1991) conducted a longitudinal study of an aphasic person whose verbal communication increased during the 18-month period of language training, while the use of body communication decreased during that period.

Aphasic word searches have been studied to some degree in a conversational context and often from an interactional point of view (Ferguson, 1994; Helasvuo *et al.*, 2004; Klippi, 2003; Laakso, 1997, 1999; Laakso & Klippi, 1999; Laakso & Lehtola, 2003; Milroy & Perkins, 1992; Oelschlaeger, 1999; Wilkinson, 1995). Based on these studies, the word searches by aphasic persons have similar features to those found in normal conversation. For instance, before the target word, different signs indicate the ongoing search. According to Laakso & Lehtola (2003), the most typical signs of an ongoing search are repetition of particles or pronouns, pauses and hesitations. They also suggest that search questions and directing gaze to the addressee seem to be the most efficient way to get the recipient to participate in the word search.

Purpose of the Study

This chapter explores the sequential development of word searching by a person with aphasia. Moreover, our interest is focused on the interactive process of word searching. We will present examples from aphasic conversations, and our aim is to analyse the following:

(1) What is the interplay between non-verbal and verbal behaviour in aphasic word searches in a conversational context?
(2) What kinds of gestures can an aphasic speaker make use of during a word search activity?
(3) How do these gestures facilitate these word searches?
(4) If a speaker fails to find the target word, or the word search is prolonged, how does a recipient react to it?

Materials and Method

A person with aphasia

PK was a 59-year-old female Finnish-speaking person with aphasia. Before her illness, she had worked as an investment advisor in a big bank. Two years earlier, she had been operated on because of a benign tumour in her left temporal lobe. Since the operation, she experienced aphasic problems. During the time of data collection, her speech was fairly fluent but she had severe word-finding problems. She constantly needed to search for words, mainly nouns but verbs as well. PK used many circumlocutions and she likewise had many hesitations and pauses in her speech.

According to the WAB-test (Kertesz, 1982, Finnish version, Lehtihalmes *et al.*, 1987), her aphasia type was conduction aphasia. Although she herself reported some paraphasias in her speech, especially immediately after the operation, they were not present in the data. It was characteristic for PK that she often used non-verbal behaviour and gesturing during her word searches. PK's scores at the time of data collection in the WAB-test are shown in Table 9.1.

Table 9.1   PK's scores in Western Aphasia Battery (Finnish version)

AQ Max. *100*	*Spont. Speech* *Max. 20*	*Comprehension* *Max. 10*	*Repetition* *Max. 10*	*Naming* *Max. 10*	*LQ Max.* *100*
69.5	17	7.05	6.8	3.9	71.6

AQ = aphasia quotient; LQ = language quotient.

Data

The data of this study is based on two videotaped conversations, consisting of a total of 80 minutes. The first conversation (59 minutes) was videotaped at PK's home, and the participants were PK, her husband and the second author (L.A.). The other conversation (21 minutes) took place at the Department of Speech Sciences at the University of Helsinki and the participants were PK and the first author (A.K.). The word searches with prominent non-verbal behaviour were then identified and transcribed according to the conventions of conversation analysis. This chapter presents a collection of the different types of word searches accompanied by gestures or other types of non-verbal behaviour.

Analysis

The excerpts were analysed according to the method of conversation analysis (see for instance Goodwin & Heritage, 1990). This approach is based on the following principles: analysis is participant-driven; conversation is orderly; sequential context is important; and quantifications are troublesome (Wilkinson, 1999; see also e.g. Klippi, 1996). In this study, the analysis focuses on the sequential development of the process of word searching. As our knowledge of non-verbal behaviour in aphasia is rather limited, our approach is qualitative. Furthermore, the present analysis has been conducted from the point of view of interaction, that is, how the person with aphasia proceeds in her turn in the case of a word-finding problem and how her addressee reacts and contributes to conversation in the next turn(s). Of particular interest are prospective indexicals preceding the target word.

Completed Word Searches with Self-Repairs

Our first example shows how PK searches for a word, and she is able to find it by herself. Transcription conventions are given in Appendix 1 and the key to glossing is given in Appendix 2 (see Figure 9.1).

Example 1: Neck

```
              T_____,,,forward_____
              points to T              sratches head
01 PK:*ja sit mul+on* *(0.7)ainaki s-tämmönen(1.2)*
       and then   I-ADE is              at least   like this
```
and then I have   **(0.7) at least s- I have this kind of**

```
              ___,,,T_____
              touches neck
02        *mulla on tää(0.5)NISka*
            I-ADE is this          neck
```
I have this   **(0.5) Neck**

```
03        (1.0)

04 T:  joo
```
yeah

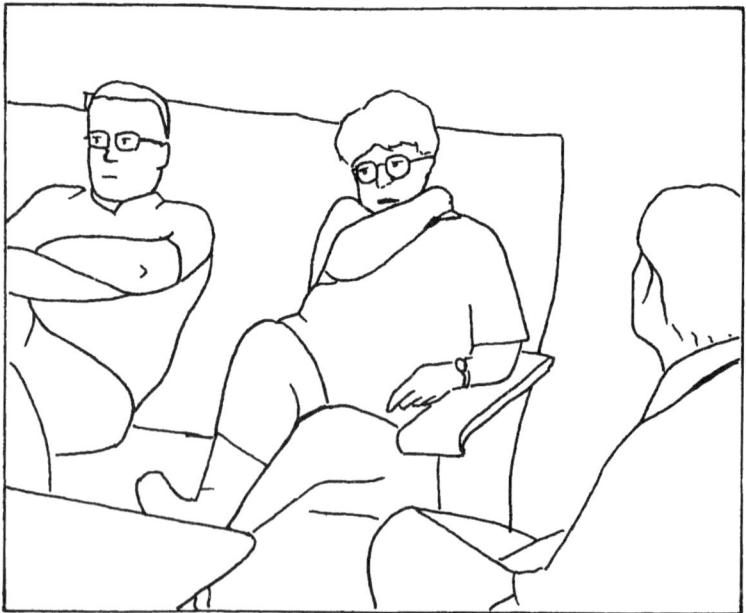

Figure 9.1

In this example, PK tells about her speech and the problems she thinks to be related to the fluency of her speech. Her impression is that her tiredness and the pain in her neck are related to her speech fluency. At the beginning of her turn, she simultaneously points to the addressee and begins to talk about the pain. However, she is unable to continue and she stops and moves her right hand to her head and scratches it while uttering '(0.7) at least s- I have this kind of *(tämmönen) (1.2)*'. Then she brings her hand to her neck and at the same time she continues by stating 'I have this *(tää) (0.5)*'. The constructions that she produces are noun phrase–constructions. According to Hakulinen *et al.* (2004), the demonstrative pronouns *tämmönen* 'this kind of' and *tämä* 'this' are used to refer to something that is near or about which the speaker is talking. *Tämmönen* is a pro-adjective, which refers to the quality or to the characteristics of the referent, but a while later PK corrects it to the *tämä*-pronoun, which indicates, however, that she is searching for a noun. During her word-search, she moves her hand from her head to her neck in order to show the localisation of the problem. This touching seems to facilitate the word finding, because by the end of her turn, she manages to find the word *niska* 'a neck' and turns her gaze back to the addressee. This example, although it is a shorter one, resembles the example presented by Helasvuo *et al.* (2004). In our example, speaker PK finds the target word while simultaneously using the touching gesture, whereas in the case presented by Helasvuo *et al.*, the speaker makes the gesture (grabs the left sleeve of her shirt) for the first time in silence and only during the second time does she manage to produce the gesture simultaneously with the verbal expression (grabs her left sleeve and says 'blouse had been made/put') (see Figure 9.2).

Example 2: Tumor

```
                              ...T_____
                           touches head           cups her hand upwards
01 PK : mu|lt ote|tt|i|i tuo|lta*(0.9) keske|ltä**niinkun (0.9) [valta]va-
        I-ABL  take-PASS-PST  that-ABL   middle-ABL   PRT           enormous
        they took from me         (0.9)  from the middle so to say like an enormous

02 H :                                                          [nii]
                                                                PRT
                                                                yeah
                            _____ ,,,forward ...T___
03 PK : valtava|n iso tuota tämmönen (0.8) kasvi*
        enormous-GEN big  PRT   like this        plant
        enormous big like this       (0.8)  tumor

04 H :=nii eli hän|hän tul|i si|itä kasvi[leikkaukse|sta]
       PRT  or  she-CLI come-PST it-ELA  plant operation-ELA
       yeah she came from  that tumor operation

05 T:                                    [ai se tul|i sellase|s]ta
                                          oh it come-PST  like that-ELA
                                          oh I see, she came from that kind of thing
```

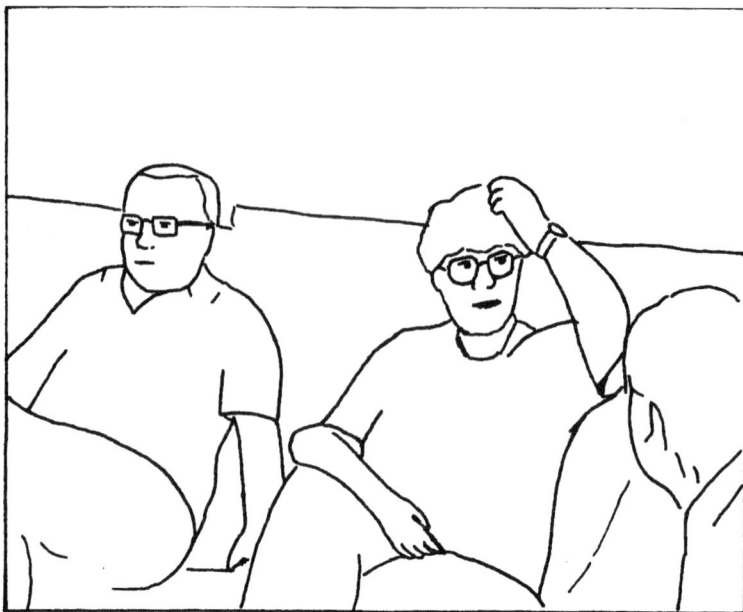

Figure 9.2

In the second example, speaker PK describes the brain tumor she had. A number of prospective indexicals occur in this example, and they reveal the word-finding problem itself. In addition, these indexicals reflect the repair process during her search. Speaker PK begins to talk about her illness and on line 1, she explains *mult otettiin tuolta* 'They took from me from there' but at that moment, she has to stop. The following pause signals the beginning of the repair process and at that time, her face shows what is referred to as the 'thinking face' (Goodwin & Goodwin, 1986) and she gazes very intensively in front of her, which evidently manifests her wish to keep the turn. At the same time, she begins to move her left hand towards her head and she touches her head. The proadverbial *tuolta* (that + ablative) she refers to the location, which usually is not in the immediate area (Hakulinen *et al.*, 2004). In this case it refers to a body part which is out of the speaker's range of vision. This touching gesture during the pause seems to facilitate her speech problem at least to some extent, because she manages to produce the construction 'from the middle', which gives further knowledge about the localisation of the referent, and at the same time, she shifts her gaze back to the addressee.

It is possible that her first gesture only partly facilitates her verbal expression because she produces the filling phrase *niinkun* 'so to say', which is regarded as a planning particle in Finnish (Hakulinen *et al.*, 2004). Thus by using *niinkun*, PK signals that her word search continues and she begins to remodel her hand posture. She then explains *valtavan iso tuota tämmönen* and all the while she not only touches her head, but she begins to cup her hand against the left side of her head. From the pronouns, *tuota tämmönen*, the first being a planning particle and the second, a pro-adjective, one can infer that she has moved from talking about the place to the quality of the referent. The gesture and the pronouns she used can be regarded as prospective indexicals because they provide important information to the interlocutor – not only where the problem has been, but also information about the form of the problem, and even maybe about the size of the problem. At this point, the target word has probably become obvious for the interlocutors, because her husband, the knowing participant, gives a short response with the *nii*–particle. However, the speaker continues her explanation 'like an enormous big like that', keeping her hand on her head. After the filling words and a short pause, she succeeds to produce the word 'tumour'. At this point, she brings her gaze back to the addressee.

Probably, because the search has been rather complicated, her husband wants to rephrase the previous turn and on line 4, he begins his explanation by using the particle combination *nii eli*. The nii–particle is used in Finnish as an alignment with the previous turn but *nii eli* is used as an initiation of a clarification after a problematic turn (Sorjonen, 2001). Furthermore, LA's reaction to this explanation begins with the particle *ai*, which typically is used in Finnish as an index for a new piece of information (Sorjonen, 2001).

Speaker PK's gestures – the touching and iconic figuring of her tumour – are parts of her successful word search process. The example shows how she first manages to localise the referent with the help of the pro-adverb and the touching gesture. After a while, she remodels her hand posture as an iconic gesture and at the same time she talks about the size of the referent, and by doing so, the participants are able to receive information about the size and the figure of the referent. Her gestures during the word search reveal that she has semantic knowledge about the referent and this slowly growing semantic knowledge evidently helps her in word finding (see Figure 9.3).

In Example 3, the speaker talks about her hobby, playing tennis, and about her neck pains due to her playing. During her first utterance, on line 1 *pitää katsoo näin* 'one must look like this' she already assumes a pantomimic position as if she were playing tennis while she looks at the addressee. She thus leans forward and hunches her shoulders up, both hands stretched forward, as if she is holding a racket in her hand. Her body position resembles a tennis player who is waiting for a serve. Her verbal utterance on line 1 is structurally vague and elliptic, as she only refers to

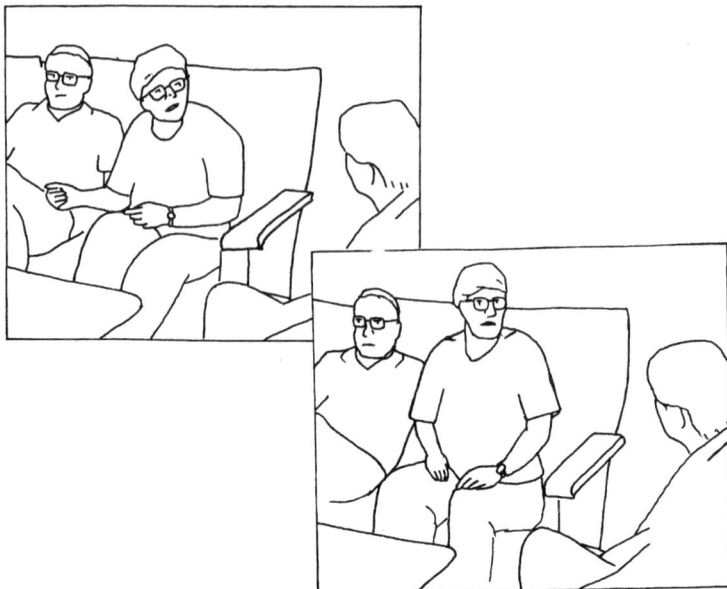

Figure 9.3

Example 3: Tennis

```
       T _____
         leans forward "with a tennis racket" in her hands
01 PK :*kato ku se tennis pitä|ä katso|o näin (0.7)*
        look  as it  tennis  must  look-INF like this
        look, as the tennis has to look like this

02 T: nii joo to[siaan]
      PRT yes  indeed
      yeah yes really

03 H :              [°(-)] [pallo°]
                           ball

                          looks forward, straightens her posture
04 PK :          [*se pitä|ä] (0.4) joo ku si|tä ei (0.4)*
                  it  must          yes  as it-PAR not
                  one must    (0.4)     yes, when one does not

05 T: joo (1.1)
      yes

       T_____
         sits with straight posture      raises her shoulders
06 PK :*pitä|s ol| ain**(.)  mu|n pitäs ol|la aina suora (0.6)*
        must-CON be(-INF) always  I-GEN must-CON be-INF always straight
        should be always   (.) I should always have good posture

07 T: joo
      yes
```

her pantomimic body position with the word *näin* 'like this'. The pronoun *näin* is a pro-adverbial and it refers to the habit of doing something. It is easy to understand that this kind of position can increase the muscle tension in her neck. She then continues her explanation on line 4 'one must' but stops her utterance and apparently tries to find the construction and the right words. Then she places her hands in her lap and she straightens her posture. From her hand position and posture, one can infer that she has changed her topic to a more general one. Her utterance 'yes, when one does not' is again very elliptic, and on line 6, she assumes an even more erect posture, raising her shoulders and producing the passive construction 'one must alw-', but she stops again. Finally, maintaining her position, she changes her verbal utterance from a passive to active construction and she utters 'I should always have good posture', which seems to be a satisfactory utterance.

In this example, speaker PK begins with very elliptic utterances and ends after several verbal self-corrections to state that she 'should always have good posture (should be straight)'. In this excerpt, her body posture changes three times: the first posture is pantomimic, the second is more related to her bearing and the third is an even more exaggerated bearing. It is interesting that from the first utterance, her verbal and non-verbal behaviour are parallel and clearly complement each other. This observation is in line with Kendon's (2000: 61) notion that gesture and speech are in partnership and gesture can be used 'as a way of exhibiting overarching units of meaning, as a way of keeping visible an aspect of meaning throughout the course of spoken utterance or even after the speech has finished'. In this excerpt, PK's body positions are very expressive and they can actually reveal many aspects which are complicated or even impossible to express exactly only through verbal means. Finally, she was also able to complete her verbal utterance.

In these three cases PK was able to produce the target word after the search. All these examples contained several of her verbal self-repairs combined with non-verbal behaviour, and she was able to complete the repair processes herself. Her gestures reveal that a speaker with aphasia has different types of knowledge about the target word. The first search (*Neck*) focused on a body part, and she could complete the search by using a touching gesture. It is possible that the kinaesthetic and the sensory feedback of the gesture helped her to find the word 'neck'. The second example (*Tumour*) shows how P illustrated the concrete referent, the tumor, which she had. She managed to offer several prospective indexicals of the referent (place, shape and even size), before she found the target word. The third example (*Tennis*) is also related to a concrete referent (postures) that could be made visible through body movements. In this example, her non-verbal and verbal expressions were closely tied together and they presented together a more complete version of the meaning than either of them could accomplish on its own.

PK used a specific strategy to progress in her word searches. The picture is clear: when she has a word-finding problem, PK relies on the process of self-repair and then begins the word search. This is in accordance with the earlier findings of everyday conversation (Schegloff *et al.*, 1977) and with conversation with persons with aphasia of Laakso (1997), who have displayed the preference of self-repair in problem turn. During the repair, the speaker recruits prospective verbal and non-verbal indexicals that reveal the one-line process of the word search. We may draw a conclusion that in these cases, the non-verbal behaviour facilitates word finding.

Collaborative Word Searches

Our data contains several examples where PK could not complete the word search on her own, although she was able to give prospective verbal and non-verbal indexicals. In the next section we will select examples from these word searches where PK's self-repair initiations did not end successfully and thereby the search became a collaborative action between the participants (see Figure 9.4).

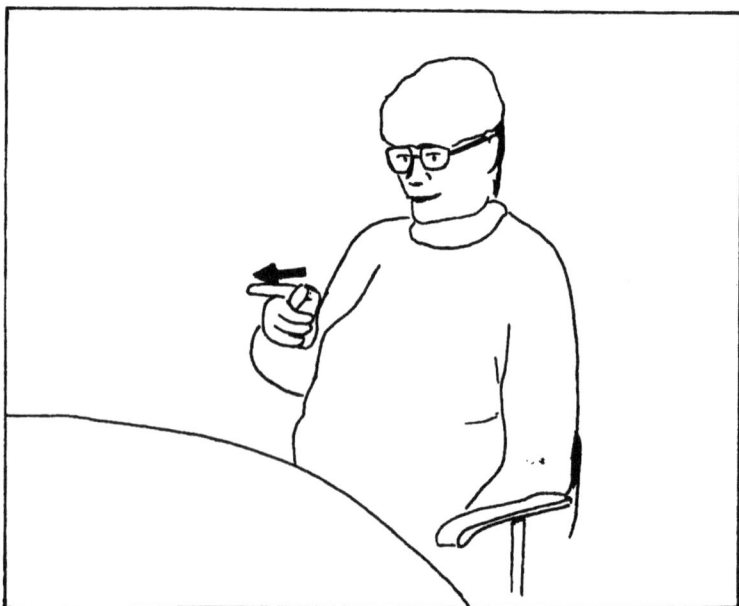

Figure 9.4

Example 4: The Round Tower

```
01 T: käytii  pyöreessä  tornissa  syömässä  ja=
      go-PAS-PST round-INE   tower-INE  eat-INE    and
```
we ate in the Round Tower and=

.
.
.

```
          T_____
          points emphatically to T
02 PK:*käytii justii siinä (0.9)*
      go- PAS-PST just     there
```
we visited just there (0.9)

```
03 T: jo[o]
      ye[ah]
```

```
          T_____
          points emphatically to T
04 PK:  [#]*>MISsä sä kävit just<*
        where-INE you  go-PST-2 just
```
where did you just visit

05 (0.6)

```
06 T: pyöree (0.3) pyö[ree] torni
      round        round    tower
```
round (0.3)   the Round Tower

```
                    T___
                    nod
07 PK:              [joo]
```
                    yeah

The topic of the fourth example is PK's town of birth, Viipuri. Both interlocutors had visited there recently, but separately. The other party (A.K.) has stated earlier in the conversation that she had lunch in a well known place in Viipuri, at *Pyöreä torni* (the Round Tower), which dates back to the 14th century. This excerpt presents PK's recollection of her visit to Viipuri. When she mentions on line 1 that she also visited *siinä* 'there', she points at the addressee and looks straight at her. This demonstrative pronoun refers to a place and probably to something that is mentioned earlier because she keeps her gaze directed to her addressee. It is evident that she cannot find the word she is looking for and she has to stop. The addressee then gives a short discourse particle *joo*, which in Finnish implies understanding and accepting the previous utterance (Sorjonen, 1999). PK continues by slightly overlapping this response and by continuing with a 'where did you just visit', pointing emphatically to the addressee.

This utterance can be regarded as being a repair initiation, because the question word *missä* 'where' refers clearly to a place and it is expressed parallel to the pointing gesture and to the personal pronoun *sinä* 'you'. For these reasons, one can interpret that she refers anaphorically to the earlier conversation as well as to something that has happened to the addressee. The intensity of her gaze and the pointing gesture give the impression of a strong orientation to interaction with the addressee (Bavelas *et al.*, 1992) and, in addition, she emphasizes the first syllable of the word *MISsä*, and slightly moves her forefinger back and forth, as if to stress the word *missä* from the point of view of the repair. The addressee clearly interprets her behaviour as an indirect request for help because she offers a candidate understanding (other-initiated repair) of what the speaker has been seeking. The place in Viipuri, *Pyöreä torni*, turned out to be the target word PK was searching for, because she confirms it with *joo* 'yes' and by nodding.

In this instance, the pointing gesture with the forefinger seemed to carry a double function. It was evidently directed to the addressee, but the verbal content of PK's utterances also connected the pointing gestures to the previous conversation, that is, to the addressee's visit in the same town and to the same place. Thus, the addressee served as a knowing co-participant, and it gave PK the opportunity to use her as an additional resource in the conversation.

The next example is taken from a longer excerpt where PK looks at a picture of milking and talks about it (Figure 9.5).

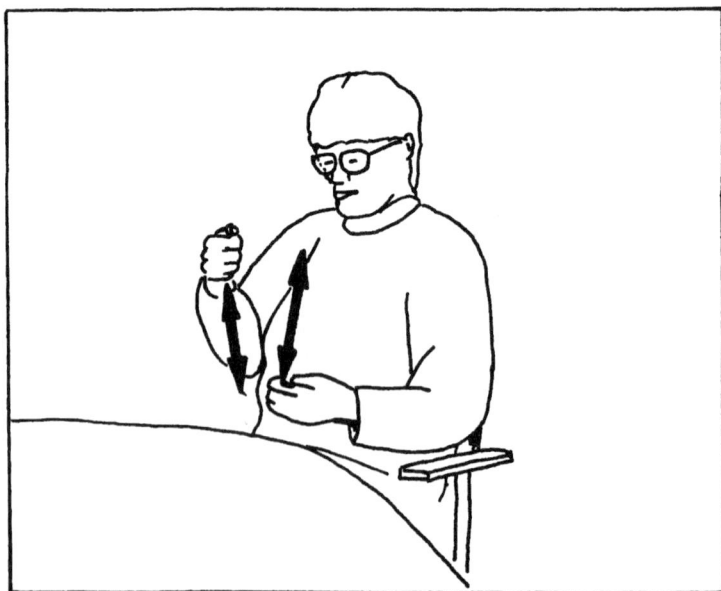

Figure 9.5

Example 5: Milking

```
            looks at paper
01 PK :  ja hän  (0.7)  alka|a  (0.7)  alka|a totanoin ##(3.0)alka|a(1.2)
         and he         begin         begin    PRT                 begin
         and she  (0.7)  begins  (0.7)  begins like                begins

                                                        ...T_____
            'milks'
02     :  mitä se *tsss tsss tsss*  (0.6)  [$mitä se tek-$  (he he)]  $ne
          what it                          what   it                  they
          what does she  tsss tsss tsss (0.6)   what is she doi-
they

03 T:                                      [$just joo$  (he he he)]
                                            PRT   yes
                                            yes yes

              T_____
04 PK:    teh|dä|än$  (he he)
          do-PAS
          do

05 T: lyp-  (0.6)
      mil-

              _T_____   ,,,paper
                              writes down
06 PK :  lypsä-  (0.6)  *lypsä-  (0.6)  [joo]  (0.8)  lyps-  (0.5)*
         milk           milk           yes           milk
         milk           milk           yes           mil-

07 T:                                   [lypsä|ä]
                                         milk

          paper_____
          nods
08 PK :*lypsä|ä maito|a*
        milk        milk-PAR
        milks milk (from the cow)
```

In line 1, PK refers to a person in the picture and begins to describe what the person is doing in the picture. However, she is unable to find the proper verb and she begins the self-repair with the particles *tota*+noin, typically used as planning particles in Finnish (Hakulinen *et al.*, 2004). In order to keep her turn, she produces several prospective indexicals, one after another, such as pauses and repetitive words. Since the self-repair does not progress, and she is still unable to produce the target word, she changes her strategy. As we see in line 2, she formulates a wh-question 'what does it' and after that, she begins to gesture. She pantomimes milking with both hands and she simultaneously produces onomato-poetic vocal effects *tsss tss tss* which is the sound that milk from a cow makes when it hits the bucket. After that she rephrases her *wh-* question, asks with a smiling voice 'what does he do', and then she begins to laugh. During her laughter she turns her gaze to the addressee. Furthermore, she makes a self-repair once again and changes the end of the question phrase into the elliptic passive construction '(What) they do'.

The addressee evidently understands the meaning of the gesturing and of the vocalising since she laughs and provides her understanding already during the gesture 'yes yes he he he' (line 3). In addition, the addressee reacts to the question and gives the first syllable of the target verb *lyp-* 'to milk'. This clearly helps PK to process the word as she begins to articulate the verb *lypsä-*, although she is unable to produce it completely. PK even writes the verb on a piece of paper and repeats the word but it nevertheless remains incomplete. At this point, the addressee makes a direct other-repair and gives the whole word *lypsää* and the aphasic speaker nods and repeats the verb adding the word *maitoa* 'milk' to her utterance.

This example shows that PK was unable to complete the word search every time on her own. She began the word search but was not able to complete it alone. However, she could make the action of milking visible to the addressee. This gesturing revealed that she had semantic knowledge of the milking action. She could even associate the sound of milking to the gesturing and produced the onomatopoetic vocal effects that served as prospective indexicals about the searched word to the addressee. In addition, the aphasic speaker turned her gaze to the addressee and formulated a request for help. This is an explicit way (and perhaps one of the most frequent ways) to make the word search a collaborative activity and thereby to involve the interlocutor in the word search (Laakso & Klippi, 1999; Laakso & Lehtola, 2003) (Figure 9.6).

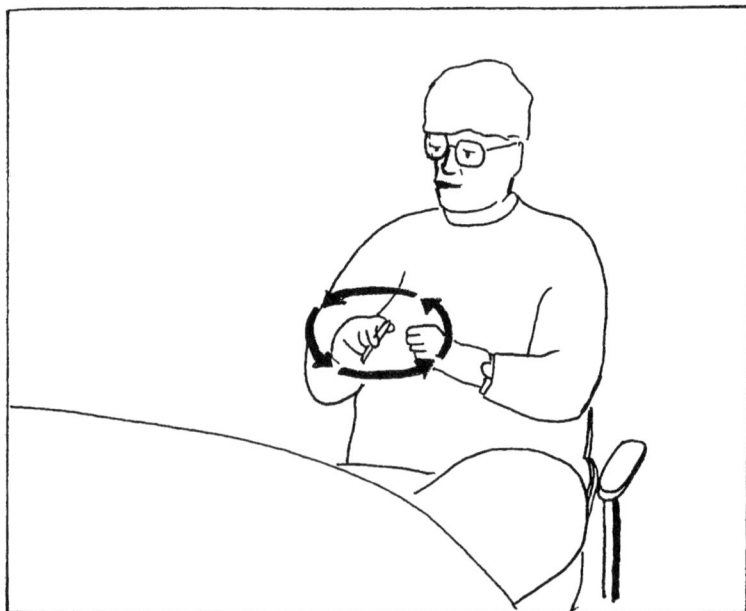

Figure 9.6

Example 6: Ice Auger

```
             looks at paper, hand in front of the mouth
01 PK:*ja sitten hän tarvitse|e se|n*(1.6)##mikä#(1.0)°mikä|s se|n
        and then  he  need    it-ACC      what        what-CLI  it-GEN
        and then he needs it        (1.6) what      (1.0) what's

02   : nimi on kun° (3.0) °kun° (0.7) °kun° (0.5) joudu|ta|an se
        name be  as          as         as        must-PAS   it
        the name as    (3.0) as    (0.7) as (0.5)  one must it

        paper _____
03   : (3.8) jää|ssä on (2.7)°si|in on jää° (0.6) ai kamala (0.4)
             ice-INE be      it-INE be ice        oh awful
             it is in the ice   (2.7) it is ice      (0.6) oh awful

04 T: m:m (.)

        looks at paper_____,,,T2_____
        hand in front of the mouth                   'drills'
05 PK:*jää|ssä on totanoin (2.9) ni TÄYty|y se**(1.6) °ra-° (0.3)*
        ice-INE be  PRT          PRT  must   it
        it is in the ice  like like (2.9) one must it   (1.6)  ?-

        looks down, scratches head
06   :*°mikä tää nyt on (0.6)*
        what  this now be
        what's this

07 T: just joo (1.0)
        PRT  yes
        yeah yes

        looks down            looks at paper
        scratches head        'holds auger'
08 PK:*°tää tää° (0.8)**ei rit- rinkka mutta ra-* (1.2) °mikä tää nyt
        this this        not      backpack but          what  this now
        this this  (0.8)  no ba- backpack but    ?-      what's this

09   ol|i° se (0.7) no häne|n täyty|y (0.8) saa|da se (0.7) ÄH (2.1)
        be-PST it       PRT he-GEN must        get-INF it       OH
        it was  (0.7) well he must        (0.8) get it  (0.7)  OH

10   : HVOI hyvä ihme (0.9)
        PRT  good wonder
        OH  good heaven

11 T: joo sä näyt|i|t se|n jo (0.4) mu|l+on (0.6) ilmein-(0.5)nyt mä
        yes you show-PST-2 it-ACC already I-ADE be        obv-    now
        yes you showed it already  (0.4) I have (0.6) obv- (0.5) now I

      (0.6) mu|l+on käsitys jo mikä si|inä [on itseasiassa]
            I-ADE be  idea     already what  it-INE be  in fact
            I already got an idea what's there
                                        _T_____
                                        'drills'
13 PK:                                  [*niin (0.7) mikä] (0.4)
                                          PRT         what
                                          yes         what

14    _____
      mikä se|n nimi [nyt] sitten on|ka tämä|n juuri (0.9)*
      what  it-GEN name now  then  be-CLI this-GEN PRT
      what's the name of this one

15 T:                  [joo]
                        yes
16 T: kai- (0.8)
      aug-

      _T___
      nods
17 PK :*kaira*
       auger
```

Example 6 resembles the previous one. The aphasic speaker wishes to talk about a man who drills and she begins to explain 'and then he needs it' but then stops for 1.6 seconds and looks at the paper on the table. She is clearly in trouble because she looks forward and produces the question word 'what' and after a pause with a low voice, 'what is the name as'. She repeats the *kun* 'as' particle a couple of times, which clearly displays that she is having trouble continuing. Next, she tries to make a new start by stating: 'one must (3.8) it is in the ice (2.7) it is ice (0.6)' and at last she utters 'oh awful'. After the addressee's short feedback *mm* with a rising pitch, PK continues 'it is in the ice (2.9) one must it (1.6) °*ra*-°'. As the verbal self-repairs do not lead to the target word, she resorts to gesturing in the search process. During the 1.6 seconds pause, she begins to pretend to be drilling and uses both hands to make iconic gesturing. It is interesting that gesturing seems to evoke some phonological knowledge about the target word because she turns her gaze to the addressee and utters *ra-* in a low voice. The produced syllable is not, however, the beginning of the target word and she stops but continues with the often heard phrase that is used for word searches: 'what is that'. Probably because the gesture of drilling has been very illustrative, the addressee gives feedback of understanding, uttering 'yeah, yeah'.

Although one could expect that this would do for the aphasic speaker, PK clearly wants to produce the target word aloud and so she continues in her word search. She looks down, scratches her head and mumbles 'this this' with a low voice. Then she puts her hands again in a drilling position and begins to speak with the excluding strategy *ei rit- rinkka mutta ra-* 'not ba- backpack but *ra-* ' and again she has to stop. This follows a search questions, 'what was it now (0.7) well he has to (0.8) to get it (0.7) OH (2.1) Oh God'. At that point, the addressee takes the turn and makes explicit that she understands the target word. PK still begins to show the drilling action and when looking at the addressee, she formulates a question by asking 'what is the name of this' and the addressee thereby provides her with the first syllable of the target word *kai-* (*kaira*, 'ice auger'). PK nods and expresses *kaira* 'ice auger'.

This excerpt features a very long and laborious word search. This passage reveals in detail how PK tried to approach the target word, first by using a general word *se* 'it', then by asking a question. First, she focused on herself as she looked down and spoke in a mumbling voice. After that, she began to expand her explanation by telling more about the circumstances of drilling and referred to ice. As none of these strategies led to the target word, she resorted to gesturing and her gesturing was so vivid that the interlocutor seemed to get the idea of drilling easily. An important notion is that gesturing evidently activated the phonological processing of the target word because PK was able to produce the last syllable of the target word. However, this was not enough for producing the whole word and at last, she had to repeat her request for help, this time by turning her gaze to the interlocutor. Through these phases, PK's word search became a collaborative activity. Word-finding became possible as PK could use gestures to express the action of drilling to the interlocutor, who for her part could give PK the needed phonological hint. Thus, PK was able to produce the name of the device needed for drilling.

In the two previous excerpts, the word searches became a collaborative action which promoted mutual understanding between the participants. In these cases, PK actively took the interlocutor as a collaborator and the word search proceeded as a mutual activity.

Discussion

We have examined how a person with aphasia conducts word searches in a conversational context with special emphasis on the use of non-verbal behaviour. The analysis aimed to illuminate and to discuss the interplay between verbal and non-verbal processes during word searches and the interactive behaviour during the word search between the person with aphasia and the interlocutor(s). The analysis has been undertaken from the point of view of repair organisation, and we have investigated these searches through the prospective indexicals, visible and auditory signs, which occur during the search process (Goodwin & Goodwin, 1986; Hayashi, 2003). We argue that various visible and auditory signs can reveal the ongoing process of the search, and some of them refer proactively to the unavailable item, giving knowledge of the searched object or action. With the help of the examples we have demonstrated that when the speaker did not succeed with word searching herself, the process could be developed collaboratively with the co-participant. The problem-indicating signs of speech, pauses, repetitions, pronouns, changing gaze orientation and mobilising gestures mutually build the context and provide resources for the next speaker to begin the collaboration.

The analysis reveals several systematic practices used by a person with aphasia and the interlocutor(s) during word searches. We will first give a summary of the sequential development of the word search. Our data show that there is a surprisingly similar pattern in the word searches of the aphasic person studied. This process can be divided into three different phases:

Phase 1: Primarily, the aphasic speaker aims to solve the word search with her verbal resources. If the speaker does not have access to the target word, the process of self-repair begins (Laakso, 1997) and by doing that, the speaker accomplishes the social organization of the conversation in the same way as ordinary speakers (Goodwin & Goodwin, 1986; Schegloff *et al.*, 1977). This process can be seen and heard by the interlocutor. Typically the speaker turns her gaze from the interlocutor and produces hesitations, repetitions and pauses. This observation confirms the result of Laakso (1997) and Laakso and Lehtola (2003). If the search cannot be completed in the first phase, the speaker enters the second phase.

Phase 2: If the verbal resources are insufficient for word finding, gestures and other non-verbal and even vocal behaviours are recruited in the word search. By these means the process of self-repair continues. For instance, the analysis showed that speaker PK used several different kinds of prospective indexicals to describe some relevant features of the target. A prospective indexical could therefore be a touch that shows the place of the referent, for example, her head or neck. It could also be an iconic gesture that illustrated the shape and perhaps even the size of the referent. Furthermore, the speaker showed the use of an object or action during the word search. These pantomimic gestures, which illustrated activities, were used when she searched for a verb, for instance, milking. In the case of a noun search (e.g. an ice auger), she used a pantomimic gesture to illustrate the use of it. Deictic gestures were used to show, for example, a point of a compass, but she also used deictic gesture anaphorically, to refer to the proper noun uttered earlier (*Pyöreä torni*). Even vocal effects could be combined with gesturing. In addition, demonstrative pronouns, such as pro-adjectives and pro-adverbs, were used during her word search. They could also serve as prospective indexicals, which provide some proactive knowledge about the searched word (Hayashi, 2003; Helasvuo *et al.*, 2004). Planning particles were also frequently used, but they gave no other information other than that the search was going on. During phase two, the speaker typically kept her gaze away from the addressee. If the search could not be completed in the second phase, the speaker entered the third phase.

In phases one and two, the verbal and non-verbal behaviours may serve as facilitators for the word search of the speaker her/himself. In addition, they serve as public practices, prospective indexicals, of the development of the search (Goodwin, 1996; Hayashi, 2003), and they may give hints of the target word for the interlocutor. Sometimes the target word also becomes evident for the interlocutor(s), even though the speaker cannot produce the word itself.

Phase 3: If the speaker could not find the target word through using non-verbal and/or vocal resources, she tried to recruit the addressee in her word search. This person with aphasia then invited the interlocutor directly or indirectly to take part in the repair. In these cases, PK typically turned her orientation and her gaze back to the interlocutor. If this was not enough to get a reaction from the interlocutor, she requested help by asking search questions such as 'What is it called?' or 'What is that?' This behaviour was also reported in the study by Laakso and Lehtola (2003). Sometimes the searched word had already been expressed earlier in the conversation and PK referred anaphorically to the earlier conversation (e.g. *Pyöreä torni*) and to the shared knowledge of the interlocutors to ask for help. This behaviour thus made the repair an interactive process. These collaborative word searches are often extended over several speaking turns of the different speakers, and they can sometimes take the form of the so-called 'hint and guess' sequences (see e.g. Laakso & Klippi, 1999; Oelschlager & Damico, 2000; Klippi, 2003). In short, collaborative word searches promote the view of conversation as an interactive process where participants orient to the ongoing verbal and bodily communicative activities.

The findings of this study confirm the results of the previous studies of aphasic word search (Laakso, 1997; Laakso & Klippi, 1999; Laakso & Lehtola, 2003; Helasvuo *et al.*, 2004), although in these studies, non-verbal behaviour has not been the main focus as it has in this study. As our study is a case study, it is not possible to generalise our results to the larger population of aphasic persons. It could be that the pattern we found related to non-verbal behaviour is typical only for the person in this study. We acknowledge that other people with aphasia may use other patterns or strategies to overcome their word-finding problems. On the other hand, some excerpts of prolonged word searches displayed in earlier studies (e.g. Laakso & Klippi, 1999; Laakso & Lehtola, 2003; Helasvuo *et al.*, 2004) seem to follow the sequential pattern observed in this study.

Non-verbal behaviour is an activity with distinctive temporal, spatial, and social properties that may have numerous different functions in talk-in-interaction. It is well known that non-verbal behaviour such as gaze direction and sometimes body and hand movements are closely related to both turn allocation activity (Goodwin, 1981) and to the flow of speech (Bavelas *et al.*, 1992; McNeill, 2000). Very little has been known about the role of non-verbal behaviour related to aphasic speech problems, for example, word searches, until the present study. In our study, the speaker with aphasia used systematically different types of non-verbal behaviour when encountering word-finding problems. Her gestures were often iconic and pantomimic, and they revealed that the speaker conceptually had the idea of the referent. Thus, one can infer that in the case of PK, the problem was primarily in her access to the phonological representations of words, or in the phonological processing itself (Lesser, 1989). It is interesting that sometimes PK produced some phonological knowledge of the word, for instance, in the example of the ice auger, but the speech processing was so slow that she was not able to complete the search herself.

Our theoretical understanding about the social organisation of language use is still rather limited in comparison to our knowledge about speech and language processing in speech language pathology. In addition, within neurolinguistics and aphasiology, the idea of modularity and accordingly, the idea of autonomous verbal processes, has been very influential (e.g. Fodor, 1983). For instance, a long-lasting trend in the literature has been to focus primarily on the process of speech and language production and verbal expression. This approach has ignored the bodily perspective and the interactive nature of human communication. On the other hand, the study of language evolution has long been interested in the gestural theory of language (e.g. Corballis, 2003). Furthermore, it is also known that in children's speech and language development, pointing gestures precede words (Capone & McGregor, 2004) and that children's expressions are bodily very comprehensive, too. In fact, there are therapy methods of manual signing and gestural activation in children with known high risks of delayed and deviant communication and speech development (e.g. Down syndrome, autism and specific language impairment) (e.g. Launonen, 1998). From the point of view of speech pathology, it is relevant to further specify the relationship between speech and gesture production systems. For the theoretical development of speech and language pathology, we also need interactive models for speech and gesture production.

Speech and language therapy aims to improve speech, language and the general communicative capacity of people with different types of communication problems. However, it is often neglected that language usage is an interactive process where participants orient and collaborate with each other. Especially if we aim to develop the pragmatic skills of our clients, we have to understand the meaningfulness of non-verbal behaviour in interaction.

The role of non-verbal behaviour in aphasia therapy has been controversial. We have examples of aphasia therapy which completely neglect non-verbal behaviour. One of the interesting examples of this tradition is an article written by Pulvermüller *et al.* (2001). This study presented a comparison of the effectiveness of two aphasia therapy methods in the treatment of chronically aphasic persons. One method was called 'constrained-induced' (CI) aphasia therapy to speech, in which non-verbal behaviour was to be suppressed in favour of verbal communication. The other method was 'conventional aphasia therapy'. The result was that CI therapy was more effective when compared to conventional aphasia therapy. However, it was not possible to answer what was the influential mechanism behind the therapy, because the therapies were administered at a different rate in such a way that the conventional aphasia therapy was stretched over a longer period. By contrast, we do have some interventions that favour the use of non-verbal behaviour in connection with verbal expression (e.g. Holland, 1991; Kagan, 1998). Some recent studies, for example, Rose *et al.* (2002) reported that iconic gestures significantly facilitate object naming in aphasic persons. In addition, Rose and Douglas (2001) found that aphasic speakers, apart from those with apraxia, are able to produce meaningful gestures in conversation and they could also compensate for their verbal expression with gestures.

Returning to our starting point: non-verbal behaviour is actively used in the organisation of interaction. Goodwin and Goodwin (1986: 72) have stated: '... while the activity can provide sense of the gesture, that relationship is reflexive; the gesture can provide detailed information about the current organization of activity'. In conclusion, if we are willing to open our eyes to consider this relationship, we will learn much more about human communicative and interactive behaviour than by ignoring it.

Acknowledgements

This study has been financially supported by the Research Council for Culture and Society of the Academy of Finland (project number 204625).

References

Ahlsén, E. (1985) *Discourse Patterns in Aphasia*. Gothenburg Monographs in Linguistics 5. University of Göteborg. Department of Linguistics.

Ahlsén, E. (1991) Body communication as compensation for speech in a Wernicke's aphasic – A longitudinal study. *Journal of Communication Disorders* 24, 1–12.

Bavelas, J.B., Chovil, N., Lawrie, D.A. and Wade, A. (1992) Interactive gestures. *Discource Processes* 15, 469–489.

Capone, N. and McGregor, K. (2004) Gesture development: A review for clinical and research practices. *Journal of Speech, Language and Hearing Research* 47 (1), 173–186.

Corballis, M.C. (2003) From hand to mouth: The gestural origins of language. In M.H. Christianse and S. Kirby (eds) *Language Evolution: The States of the Art* (pp. 201–218). Oxford: Oxford University Press.

Ferguson, A. (1994) The influence of aphasia, familiarity and activity on conversational repair. *Aphasiology* 8, 143–157.

Fex, B. and Månsson, A-C. (1998) The use of gestures as a compensatory strategy in adults with acquired aphasia compared to children with specific language impairment (SLI). *Journal of Neuroliguistics* 11, 191–206.

Feyereisen, P. (1983) Manual activity during speaking in aphasic subjects. *International Journal of Psychology* 18, 545–556.

Feyereisen, P., Barter, M., Goossens, M. and Clerebaut, N. (1988) Gestures and speech in referential communication by aphasic subjects: Channel use and efficiency. *Aphasiology* 2, 21–32.

Fodor, J. (1983) *The Modularity of Mind*. Cambridge MA: MIT Press.

Goodwin, C. (1981) *Conversational Organisation: Interaction between Speakers and Hearers*. New York: Academic Press.

Goodwin, C. (1996) Transparent vision. In E. Ochs, E.A. Schegloff and S.A. Thomson (eds) *Interaction and Grammar* (pp. 370–404). Cambridge: Cambridge University Press.

Goodwin, M.H. and Goodwin, C. (1986) Gesture and coparticipation in the activity of searching for a word. *Semiotica* 62, 51–75.

Goodwin, C. and Heritage, J. (1990) Conversation analysis. *Annual Review of Anthropology* 19, 283–307.

Hadar, U. (1991) Speech-related body movement in aphasia: Period analysis of upper arms and head movement. *Brain and Language* 42, 339–366.

Hadar, U. and Butterworth, B. (1997) Iconic gestures, imagery, and word retrieval in speech. *Semiotica* 115, 147–172.

Hadar, U. and Yadlin-Gedassy, S. (1994) Conceptual and lexical aspects of gesture: Evidence from aphasia. *Journal of Neurolinguistics* 8, 57–65.

Hakulinen, A., Vilkuna, M., Korhonen, R., Koivisto, V., Heinonen T.R. and Alho, I. (2004) *Iso suomen kielioppi [Comprehensive Finnish Grammar]*. Finnish Literature Society. Hämeenlinna: Karisto.

Hanlon, R.E., Brown, J.W. and Gerstman, L.J. (1990) Enhancement of naming in nonfluent aphasia through gesture. *Brain and Language* 38, 298–314.

Hayashi, M. (2003) Language and the body as resources for collaborative action: A study of word searches in Japanese conversation. *Research on Language and Social Interaction* 26 (2), 109–141.

Helasvuo, M-L., Laakso, M. and Sorjonen, M-L. (2004) Searching for words: Syntactic and sequential construction of word search in conversations of Finnish speakers with aphasia. *Research on Language and Social Interaction* 37 (1), 1–37.

Herrmann, M., Koch, U., Johannsen-Horbach, H. and Wallesh, C-W. (1989) Communicative skills in chronic and severe nonfluent aphasia. *Brain and Language* 37, 339–352.

Holland, A. (1991) Pragmatic aspects of intervention in aphasia. *Journal of Neurolinguistics* 6, 197–211.

Kagan, A. (1998) Supported conversation for adults with aphasia: Methods and resources for training conversation partners. *Aphasiology* 12 (9), 816–830.

Kendon, A. (2000) Language and gesture: unity or duality. In D. McNeill (ed.) *Language and Gesture* (pp. 47–63). Cambridge: Cambridge University Press.

Kertesz, A. (1982) *The Western Aphasia Battery*. New York: Grune & Stratton (Finnish version Lehtihalmes, M., Klippi, A. and Lempinen, M., 1987).

Klippi, A. (1996) *Conversation as an Achievement in Aphasics*. Studia Fennica Linguistica 6. Helsinki: Finnish Literature Society.

Klippi, A. (2003) Collaborating in aphasic group conversation: Striving for mutual understanding. In C. Goodwin (ed.) *Conversation and Brain Damage* (pp. 117–143). New York: Oxford University Press.

Laakso, M. (1997) *Self-Initiated Repair by Fluent Aphasic Speakers in Conversation*. Studia Fennica Linguistica 8. Helsinki: Finnish Literature Society.

Laakso, M. (1999) Afaattisten puhujien sananlöytämisvaikeudet keskustelussa (Aphasic speakers' word searches in conversations). *Suomen Logopedis-Foniatrinen Aikakauslehti* 19 (3), 109–123.

Laakso, M. (2003) Collaborative construction of repair in aphasic conversation: An interactive view on the extended speaking turns of Wernicke's aphasics. In C. Goodwin (ed.) *Conversation and Brain Damage* (pp. 163–188). New York: Oxford University Press.

Laakso, M. and Klippi, A. (1999) A closer look at the 'hint and guess' sequences in aphasic conversation. *Aphasiology* 13 (4/5), 345–363.

Laakso, M. and Lehtola, M. (2003) Sanojen hakeminen afaattisen henkilön ja läheisen keskustelussa. (Word searches in conversations between people with aphasia and their spouses). *Puhe ja kieli* 23 (1), 1–24.

Larkins, P. and Webster, E. (1981) The use of gestures in dyads consisting of an aphasic and a nonaphasic adult. In R. Brookshire (ed.) *Clinical Aphasiology Conference Proceedings* (pp. 120–126). Minneapolis: BRK Publishers.

Launonen, K. (1998) *Eleistä sanoihin, viittomista kieleen. Varhaisviittomisohjelman kehittäminen, kokeilu ja pitkäaikaisvaikutukset Downin syndrooma -lapsilla [From Gestures to Words, from Signs to Language. Development, Application, and Long-Term*

Effects of an Early Signing Programme in the Early Intervention of Children with Down Syndrome]. FAMR Research Publications, No. 75. Helsinki: Kehitysvammaliitto ry.

Le May, A., David, R. and Thomas, A. (1988) The use of spontaneous gesture by aphasic patients. *Aphasiology* 2, 137–145.

Lesser, R. (1989) Aphasia: theory based intervention. In M.M. Leahy (ed.) *Disorders of Communication: The Science of Intervention* (pp. 189–205). London: Taylor and Francis.

McNeill, D. (2000) Introduction. In D. McNeill (ed.) *Language and Gesture* (pp. 1–10). Cambridge: Cambridge University Press.

Milroy, L. and Perkins, L. (1992) Repair strategies in aphasic discourse: Towards a collaborative model. *Clinical Linguistics & Phonetics* 6, 27–40.

Nickels, L. (ed.) (2002) Special Issue: Rehabilitation of spoken word production in aphasia. *Aphasiology* 16 (10/11).

Oelschlaeger, M.L. (1999) Participation of a conversation partner in the word searches of a person with aphasia. *American Journal of Speech-Language Pathology* 8, 62–71.

Oelschlaeger, M.L. and Damico, J. (2000) Partnership in conversation: A study of word search strategies. *Journal of Communication Disorders* 33, 205–225.

Pulvermüller, F., Neininger, M.A., Elbert, T., Mohr, B., Rockstroh, B., Koebbel, P. and Taub, E. (2001) Constraint-induced therapy of chronic aphasia after stroke. *Stroke* 32, 1621–1626.

Rauscher, F.H., Krauss, R.M. and Chen, Y. (1996) Gesture, speech and lexical access: The role of lexical movements in speech production. *Psychological Science* 4, 226–231.

Rose, M. and Douglas, J. (2001) The differential facilitatory effects of gesture and visualization processes on object naming in aphasia. *Aphasiology* 15, 977–990.

Rose, M., Douglas, J. and Matyas, T. (2002) The comparative effectiveness of gesture and verbal treatments for a specific phonologic naming impairment. *Aphasiology* 16, 1001–1030.

Schegloff, E., Jefferson, G. and Sacks, H. (1977) The preference of self-correction in the organisation of repair in conversation. *Language* 53, 361–382.

Sorjonen, M-L. (1999) Dialogipartikkelien tehtävistä [On the use of response words]. *Virittäjä* 2, 170–194.

Sorjonen, M-L. (1996) On repeats and responses in Finnish conversations. In E. Ochs, E.A. Schegloff and S.A. Thompson (eds) *Interaction and Grammar.* Cambridge: Cambridge University Press.

Sorjonen, M-L. (2001) *Responding in Conversation.* A study of response particles in Finnish. Amsterdam: Benjamins.

Smith, L. (1987) Nonverbal competency in aphasic stroke patients' conversation. *Aphasiology* 1, 127–139.

Whitehouse, P., Caramazza, A. and Zurif, E. (1978) Naming in aphasia: Interacting effects of form and function. *Brain & Language* 6, 63–74.

Wilkinson, R. (1995) Aphasia: conversation analysis of a non-fluent aphasic person. In M. Perkins and S. Howard (eds) *Case Studies in Clinical Linguistics* (pp. 271–292). London: Whurr.

Wilkinson, R. (1999) Introduction to special issue: Conversation analysis. *Aphasiology* 13, 251–258.

Appendix 1

Key to transcription conventions

Gaze:	T_____
Non-verbal behaviour:	points to T
Original Finnish talk:	01 PK:*ja sit mul+on*
English gloss:	and then I-ADE is
Translation into English:	**and then I have**

Gaze: looking T is noted by marking T_____
Gaze: turning gaze to T is noted by marking ...T
Pauses are given in brackets in seconds (1.3)
Square brackets indicate [over]lapped speech, for example
[speech]
Non-verbal behaviour occurs within stars *   *
Falling intonation is indicated by.
Low voice is indicated by °degree symbols around the relevant words°
Laughing voice is indicated by $dollar symbols around the relevant words$
Cut offs are indicated by a dash, for example: lypsä-
Out breath is indicated by hhh.
Adjacent utterances without a pause between them are indicated by =
Sounds that are stretched are indicated by colons; for example, nii:i
Words uttered together are indicated by +; for example, muistaks+mä
Faster speech occurs between ><

Appendix 2

Principles and abbreviations used in glossing

(modified from Sorjonen, 1996)

In the gloss, morphemes have been separated from the root word with a vertical (|). The following have been treated as unmarked forms, not indicated in the glossing:

- nominative case
- singular
- third person singular (except when there are special reasons for indicating it)
- active voice
- present tense

Abbreviations used in glossing are:

(1) 1st person ending
(2) 2nd person ending
(3) 3rd person ending

Case endings

Case	Abbreviation	Approximate meaning
accusative	ACC	object
genitive	GEN	possession
partitive	PAR	partitiveness
inessive	INE	'in'
elative	ELA	'out of'
adessive	ADE	'at, on'
ablative	ABL	'from'

Other abbreviations

CLI	clitic
CON	conditional
INF	infinitive
PAS	passive
PRT	particle
PST	past tense

Part 4

The Development of Speech and Language in Hearing Disorders, Sign Language and Cochlear Implant

Chapter 10

The Acquisition of Finnish Sign Language

RITVA TAKKINEN

Introduction

Despite the fact that the mode of signed languages is different from that of spoken languages, the course and timing of first language acquisition is very similar. This conclusion has been drawn from the literature, although the acquisition of signed languages has not yet been studied in depth (Bonvillian & Folven, 1990; Caselli, 1983, 1987; Newport & Meier, 1985; Petitto, 1996). Some research has been conducted on lexical acquisition (Bonvillian & Folven, 1990; Bonvillian *et al.*, 1983), phonology (Boyes-Braem, 1990; Marentette, 1996; Takkinen, 1994, 1995, 2002), grammar (Kantor, 1980; Newport & Meier, 1985; Newport & Supalla, 1980; Schick & Gale, 1996) and interaction (Ackerman & Woll, 1990). Some assessment methods or tests of sign language acquisition have been developed for ASL (American Sign Language), such as Maller *et al.*'s (1999) test, designed for children between six and 12 years of age, and Hoffmeister's (1998) and Prinz and Strong's (1998) assessments for school-age children. Herman *et al.* (1998) developed a test of BSL (British Sign Language) for children between the ages three and 11 years. The GSL (German Sign Language) test developed by Fehrmann *et al.* (1995a, 1995b) is designed for adult sign language users (for a more detailed review of assessment methods, see Haug, 2005). For several signed languages there is a need for a test to assess early acquisition and sign language development at school age. In order to create a test to assess sign language acquisition a certain body of basic research is needed on the sign language in question. For most sign languages this basic knowledge is still missing.

Sign language users always belong to a linguistic minority in their environment. Therefore it is important for them to also learn the majority language of their community. Research into the bilingualism of deaf sign language users has shown that the better deaf people know their first language, sign language, the better they learn the spoken language of their environment (at least in its written form) (Hoffmeister, 2000; Padden & Ramsey, 2000). Good skills in the first language provide a strong basis for learning other languages. To be able to support the sign language acquisition of all deaf children, whether born to deaf or hearing parents, it is important to know the developmental course of sign language acquisition as a first language.

The Structure of Finnish Sign Language

Finnish Sign Language (FinSL), like other sign languages, can be examined on the levels of lexicon, phonology, morphology, syntax, semantics and pragmatics (Jantunen, 2003; Pimiä & Rissanen, 1987; Rissanen, 1985; Takkinen, 2002; see also Emmorey, 2002; Sutton-Spence & Woll, 1999; Valli & Lucas, 1995, 2000). FinSL has lexicalised signs, which can be put in a dictionary according to their basic forms. The signs are composed of basic parameters: handshapes, orientations of the fingers and the knuckles, articulation places, articulation movements and non-manual elements. In fluent signing there appear several modifications in the basic forms of the signs. These modifications are called *phonological processes* (Liddell & Johnson, 1989), and they are phenomena of the *phonological level*.

In addition to *lexicalised signs,* signers very frequently also use productive signs (*polysynthetic signs*; Takkinen, 2002) in discourse which have no basic form but are generated in a signing situation. Combined parameters can each bring a separate meaning to a productive sign. These signs are iconic, and they depict visual-geometric properties, as well as the motion and location of an entity. The handshape (also called a *classifier handshape*; e.g. Supalla, 1986) is chosen according to the visual-geometric properties of the object in question. The movement of the hand represents the motion of the object or depicts its form. The location represents the location, and the orientation represents the orientation of the object in space. The non-manual parameter defines the quality of the motion or the object's visual-gestural property (see also Wallin, 1994, 2000).

Signed languages, in general, have a rich *morphology*, and that is also the case with FinSL. The morphological processes can be divided into *derivation* and *inflection*. There are several ways to derive new signs. In the case of some verbs negative derivatives can be produced by attaching a negative affix to the basic verb (e.g. TIETÄÄ/EI-TIETÄÄ 'know'/'not-know') (see Figure 10.1).

It is possible to produce agentive derivatives from verbs (OPISKELLA/ OPISKELIJA 'to study'/'a student'), by attaching an affix to the verb sign (as in Figure 10.2).

By incorporating a numeral handshape in the case of certain nouns, numeral derivatives can be produced (VUOSI/YHDEKSÄN-VUOTTA

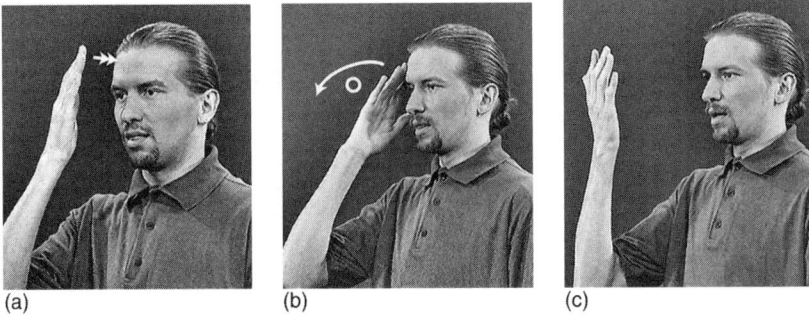

Figure 10.1 (a) TIETÄÄ 'know'; (b)–(c) EI-TIETÄÄ 'not-know'

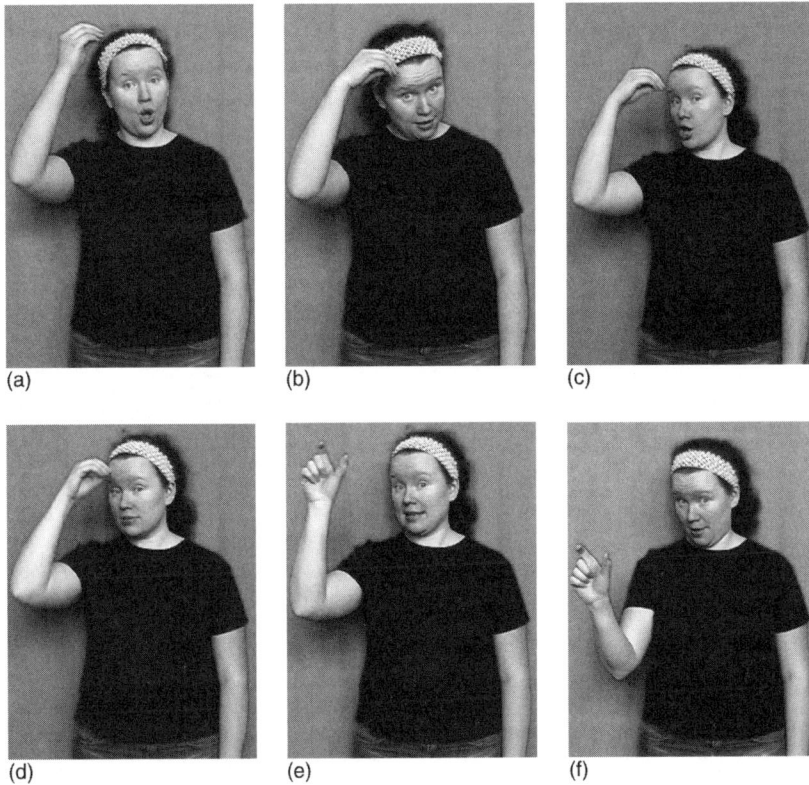

Figure 10.2 (a)–(b) OPISKELLA 'study'; (c)–(f) OPISKELIJA 'student'

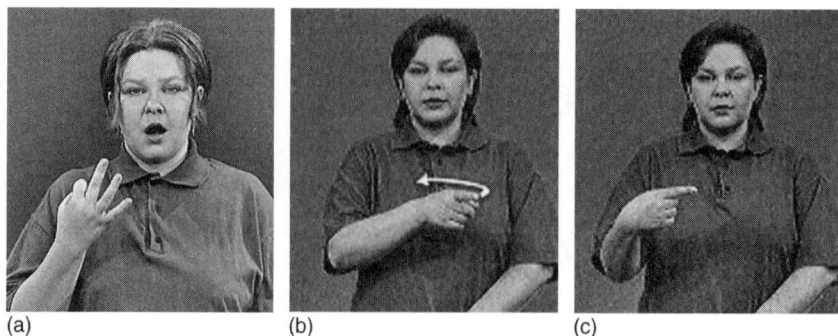

(a)   (b)   (c)

Figure 10.3 (a) KAHDEKSAN 'eight'; (b)–(c) KERROS 'floor'

'year'/'nine-years', KERROS/KAHDEKSAS-KERROS 'floor'/'eighth-floor'), as in Figures 10.3 and 10.4.

A new sign can be also derived by incorporating a new handshape, for example, in the signs for the days of the week (m for MAANANTAI 'Monday', k for KESKIVIIKKO 'Wednesday', etc.; see Figure 10.5).

Compounds are new derivatives from two or sometimes more signs including a phonological reduction in the basic forms of the contributing signs (SYNTYÄ + PÄIVÄ/SYNTYMÄPÄIVÄ 'be born' + 'day'/'birthday'), PYÖREA + PAISTAA/AURINKO 'round' + 'shine'/'sun', as in Figures 10.6 and 10.7).

Polysynthesis is another way of creating new signs, and it is a very productive means in signed discourse. In these signs each of the basic

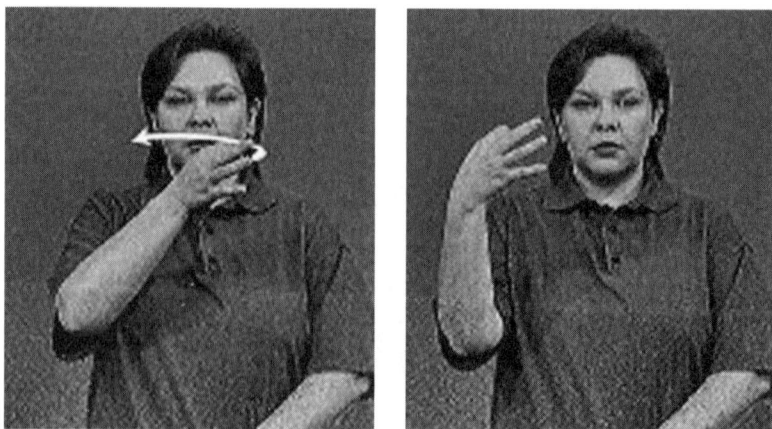

Figure 10.4 KAHDEKSAS-KERROS 'eight-floor'

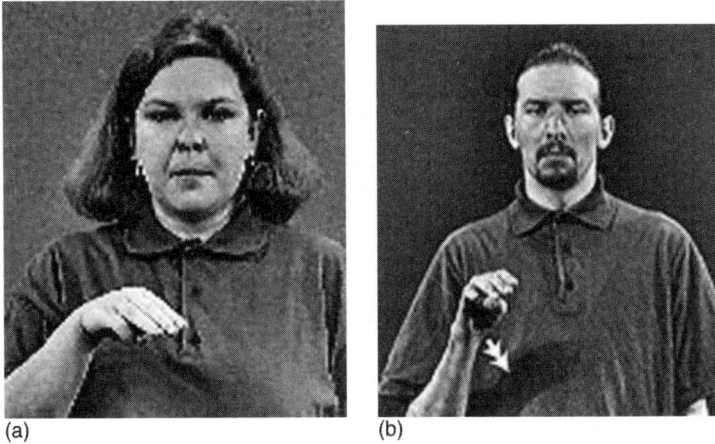

Figure 10.5 (a) m 'm'; (b) MAANANTAI 'Monday'

parameters of the sign can bring its own meaning to the sign (see the previous paragraph, and Jantunen, 2003).

Some verbals (verbs and adjectives) can be *inflected aspectually*, that is, the movement can be modified so that it expresses, for example, durative aspect (LUKEA 'read'/LUKEA 'read' + durative modification of the movement; meaning to read for a long time), or frequentative aspect (TAVATA 'tavata'/TAVATA 'meet' + frequentative modification; meaning to meet regularly); see Figure 10.8 (for more details, see Rissanen, 1985).

Verbals can be inflected in an adverbial manner by modifying the movement and adding a facial expression, for example, KAUAN '(to wait) a long time'/KAUAN + adv. modification + facial expression '(to wait) a very long time', or to write very carefully (KIRJOITTAA 'write' + adv.modification + facial expression; see Figure 10.9).

Plural forms in FinSL can be produced in several ways, for example, by repeating the noun, iterating the movement in the predicate verb, using an iterated or wiping point, by lexical means, that is, by adding a number or other sign referring to quantity, or by using polysynthetic constructions. Some verbs can be inflected to contain information as to the object or the object and subject of the action by using the signing space (MINÄ-OPETAN-JOTAKUTA 'I teach somebody'/JOKU-OPETTAA MINUA 'somebody teaches me') This process is called *verb agreement* (Padden, 1990; Valli & Lucas, 1995). These verbs are also called *directing verbs* (e.g. Emmorey, 2002), or *indicating verbs* (Liddell, 2003).

Syntax is the area of sign language research which examines what kinds of sign orders are possible in a particular sign language, what kind of

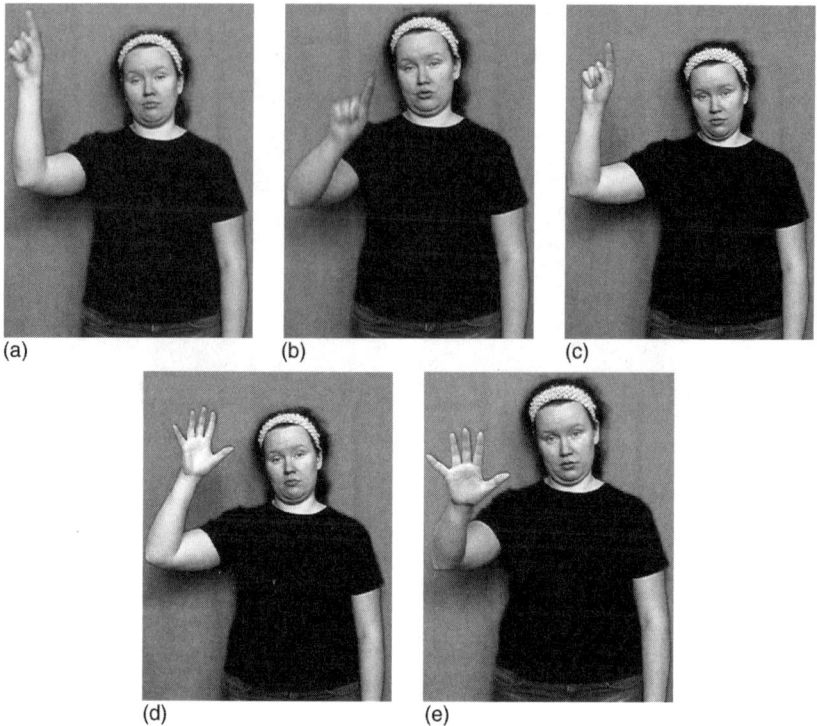

(a)   (b)   (c)

(d)   (e)

Figure 10.6 (a)–(c) PYÖREÄ 'round'; (d)–(e) PAISTAA 'shine'

markers (manual and/or non-manual) there are at the boundaries of sentences and constituents, how the different sentence types are marked, and what kinds of sign categories exist in a particular sign language.

In *semantics* sign meanings can be examined (e.g. relations between signs) as well as sentence meanings and how they are composed. *Pragmatics* examines language use: for what functions language can be used; what kinds of norms there are, for example, in FinSL; how the language varies between different areas, between signers of different ages and genders; how education affects language use, and what different registers are used in FinSL. Another aspect of research into FinSL is how it has changed during its fairly short known and documented history.

The Acquisition of Finnish Sign Language

This chapter is based on a study of the acquisition of FinSL in deaf children of deaf signing parents and deaf children of hearing parents who use sign language in communication with their child (see Takkinen, 1999,

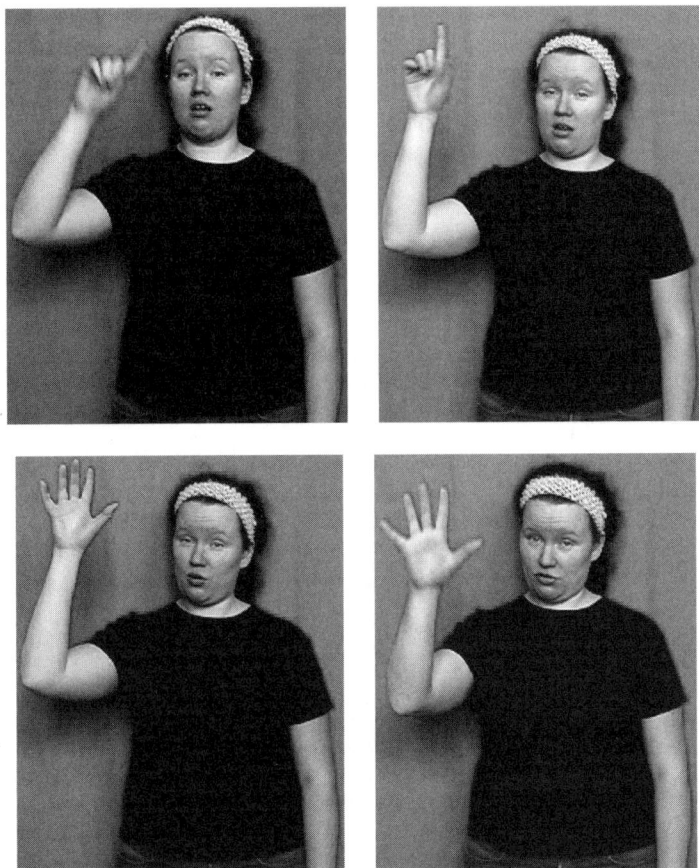

Figure 10.7 AURINKO 'sun'

2003; Takkinen *et al.*, 2000 for more detail). This multi-case study was concerned with sign language acquisition at the ages of 1;6, 2, 3, 4 and 5 years. Because the children were of different ages at the beginning of the study, and because the study was longitudinal, the data totals are different for different age groups. The children in the native category were deaf children born to deaf signing parents, and they had been exposed to sign language from birth. The children in the non-native category were deaf children whose parents are hearing but started to study sign language when their children were about 1 year-old and use it in communication with their deaf children. Thus the children in the second category were not native signers. Data were obtained for three children in the 1;6 year age group (one native and two non-native), four 2-year-olds (two native and two non-native), six 3-year-olds (two native and four non-native), seven

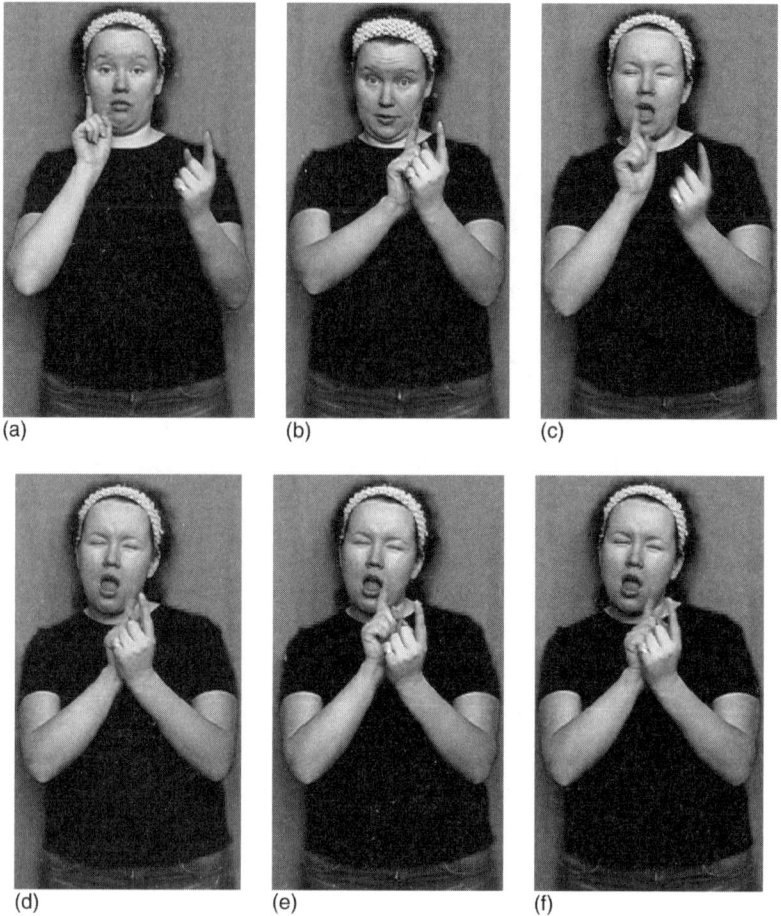

Figure 10.8 (a)–(b) TAVATA 'meet'; (c)–(f) TAVATA + frekv. aspekti 'meet + frequentative aspect'

4-year-olds (three native and four non-native), and four 5-year-olds (two native and two non-native). All the children were girls (see Table 10.1).

The study covered three areas: (1) sign language production, (2) sign language comprehension and (3) interaction. Assessments included phonological, morphological, syntactic and lexico-semantic items. Phonological assessment targeted handshapes, orientation, places and movements, and was designed to test when these parameters are produced correctly and, on the other hand, what kind of variation appears.[1] The lexico-semantic items included for example, the kind of signs the child used. The vocabulary of these children was studied by applying a short

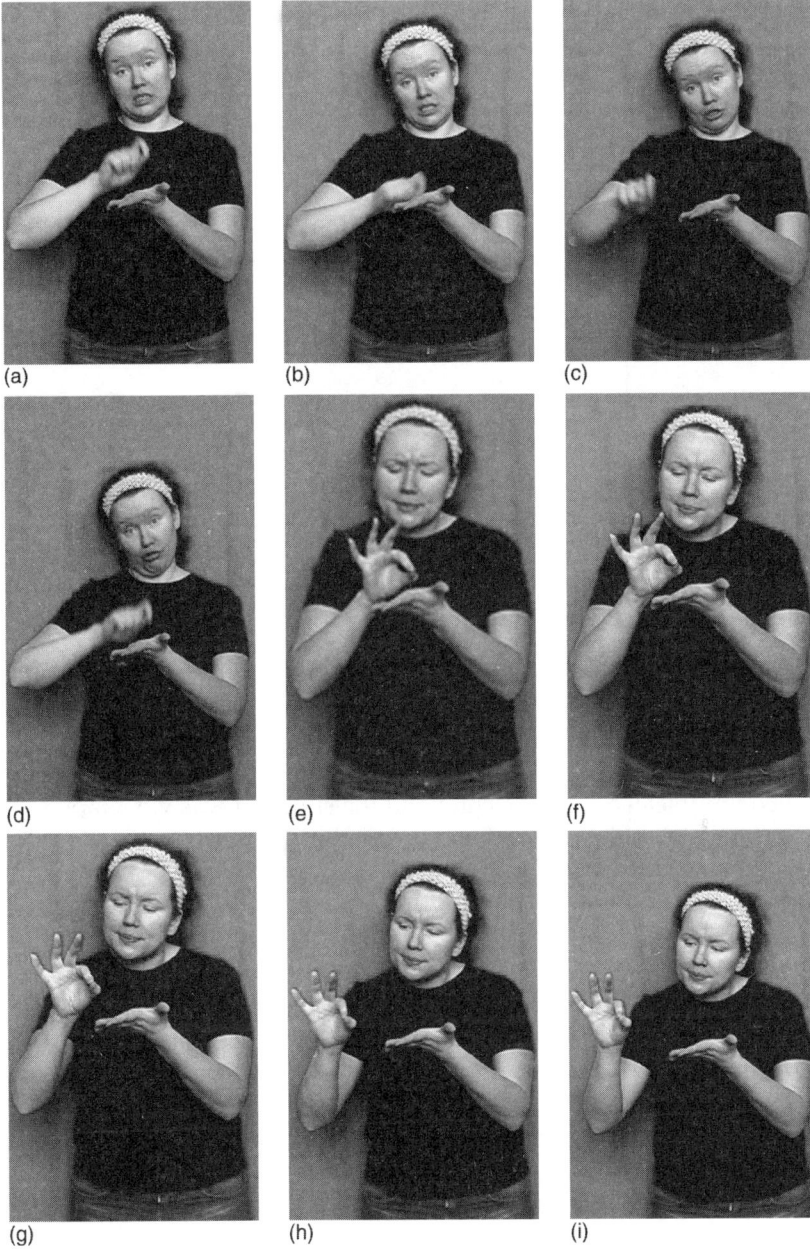

Figure 10.9 (a)–(d) KIRJOITTAA 'write'; (e)–(i) KIRJOITTAA-HUOLELLISESTI 'write-carefully'

Table 10.1 Native and non-native signers and age-groups

Age	Native	Non-native
1; 6	1	2
2	2	2
3	2	4
4	3	4
5	2	2

picture test for spoken languages (Ege, 1985) which is not standardised for FinSL. In the description of morphological development the use of possessive forms, plurality, modification of verbs, agreement of verbs, negative and numerals derivatives were studied. The syntactic items included the length of sentences, the types of sentences and word order. The comprehension items for the earlier ages included, among others, tasks where the child had to act on the teacher's instructions, and to identify a similar toy or picture to one the tester had shown. The comprehension of questions as well as the relation of cause and effect were also studied. Interaction items included gaining attention, eye contact and turn-taking, as well as the functions the children used language for.

The children were observed every six months. A deaf teacher played and communicated with the child and the situation was videotaped. The materials used in these situations consisted of pictures, picture books and toys. Some of the material was partly structured in the form of pictures that elicited certain handshapes or movements, or verb agreement. The interaction also contained free discussion between the child and a deaf adult. The video recordings lasted about 30 minutes per session. At the age of 1;6 the recording was less than 30 minutes per child. At the other ages two recordings were made, which resulted in approximately 60 minutes of data per child at each age.

Development of Interaction and Language Comprehension

According to Ackerman's and Woll's (1990) findings, deaf parents systematically use visual and tactile channels when they want to get their baby's attention and communicate with him/her. They naturally guide their child towards visual communication and catching another person's attention by tactile and visual means, and towards understanding the importance of eye gaze during communication. When the child is less than one year old, the parents sign at the place the child is looking at (Ackerman & Woll, 1990). Thus, deaf parents also use the joint attention strategy that is seen in the communication of hearing parents with their hearing children (Tomasello, 1995). When the child is about 1 year old, parents catch his/her attention by tapping him/her on the arm (Ackerman & Woll, 1990). The child realises that he/she has to look at the parent because the parent has something to say to him/her. The getting and maintaining of eye-gaze is a crucial point in the development of the communication of deaf as well as of hard-of-hearing children.

Deaf children acquiring FinSL (Takkinen, 2003; Takkinen *et al.*, 2000) show the same trend in their acquisition as described above. At the age of a year and a half the children taking part in this study knew how to get other people's attention by tapping them. They had also learnt the meaning of eye-gaze in communication and were able to maintain eye contact with their interlocutor for a while.

At the age of two the basic interaction skills of the deaf children in this study were estimated to be good. The children knew how to get another person's attention (by tapping them on the knee or shoulder), they knew the importance of eye contact during communication and they could maintain it, as well as wait for their turn. The children followed short instructions, identified a similar object to one that the tester had shown them, and understood easy questions.

It was generally observed, however, that the interaction skills of the children of deaf parents (native) were better developed than those of the children of hearing parents (non-native). The native signers conversed actively, answered questions and commented on their observations about the pictures. They introduced more new topics into the conversation, for example, by pointing to a picture or by signing. Their expressions were longer than those of the non-native signers.

At the age of three interaction with a deaf adult was, in general, more fluent in the native signers. These children also understood the signing of the adult better. All the children, though, followed short instructions and understood easy questions, as well as concepts of time.

All the children used language for informing and for getting something. The native signers also used it socially and in imaginative ways. One child even showed emergence of phonological awareness, in that she was comparing two namesigns (namesign is a sign language name for a person) of her friends which were much alike. She also informed the deaf adult how to sign correctly the namesign of one nurse in the kindergarten. In general, the non-native signers signed less than native signers.

At four years of age all the children understood questions and simple relations of cause and effect. Both the production and comprehension of sign language were still more advanced in the native signers. These children were signing more and interaction was easier with them than with the non-native signers. They were able to converse in a small group of children. They also showed awareness of polite ways of signing.

At the age of five the children understood versatile and fluent signing. All of them showed expressive, instrumental, social and imaginative functions of language use. The native signers could, for example, tell fairy-tales expressively. They also showed metalinguistic knowledge on the phonological level by talking about how to sign two different signs which closely resembled each other.

The general observation was that the children in the non-native group were not as used to communicating in sign language as the native signers. Therefore, the deaf adult had to sign a little more slowly to these children and sometimes to repeat his comments or questions. However, by the age of five, the interaction, comprehension and signing of the non-native signers had developed considerably.

Development of Sign Language Production

Early acquisition

The speech development of hearing children starts by vocalisation and by combining different speaking sounds to form syllables and longer chains of syllables. The same development occurs in deaf children in a manual mode. Petitto and Marentette (1991) have analysed the manual babbling of deaf and hearing children. They have observed that hearing children, too, babble with their hands at the age of 10–14 months although they have less manual babbling than deaf children. The vocal babbling of hearing children develops more strongly and then transitions to speech, but deaf children develop manual babbling further and then make the transition to manual signs.

Petitto and Marentette (1991) have defined manual babbling to consist of a restricted number of phonetic units, which are organised like syllables in signed language but do not have linguistic meaning. The following six handshapes, 👋 ✌ 🤏 👆 🤟 👌, represented 75% of the handshapes the children used in babbling. The most common movements of the hands in manual babbling were closing of the handshape, movement towards the body and movement up and down. Most of the babbling occurred in a restricted area in front of the body. Meier and Willerman (1995) have observed repeated movements like bending the arm at the elbow, rotating the wrist or repeated inner movement of the hand.

The children in Petittos's and Marentette's study (1991) repeated the handshapes and movements in their manual babbling, and at the age of 10 months they were at the phase of syllabic babbling. The deaf children progressed at the same pace as hearing children in vocal babbling, and produced jargon babbling at the age of 12–14 months (Petitto & Marentette, 1991). In FinSL this kind of research has not been carried out, but some deaf parents of deaf children have reported roughly the same kind of features: opening and closing the handshape, bending the hand at the elbow and rhythmically producing 'sentence-like' sequences which do not contain any meaning.

Phonological acquisition

The parameters of a sign are handshape, orientation of the palm and the knuckles, movement of the signing hand, place of articulation and non-manual signal. The number of the primes in the parameters is much larger than the number of speech sounds (phonemes) in spoken language, in general. For the children exposed to sign language the easiest parameter to acquire is the place of articulation. Handshapes and movements are fairly inaccurate between the ages of one and three. This has been observed in FinSL (Takkinen, 1988, 1994, 1995) as well as in ASL (Conlin *et al.*, 2000; Marentette, 1996; Siedlecki & Bonvillian, 1993).

In their first signs children use only a small number of *handshapes* of the sign language they are acquiring. The handshapes that are acquired first are basic handforms which often substitute for more marked handshapes (Siedlecki & Bonvillian, 1993; Takkinen, 1988, 1990, 2002). In the early handshapes the fingers are extended or closed. If there are two different handshapes in a sign or if the signs are signed with two hands, the handshapes tend to be less accurately produced (Takkinen, 2002).

Takkinen (2002) observed an increase in the number and accuracy of handshapes as children get older. At the age of two there is much variation in the way children produce even the same handshape in different signs. This also happens with hearing children's speech: the surrounding phonemes affect the way children pronounce a certain phoneme in different words. At the age of three, children can better control the individual functions of the fingers. Children acquire different degrees of finger extension, for example, extension of the fingers from the proximal phalanx and rounding of the fingers. The correct thumb position appears in many handshapes.

The handshapes seem to be mainly acquired by the age of five or six (Takkinen, 1994, 1995, 2002). All the extension degrees of all the joints are mastered at this age, as well as the different kinds of finger arrangement (linear and non-linear). At this age there are still some handshapes which differ from the target handshape. However, two-handed signs no longer cause any difficulties, and even signs with a handshape change are mostly correct.

The inner features of handshapes[2] – the degree of extension of the fingers, the spreading and non-spreading of the fingers, the position and the degree of extension of the thumb, the number of selected fingers – are acquired by the age of seven and the handshapes are mostly accurate.

Of course, the signing situation affects the accuracy of signing as it does also among adult signers (Takkinen, 2002).

The *movements* in the first signs of young children are inaccurate to a large extent. At the age of one and a half, children's movements are simple. Siedlecki and Bonvillian (1993) observed in their research on ASL that two-thirds of the movements produced by children at this age consist of only one single movement. After this age the movements become more versatile (Takkinen, 1988, 1990). Conlin *et al.* (2000) observed that children between seven and seventeen months tend to proximalise movements. Because the control of the articulators close to the body (shoulder) is better than that of the more distant articulators (elbow, wrist and fingers), children substitute movements of the joints closer to the body (proximal movements) for movements of the joints further from the body (distal movements) (see also Marentette & Mayberry, 2000).

The movements of children at the age of two and three are still inaccurate. Coordination of the hands is more difficult in two-handed signs than in one-handed signs. Children acquire straight movements earlier than circular movements. Inner movements of the hands (distal movements, micro movements) are still more difficult to produce at the age of two and three than the proximal movements (movements of the whole arm). If a sign includes both distal and proximal movements, one or the other is often omitted. In signs with complex movements the form or the direction of the movement may be vague (Takkinen, 1988, 1990).

Articulation movements become much clearer when children reach the age of five or six (Takkinen, 1994, 1995). The movements in two-handed signs can still cause some problems but the movements in one-handed signs are well established. The co-ordination of distal movements and proximal movements may vary a little. Even at school age movements may vary because of stylistic variation or careless articulation although the motor, perceptual and cognitive functions may be well developed.

The production of *articulation place* does not demand such finely controlled motor skills as the production of handshapes and articulation movements. Therefore the place of articulation is acquired considerably earlier than movements and handshapes. The acquisition of articulation place between the ages of 6 and 16 months has been studied by Bonvillian and Siedlecki (1996). In this study children started in the first phase to use places that are clearly distinct from each other, neutral space, body, and the chin and the forehead (see also Conlin *et al.*, 2000). In the next phase they acquired the non-dominant hand with handshape 5 (👋), and the cheek. Then they acquired the middle of the face, the back of the wrist, the neck, the whole head and handshape B (🖐) in the non-dominant hand. In the fourth phase they started to use the forearm. In the fifth phase they used several more handshapes as an articulation place.

The places acquired first by children are also frequent in adults' signing. The places that are less frequent and the handshapes of the non-dominant hand, which demand more fine-tuned motor skills, are acquired later. They demand better visual perception of the handshape and the contact point. In two-handed signs the different handshapes in the different hands demand a well developed co-ordination of both hands (Bonvillian & Siedlecki, 1996; Takkinen, 2002). It is important that the schema of the body is well developed in the child when he/she is acquiring articulation place (Marentette & Mayberry, 2000).

At the age of two or three years, places are more accurately produced than handshapes and movements. There occurs some typical variation in places: the articulation place can move from the body to neutral space, from the face or in the neutral space downwards, or from the face to the side. This feature can also occur between the ages of five and seven, as well as in adult signing (Takkinen, 1988, 1990).

The *orientation* of the palm and the knuckles is interlinked essentially with handshape. According to Takkinen (1988, 1990, 1995) the orientation of a sign diverges more easily from the correct one at the age of three if the sign includes a complex handshape and/or movement, and if the place of articulation and movement are outside the child's visual field. The changes in palm orientation, and knuckle orientation are mostly of 90 degrees. A change of 180 degrees is rare and mostly occurs in palm orientation. Changes in orientation occur mostly in order to make the articulation of a sign easier. By the age of five or six, the orientation of signs is mostly correct. If changes in orientation occur it is caused by fast and careless articulation.

Two-handed signs are difficult for young children to sign correctly. The visual-motor control of two-handed signs is very demanding. At the ages of one and two years, children do not use many two-handed signs, and if they use them, they sign them mostly with one hand, especially if the hands act in the same way in the sign. Therefore, the signs do not lose much information. When the other hand is a place of articulation, children do not omit it as often. Many variations in parameters occur if young children use two hands when signing them (Bonvillian & Siedlecki, 1996; Takkinen, 2002).

Lexico-semantic acquisition

Children who acquire a sign language produce their first signs at the age of approximately one, like hearing children acquiring a spoken language (Bonvillian & Folven, 1990; Caselli, 1983, 1987; Petitto & Marentette, 1991). Early studies (Bergmann 1980; Bonvillian *et al.*, 1983) concluded that children already start to sign at the age of eight months, that is, earlier than hearing children start to speak. It has since been shown, however, that those signs were not used in a symbolic way but in ritual situations in which certain signs are repeatedly produced in association with certain actions, for example, eating and bathing (Bonvillian & Folven, 1990). The meaning of the first signs is broad, just like the meaning of the first words in hearing children acquiring spoken languages: one sign can be used for all the referents whose meaning is close to each other. Children can also express a statement or a demand with one sign, in which case the sign has the meaning of a sentence (Caselli, 1983; Takkinen *et al.*, 2000).

The rate of sign vocabulary expansion is individual, as is the emergence of the first signs. Bonvillian *et al.* (1983) observed that at the age of one, children had approximately 10 signs, and at the age of one and a half approximately 50 signs. The vocabulary of deaf children of hearing parents can also develop quickly if the parents start to sign early. Takkinen (2002) observed that when the parents had started to learn sign language when the children were under 1 year old the children had a vocabulary of 40–50 signs by the age of one and a half. Thus, the emergence of signs and the enlargement of vocabulary at an early age does not demand native-like input of sign language. Parents who have just started to learn sign language and who use those signs they have learned can be good models for their deaf children at the beginning of sign language acquisition.

At the age of one and a half children's vocabulary mainly consists of nouns (e.g. TYTTÖ 'girl', AUTO 'car'), and clear verbs are infrequent (e.g. ITKEÄ 'cry', KEINUA 'swing') (Takkinen, 1999, 2003; Takkinen *et al.*, 2000). At this age children make no clear distinction between close noun–verb pairs in their signing. At the age of two, in addition to nouns (e.g. BANAANI 'banana', KENKÄ 'shoe', NUKKE 'doll'), and verbs (HAKEA 'fetch', HALUTA 'want', PELÄTÄ 'be afraid') also adjectives (KAUNIS 'nice', SININEN 'blue', SURULLINEN 'sad'), pronominal points (MINÄ 'I', SINÄ 'you', HÄN 'he/she'), locative points (TÄSSÄ 'here', TUOLLA 'there') and some numerals (YKSI 'one', KAKSI 'two') appear in children's vocabulary. At this age also some adverb-like signs (PALJON 'much', PIAN 'soon', KYLLÄ 'yes', LOPPU 'finished', 'out of something') appeared.

By the age of three the vocabulary has increased both quantitatively and qualitatively. When assessed using the Bo Ege picture vocabulary test (Ege, 1985) the native signers were 3–12 months ahead of the standard age for Finnish-speaking children, and the non-native signers were 0–3 months ahead. This finding gives some idea of the growth of vocabulary in general, and also between these two groups. All the children used signs of all categories: nouns (RANTA 'shore', RAPU 'crayfish', SIMA 'mead', RUUSU 'rose'), verbs (TUULLA 'blow', KERTOA 'tell', OSATA 'know/can', MENNÄ-SISÄLLE 'go-in'), adjectives (SAMANLAINEN 'similar', VAARALLINEN 'dangerous', KILTTI 'good/nice', KYLMÄ 'cold', SÖPÖ 'sweet/cute'), numerals (1, 2, 3) and adverbs (of time and manner) (MYÖHEMMIN 'later', JÄLKEEN 'after', VARMA 'sure', VÄHÄN '(a) little'). Concepts of quantity (PALJON 'much', VÄHÄN 'little') and time (NYT 'now', MYÖHEMMIN 'later', PIAN 'soon', JÄLKEEN 'after') were more frequent than earlier. The concept of colour was developed, and children could produce signs for several colours.

At the age of four sign language started to become more abstract, with abstract signs (MATEMATIIKKA 'maths', TÄRKEÄ 'important'), hypernyms (e.g. toy, clothes, food), and broader concepts of time and numerals. The vocabulary was 10–24 months ahead of the age standard in both groups. This shows that the lexicalised vocabulary had grown well also in the non-native signers. It is important to notice that the test does not measure the use of productive lexicon (polysynthetic signs) which is a resource very much used in signed discourse. The native signers were more competent than the non-native ones in using that part of the lexicon.

At the age of five the abstract signs became more frequent, and vocabulary became more versatile in both groups. According to the Bo Ege test (1985) the vocabulary of all the children was from half to one year above the age standard. Thus, the development of lexicon was very even among the children.

Morpho-syntactic acquisition

At the age of one and a half three of the children in this study mostly used expressions of one sign (VAUVA 'baby', HEVONEN 'horse', ITKEÄ 'cry'), or one sign and a point (PUPU os. kuva 'bunny' + 'point to the picture' os. kuva LINTU 'point to the picture' + 'bird). Two of them also combined two signs (LAMMAS NUKKUA 'sheep sleep', os. + PALLO HEITTÄÄ 'point' + 'ball throw'). There was no indication of morphological development at this age, an observation also found in research on the development of ASL (Newport & Meier, 1985; Newport & Supalla, 1980).

At the age of two both of the children in the native group and both of the children in the non-native group used sentences composed of two and three signs, the native signers even four signs. (In the examples, the Finnish glosses, in upper case indicate the signs that the child has signed; these are followed by glosses in English, written in lower case; and then by a semantic coding in English, in parentheses. N refers to native signer and Nn non-native signer.)

(1) TYTTÖ NUKKUA 'girl sleep' (The girl is sleeping.) (Nn)
(2) PIAN HAKEA 'soon fetch' ([He] soon fetches [me].) (Nn)
(3) ODOTA HAKEA 'wait fetch' (Wait I will fetch [it].) (N)
(4) NUKKUA VÄSYNYT 'sleep tired' (He is sleeping. He is tired.) (N)
(5) BANAANI HALUTA 'banana want' (I want a banana.) (N)
(6) MINÄ HALUTA SAMA 'I want same' (I want the same.) (N)
(7) MINÄ SAMA PALJON 'I same much' (I have much the same kind [of things].) (N)

(8) NUKKUA$_{P_1}$ NUKKUA$_{P_2}$ NUKKUA$_{P_3}$ 'sleep$_{P_1}$³ sleep$_{P_2}$ sleep$_{P_3}$' (Many are sleeping.) (N)

All children used mainly affirmative sentences, the negative expressions being composed of one sign (EI-VOI 'not-able', EI-MITÄÄN 'nothing') or a head shake. Also some imperative forms appeared as seen in Example 3 above. On one occasion the child had a two sentence expression including only one verbal in each sentence (Example 4). Example 8 gives a cue of plural form. The child has in her mind an idea of plurality but the expression is not correct at this stage. She repeats the lexical verb NUKKUA 'sleep' in different places instead of using the lexical verb NUKKUA 'sleep' + a polysynthetic verb in the way the expression would be signed by adult signers.

At the age of three the two groups differed even more in their language skills than at the age of two. The expressions of the native signers were longer and more complex than those of the non-native signers.

(9)   VÄHÄN SATTUA 'little hurt' (It hurts a little.) (Nn)
(10) TYTTÖ KEINUA 'girl swing' (The girl is swinging.) (Nn)
(11) RUOKA JÄLKEEN SINÄ LÄHTEÄ MINÄ NUKKUA 'eating after you go I sleep' (After lunch you will go away and I will go to sleep.) (N)
(12) HEI/SIILI NÄLKÄ HALUTA ULKONA SYÖDÄ/ANTAA-KUPPI LIPITTÄÄ VIEDÄ-KUPPI-POIS LÄHTEÄ POIS 'att.*/hedgehog hunger want outside eat/give-dish lap take-dish-away go away' (Att. A hedgehog is hungry, it wants to eat outside. I give it a dish and it laps [the milk]. Then I take the dish away and the hedgehog goes away.) (N)
(13) NYT TÄMÄN-KOKOINEN/SYÖDÄ PALJON KASVAA SAMAN-KOKOINEN 'now this-tall eat much grow as-tall-as-the-other' (Now I am this tall but when I eat a lot I will grow as tall as she is.) (N)
(14) HÄIKÄISTÄ-MINUA AURINKO 'dazzle-me sun' (The sun dazzles me.)
(15) HÄMÄHÄKKI os-4a/MINÄ VAHVA LYÖDÄ-4a/KUOLLUT os-4a HÄMÄHÄKKI KUOLLUT 'spider-4d (d = down) I strong hit-4d dead point 4d spider dead' (On the floor there was a spider. I am strong, I hit the spider and now it is dead.) (N)
(*)   Att. = attention getting, e.g. waving

The children in both groups used affirmative, negative and interrogative sentences. The word order of the non-native signers was mainly SV. Their sentences were, as a rule, shorter than the native signers', mostly composed of one, two or three signs. The word order varied in the signing of the native signers, and they even used signing space to some extent in sentence formation. Both groups used many sentences consisting of two signs, and the order was mainly subject–verb (POIKA ISTUA 'boy sit', HEVONEN LAUKATA 'horse gallop', MINÄ PIIRTÄÄ 'I draw'), sometimes verb–subject in a non-native signer (KEITTÄÄ ÄITI 'cook mother'). The object–verb order was used sometimes by native signers (SUKLAA SYÖDÄ PANNA-PALA-SUUHUN 'chocolate eat put-a-piece-into-mouth'), as well as by the non-native signers (SIENI ETSIÄ 'swamp seek', LAHJA ANTAA 'present give'). The object–subject–verb order appeared in native signers (LEHMÄ MINÄ NÄHDÄ JO MINÄ 'cow I see already I', LUSIKKAxx HAARUKKAxx VEITSIxx MINÄ OLLA 'spoons forks knives I have'). When the object was transferred to the beginning of the expression it was mostly not accompanied with a facial expression as it occurs in adult language. Other sign orders also appeared but this is natural in conversation where sentences, in general, are not complete. In their research on the acquisition of sign order in ASL, Schick and Gale (1996) observed that sign order varied, and that children made little use of verb inflection at an early age. The context helped to clarify ambiguous expressions.

In research on the acquisition of FinSL (Takkinen, 1999, 2003; Takkinen *et al.*, 2000) the emergence of verb agreement (e.g. a verb which shows the goal or the goal and the source of the action in its form) was only seen in the signing of the native signers. In Example 14 the hand orientation in the verb HÄIKÄISTÄ 'dazzle' shows that the dazzling starts from the sun and is directed to the signer (me). Example 15 also shows the constancy of the first chosen locus in the signing space throughout the signed expression. The child first signs the sign for spider and points to locus 4a. Then she directs the verb for hit towards that locus (4a). After that she signs the sign for dead and points to locus 4a.

Unlike the non-native signers, the native signers used compounds, such as: VIIKONLOPPU 'weekend', JÄÄTELÖKAKKU 'ice-cream cake', SAAPAS 'boot ', AURINKO 'sun'. The children in both groups used possessive forms (OMA-1 'my', OMA-2 'your', OMA-3 'his/her'). There also appeared some instances of **plural forms:** PALJON ULKONA KIVI 'a-lot-of outside stone', TALO VIISI 'house five', LUSIKKA HAARUKKA VEITSIxx[4] MINÄ OLLA 'spoon fork knife xx I have'. In the first two examples of plural forms there is a sign indicating amount (a-lot-of, five) in connection with the noun, and in the last example the last noun was repeated several times.

The children in both groups already used **negative derivatives,** signs with a special negative morpheme affixed to them, (see e.g. Zeshan, 2004), a verb like EI-HALUTA 'want-not,' EI-SAA 'not-allowed', EI-TIETÄÄ 'know-not'. **Numeral derivatives,** signs with incorporated number handshape in a nominal (KOLME-VUOTTA 'three-years'), appeared only in the native group.

One clear difference between these two groups was the use of the productive lexicon, that is, polysynthetic signs, which are morphologically complex forms. The children in the native group were beginning to use them, while the non-native signers used only a few very simple polysynthetic forms. Mostly these sign forms were not yet correct but the emergence of the idea of using the productive lexicon could clearly be seen.

(16) PERHONEN KILTTI AMPIAINEN TUHMA AINA PISTÄÄ KÄSI-TURVOTA + posk.pullistus 'butterfly good wasp bad always sting hand-swell + the cheeks puffed up' (Butterflies are good but wasps are bad because they always sting and then the hand will swell a lot.) (N)

(17) HIIRI HIIPIÄ MENNÄ-MAAN-ALLE RAAPIA RAAPIA-NAAMA OLLA-EI KYNSIxx 'mouse creep go-under-ground scratch scratch-face have-no nail' (A mouse creeps, goes under the ground. It scratches my face. It has no nails.) (N)

(18) MINÄ   SUKELTAA-KÄDET-LEVÄLLÄÄN   SUKELTAA-ALAS-NOUSTA-PINTAAN 'I dive-with-arms-open dive-down-come-to-the-surface' (I dive with my arms open and then I come up.) (N)

In Example 17 the handshape of the sign HIIPIÄ 'creep' is not correct when referring to a mouse. The child uses handshape 5 (🖐) (extended, separated fingers) instead of G (☝) (index extended). In Example 18, in the first polysynthetic sign of the expression (dive-with-arms-open) the hand went first as if the diver were diving head first. However, in the following sign (dive-down) the fingertips were oriented downwards as if the diver were diving feet first. Thus, the morphemes of the verbs were not combined correctly because the hand orientations of these two polysynthetic verbs conflicted with each other.

At the age of four both the production and comprehension of sign language were more advanced in the native group than in the non-native group. These children were signing more, and interaction with an adult deaf signer was smoother for them than for the non-native signers. Some examples of the expressions produced by the children are given below.

The expressions of the non-native signers had also become longer and more developed than at the age of three. All children used affirmative, negative, and interrogative expressions; one imperative expression (Example 21 below) also occurred. The word order varied in different sentences. In short expressions the order subject–verb appeared naturally (ÄITI LEVÄTÄ 'mother rest', TYTTÖ ISTUA 'girl sit', AURINKO PAISTAA 'sun shine'). In some expressions the manually coded object was omitted (HAKEA TOINEN 'fetch another') but it was expressed by the eyes (Fetch another [book]!). On the other occasion the subject, the first person, I, was omitted (HALUTA TOINEN 'want another'). The order object–verb appeared, for example, in expressions PUPU AMPUA 'bunny shoot', KUKKA KASTELLA 'flower water'. In addition, the order subject–verb–object appeared (ÄITI KASTELLA KUKKA 'mother water flower', ISÄ JUODA MAITO 'father drink milk').

Moreover, the children in the non-native group used the signing space, for example, by using polysynthetic signs to form sentences but the children in the native group did so in a more developed and effective way.

(19) A-viittomanimi KUUSI-VUOTTA TAMMIKUU 'A-namesign six-year January' (A ... will be six in January.) (Nn)

(20) TÄNÄÄN HUOMENNA KOULU EI-OLLA EI-OLLA/TÄÄLLÄ TÄNÄÄN TÄÄLLÄ 'today tomorrow school have-not have-not, here today here' (Today and tomorrow I don't go to school, I am here today.) (Nn)

(21) HEI/os. r-kirjain JO/SINÄ ANTEEKSI SINÄ 'att. (point to letter-r) already/you apologize you' (Att. I have already fingerspelled the letter r. You must apologize.) (N)

(22) KIRJA ERITTÄIN-MIELENKIINTOINEN MISSÄ KIRJA MISSÄ 'book very-interesting where book where' (Where is the book which is very interesting? Where is it?) (N)

(23) HEI N-viittomanimi OLLA KIRJA UUSI MATEMATIIKKA KIRJA HARMAA VÄRI 'Att. N-namesign have book new maths book grey colour' (Att. N ... has got a new math book. It is grey.) (N)

(24) KISSA SÖPÖ RUOKA PUUTTUA KISSA-KÄVELLÄ 'cat cute food missing cat-is-walking' (What a cute cat. There isn't any food. The cat is walking around.) (N)

The children in both groups used *compounds*, for example, VIITTOMAKIELI 'sign language', ILTAPALA 'evening snack', ILMAPALLO 'balloon', PÄIVÄKOTI 'kindergarten'. The children also expressed *plurality* in different ways: repeating the noun, for example, KUKKAxx 'flower xx', connecting a numeral or another sign indicating amount with the noun, like MONTA SIMPUKKA 'many shell', LUSIKKA VEITSI HAARUKKA ERILAINENxx 'spoon fork knife different-kinds', or using polysynthetic signs, for example, TÄHTI PALJON-TÄHTIÄ-TAIVAALLA 'star many-star-in-the-sky'. All the children used possessive forms (OMA-1 'my', OMA-2 'your', OMA-3 'his/her').

The children in the native group used numeral derivatives, signs with incorporated number handshape in a noun, for example, NELJÄ-VUOTTA 'four-year', KAKSI-KAPPALETTA 'two-' and negative derivatives, for example, EI-HALUTA 'not-want', EI-OLLA 'not-have', EI-TIETÄÄ 'not-know', EI-MUISTAA 'not-remember'. The children in the non-native group used some of these forms but in a more restricted way.

At the age of four the children in the non-native group also started to use *polysynthetic signs*. They were not correct in form but the idea was gradually emerging. In Examples 25 and 26 the children used two hands in the polysynthetic signs but both hands represented the same object in each construction. The children in the native group used these morphologically complex signs more and in a more developed manner, but still not quite correctly. The main sign, the subject of the sentence, to which the polysynthetic predicate refers, was sometimes omitted. In Example 27 'plaits-on-both-side-of-the-head' refers to a girl, who has plaits and who is swinging but the sign TYTTÖ 'girl' is omitted. The child used two hands to represent two plaits. In Example 28 the child used handshape 5 (🖐) in both hands to refer to many animals. In Example 29 the child referred to many persons with both hands (H handshape 🖐) and located them in different places by repeating the placement.

One native child simultaneously used different handshapes in both hands (Example 30), the non-dominant hand referring to one object, on this occasion the bed, and the dominant hand to the other object, a person sitting under the bed.

> SÄNKY 'bed' (left hand): handshape 🖐-SÄNKY-YLHÄÄLLÄ 'bed-on-upper-level'
>> (right hand): handshape 🖐 ISTUA-ALAPUOLELLA 'sit-under-bed'

To use two hands simultaneously referring to different referents is a complex and more demanding form.

(25) KOTONA   VETO-LAATIKKO   MONTA-LAATIKKOA-PÄÄLLEK-KÄIN 'home dresser many-drawers-one-upon-another' (At home there is a dresser with many drawers one above another.) (Nn)

(26) KOIRA MAATA-SELÄLLÄÄN 'dog lying-on-its-back' (The dog is lying on its back.) (Nn)

(27) LETIT-MOLEMMIN-PUOLIN PÄÄTÄ KEINUA 'plaits-on-both-side-of-the-head swing' ([A girl with] plaits on both sides of the head is swinging.) (N)

(28) NORSU MONTA-KÄVELLÄ-JONOSSA 'elephant many-go-in-line' (Many elephants are going in line.) (N)

(29) MONTA-SEISOA-ERI-PAIKOISSA 'many-stand-in-different-places' ([People] are standing in different places.) (N)

(30) SÄNKY SÄNKY-YLHÄÄLLÄ-ISTUA-ALHAALLA 'bed bed-on-upper-level sit-under-bed' ([A person] is sitting under the bed which is higher up.) (N)

At the age of five the children's signing was quite intelligible even for unfamiliar people. The non-native signers signed more fluently than at the age of four. This age seemed to be a fast phase of development for the non-native signers. Comprehension of signing had become better and thus interaction with an adult deaf signer had become smoother and more active.

All the children showed expressive (e.g. story telling), instrumental, social and imaginative functions of language use. They all used affirmative, negative and interrogative sentences. In addition imperative sentences were employed by all children but one. Word order varied in both groups but other devices in syntactic structure, the use of space and non-manual signals, were employed in a more advanced way by the children in the native group. Even the non-native signers had started to use agreement verbs (i.e. verbs which show the goal or the goal and the source of the action in their form). There are examples of this below.

(31) MUMMO UKKI ANTAA-1 'grandma grandpa give-1' (Granma and grandpa give to me.) (Nn)
(32) MENNÄ-LUO-3 'go-to-3' (... to go to someone.) (Nn)
(33) R-viittomanimi OMA-1 KOTI KÄYDÄ-1 'R-namesign own-1 home go-to-1' (R ... will come to my home.) (Nn)
(34) ISKEÄ-3 'hit-3' (... to hit him). (N)
(35) KISSA RUOKA ANTAA-3a 'cat food give-3a' (I give food to the cat.) (N)

The children in the native group used different plural forms. Once even a dual form appeared, for example, KAKSI-KATSELLA-YMPÄRILLE 'two-look-around'. One of the children in the non-native group also used a dual form but it was not quite correct, SÄNKY KAKSI-PÄÄLLEKKÄIN 'bed two-upon-another'. Both non-native signers in this group employed several kinds of plural forms but not in such a rich way as the native signers.

The children in both groups employed negative derivatives. They could form numeral derivatives, signs with incorporated number handshape in a noun, in a more advanced way than at the age of four. They employed forms such as KAKSI-YHDESSÄ 'two-together', NELJÄSTÄÄN 'we-four', KOLMEN-PÄIVÄN-PÄÄSTÄ 'three-day-later'.

Adverbial inflection of verbs was emerging in the signing of the children in the non-native group. They used forms such as

LASKETELLA-SUJUVASTI 'slalom-ski-smoothly'
LASKETELLA-KOVALLA-VAHDILLA 'slalom-ski-at-a-high-speed'

The use of polysynthetic signs had developed in both groups. The children in the native group, however, used them in a more advanced manner (see Examples 36–41). A noun functioning as a subject is often omitted from the expression. In adult signing an object (entity) that is described with polysynthetic signs should be presented at the beginning of a longer expression that is describing the same situation with several plysynthetic verbs.

(36) KAKSI-LASKETELLA-VIEREKKÄIN 'two-slalomski-side-by-side' (Nn)
(37) AUTO -LUISUA-ALASPÄIN 'car-slide-downhill' (Nn)
(38) KAKSI-KATSELLA-YMPÄRILLE 'two-look-around' (N)

(39)   ISTUA-KAARESSA 'sit-in-arch' (N)
(40)   TUOLEJA-PöYDÄN-YMPÄRILLÄ 'chairs-around-table' (N)
(41)   ULKONA LEIKKIÄ LIIKKUA-YMPÄRIINSÄ 'out-of-doors play move-around' (N)

One of the non-native signers used only simple polysynthetic expressions but the other one already used more complex ones. The use of signing space had also developed in both groups in other respects.

Discussion

Research on sign language acquisition has shown that the timing of when a child achieves a certain milestone is strikingly similar to that in the development of spoken languages. This shows that the nature and function of signed languages are similar to those of spoken languages despite their different modality. Even at the pre-linguistic phase the developmental features – the transition from sounds to babbling with its different phases, and from gestures to manual babbling – resemble each other in spoken and signed languages. Manual babbling and its change to symbolic elements, that is, the first signs in signing children, is analysable in the same way as vocal babbling and its change to words in hearing children.

In research on the acquisition of FinSL (Takkinen, 1999, 2003; Takkinen *et al.*, 2000) children living in a native signing environment and children living in a non-native signing environment (deaf children born to hearing parents who used FinSL with their children) were studied. The children in the native group had been surrounded by sign language from birth, and their model of language was rich and developed. Therefore, it is easy to understand that their language and interactive skills were more advanced than those of the non-native signers. The families of non-native signers had started to learn sign language and familiarise themselves with deaf adults and the deaf community when their deaf child was about one year old. Their children started to acquire signs soon after that. By the ages of one and a half and two they were, regarding language acquisition, not very far behind the children in the native group. However, once grammatical acquisition emerged, the difference between these groups increased. At the ages of three and four the children in the non-native group did not sign very much and their grammar was simple. The most interesting finding of this study was that in the non-native group at the age of five years a rapid phase of development was seen in all areas. Appendix 1 summarises the course of acquisition.

Sign vocabulary was good in both groups of children. The test used (Ege, 1985) assessed only lexicalised signs, not the ability to use productive signs. Although the vocabulary of the non-native signers was good, grammatical structure and fluency of signing were less developed. It seems that hearing parents are able to develop vocabulary more effectively than grammar or fluency of signing.

One explanation for the delay in grammar acquisition and the poor fluency in signing could be the fact that the parents themselves were starting to learn sign language. Therefore, their own grammar and fluency were not yet far advanced. However, by the age of five their children had for the most part acquired the core substance of the developmental tasks expected for this age group, even though their expressive and receptive skills were not as sophisticated as those of the children living in the native language environment. Their communication skills were, however, good; they were able to talk about their own life and understand what others were signing. By that time the sign language skills of their parents had developed greatly. On the other hand, the children probably had more contact with adult signers and other deaf children so they had seen quite a lot sign language used also outside their home, for example, in the kindergarten and in other activities with signing persons. An interesting question is how their sign language skills on the grammatical and pragmatic levels will develop later on at school age. The research completed so far on the acquisition of FinSL cannot answer this question yet, but it will be continued using the data for these children collected when they were of school age between six and 10.

Knowledge about sign language acquisition is important for parents, both deaf and hearing, so that they can support the language development of their children appropriately. This knowledge is also important for the assessment of the language skills of people using sign language, and when developing assessment methods or tests for the evaluation of sign language skills. Speech therapists are responsible for assessing language acquisition in general. They have an urgent need for an assessment tool for sign language, something which is lacking from most sign languages, including FinSL. In addition, if the speech therapist is not a native signer or otherwise a good signer, he/she needs a skilled signer to help with the evaluation of language acquisition. There are cases where the language skills of a child using sign language have not been evaluated successfully: skills have been underestimated, or signs of language problems have not been observed. In both cases the family and the child do not receive appropriate guidance. The same issue arises at school, namely how to evaluate and properly support sign language development.

Knowledge about sign language acquisition is important also for others who are concerned with the development of deaf or other signing children, for example, teachers, psychologists and doctors. What is very important is the basic understanding that signed languages function as well as spoken languages in developing children's language, cognitive, emotional and social skills, and in creating a good basis for learning in general, and the learning of other languages. Bilingualism, or multilingualism, is important to everyone in the present world but exceptionally so to those whose native language is a minority language, for example sign language users. Research has shown (Hoffmeister, 2000; Padden & Ramsey, 2000; Strong & Prinz, 2000; Singleton *et al.*, 1998) that for those who acquire a sign language early and develop strong skills the learning of other languages (at least in written form) is easier and more successful.

How is a good sign language environment to be created for deaf or hard of hearing children born to hearing parents? The most basic contribution to harmonious social, psychological, cognitive and linguistic development is that the parents approve of the deaf child as he/she is and of themselves as complete parents to their deaf child. It is also important to create good opportunities for hearing families to study sign language and get acquainted with the deaf community and deaf adults. Of course, it is important that hearing loss is discovered as early as possible. Then the parents should be guided to learn sign language and communicate visually with the child. It is important that signing children can meet other deaf children and adults so that they have opportunities to see rich sign language and also models of identity. The parents need to know what it is like to live as a sign language user, and a bilingual person when the other language is a signed language. Then it will be easier for them to support the bilingualism (or multilingualism) of their deaf or hard of hearing child.

Notes

1. The description of the phonological acquisition of FinSL in this chapter is mainly based on other case studies: acquisition of handshapes, orientations, articulation places and movements (Takkinen, 1995) and acquisition of handshapes (Takkinen, 2002), both in deaf children of deaf parents.
2. The inner features of handshapes are analysed according to the phonetic description of signs developed by Johnson and Liddell (1996).
3. p1, p2, p3 refer to different places where the sign sleep was signed.
4. xx refers to the repetition of the sign and is the plural form.

References

Ackerman, J. and Woll, B. (1990) Deaf and hearing children learning to sign and to speak: From birth to three years. In J. Kyle (ed.) *Deafness and Sign Language into the 1990's* (pp. 54–61). Bristol: Deaf Studies Trust.

Bergmann, R. (1980) Tegnsprog som modersmål. *Døvebladet* 4, 12–13.

Bonvillian, J.D. and Folven, R.J. (1990) The onset of signing in young children. In W.H. Edmondson and F. Karlsson (eds) *SLR '87. Papers from the Fourth International Symposium on Sign Language Research.* Lappeenranta, Finland July 15–19, 1987 (pp. 183–189). Hamburg: Signum-Verlag.

Bonvillian, J.D., Orlansky, M.D. and Novack, L.L. (1983) Early sign language acquisition and its relation to cognitive and motor development. In J. Kyle and B. Woll (eds) *Language in Sign* (pp. 116–125). London: Croom Helm.

Bonvillian, J.D. and Siedlecki, T. (1996) Young children's acquisition of the location aspect of American sign language signs: Parental report findings. *Journal of Communication Disorders* 29, 13–35.

Boyes-Braem, P. (1990) The acquisition of the dez (handshape) in American sign language: A preliminary analysis. In V. Volterra and C. Erting (eds) *From Gesture to Language in Hearing and Deaf Children* (pp. 107–127). Springer Series in Language and Communication 27. Berlin: Springer Verlag.

Caselli, M. (1983) Communication to language. Deaf children's and hearing children's development compared. *Sign Language Studies* 39, 113–144.

Caselli, M. (1987) Language acquisition by Italian deaf children: Some recent trends. In J. Kyle (ed.) *Sign and School* (pp. 44–53). Clevedon: Multilingual Matters.

Conlin, K.E., Mirus, G.R., Mauk, C. and Meier, R.P. (2000) The acquisition of first signs: Place, handshape, and movement. In C.D. Chamberlain, J.P. Morford and R. Mayberry (eds) *Language Acquisition by Eye* (pp. 51–69). Hillsdale, NJ: Erlbaum.

Ege, B. (1985) *Sproglig Test 1*. Herning: Special-pædagogisk forlag.

Emmorey, K. (2002) *Language, Cognition, and the Brain: Insights from Sign Language Research*. Mahwah, NJ: Lawrence Erlbaum.

Fehrmann, G., Huber, W., Jäger, L., Sieprath, H. and Werth, I. (1995a) Linguistische Konzeption des Aachener Tests zur Basiskompetenz in Deutscher Gebärdensprache (ATG). Unpublished Report, RWTH-Aachen, Germanistisches Institut & Neurologische Klinik, Projekt DESIRE.

Fehrmann, G., Huber, W., Jäger, L., Sieprath, H. and Werth, I. (1995b) Aufbau des Aachener Tests zur Basiskompetenz in Deutscher Gebärdensprache (ATG). Unpublished Report, RWTH-Aachen, Germanistisches Institut & Neurologische Klinik, Projekt DESIRE.

Haug, T. (2005) Review of sign language assessment instruments. *Sign Language & Linguistics* 8 (1/2), 61–98.

Herman, R., Holmes, S. and Woll, B. (1998) Design and standardization of an assessment of British sign language development for use with deaf children: Final report, 1998. Unpublished Report, Department of Language & Communication Science, City University London, London.

Hoffmeister, R.J. (1998) American Sign Language Assessment Instrument (ASLAI). Unpublished Paper, Center for the Study of Communication & the Deaf, Boston University, Boston.

Hoffmeister, R. (2000) A piece of the puzzle: ASL and reading comprehension in deaf children. In C. Chamberlain, J. Morford and R. Mayberry (eds) *Language Acquisition by Eye* (pp. 143–163). Mahwah, NJ: Lawrence Erlbaum.

Jantunen, T. (2003) *Johdatus suomalaisen viittomakielen rakenteeseen [Introduction to the Structure of Finnish Sign Language]*. Helsinki: Finn Lectura.

Johnson, R. and Liddell, S. (1996) ASL phonology: The phonological description of hand configuration. Unpublished manuscript.

Kantor, R. (1980) The acquisition of classifiers in American Sign Language. *Sign Language Studies* 28, 193–208.

Liddell, S. (2003) *Grammar, Gesture, and Meaning in American Sign Language*. Cambridge: Cambridge University Press.

Liddell, S. and Johnson, R. (1989) American Sign Language: The phonological base. *Sign Language Studies* 64, 195–177.

Maller, S.J., Singleton, J.L., Supalla, S.J. and Wix, T. (1999) The development and psychometric properties of the American Sign Language Proficiency Assessment (ASL-PA). *Journal of Deaf Studies and Deaf Education* 4 (4), 249–269.

Marentette, P.F. (1996) The emergence of phonology in American Sign Language: A case study. Paper presented at the *Fifth International Conference on Theoretical Issues in Sign Language Research*, September, Montreal, Canada.

Marentette, P.F. and Mayberry, R. (2000) Principles for an emerging phonological system: A case study of early ASL acquisition. In C.D. Chamberlain, J.P. Morford and R. Mayberry (eds) *Language Acquisition by Eye* (pp. 71–90). Hillsdale, NJ: Erlbaum.

Meier, R. and Willerman, R. (1995) Prelinguistic gesture in deaf and hearing infants. In K. Emmorey and J. Reilly (eds) *Language, Gesture, and Space* (pp. 392–409). Hillsdale, NJ: Erlbaum.

Newport, E.L. and Meier, R.P. (1985) The acquisition of American Sign Language. In D.I. Slobin (ed.) *The Crosslinguistic Study of Language Acquisition: Volume 1; The Data* (pp. 881–938). Hillsdale, NJ: Lawrence Erlbaum.

Newport, E.L. and Supalla, T. (1980) Clues from the acquisition of signed and spoken language. In U. Bellugi and M. Studdert-Kennedy (eds) *Sign and Spoken Language: Biological Constraints on Linguistic Form* (pp. 187–221). Weinheim: Verlag Chemie.

Padden, C. (1990) The relation between space and grammar in ASL verb morphology. In C. Lucas (ed.) *Sign Language Research: Theoretical Issues* (pp. 118–132). Washington, DC: Gallaudet University Press.

Padden, C. and Ramsey, C. (2000) American Sign Language and reading ability in deaf children. In C. Chamberlain, J. Morford and R. Mayberry (eds) *Language Acquisition by Eye* (pp. 165–189). Mahwah, NJ: Lawrence Erlbaum.

Petitto, L. (1996) How does early human language acquisition begin: Evidence from studies of signed and spoken languages. Paper presented at the *Fifth International Conference on Theoretical Issues in Sign Language Research*, September, Montreal, Canada.

Petitto, L. and Marentette, P.F. (1991) Babbling in the manual mode: Evidence for the ontogeny of language. *Science* 251, 1493–1496.

Pimiä, P. and Rissanen, T. (1987) *Kolme kirjoitusta viittomakielestä [Three essays on sign language].* Yleisen kielitieteen laitoksen julkaisuja 17. University of Helsinki, Helsinki.

Prinz, P. and Srong, M. (1998). ASL proficiency and English literacy within a bilingual deaf education model instruction. *Topics in Language Disorders* 18 (4), 47–60.

Rissanen, T. (1985) *Viittomakielen perusrakenne [Basic Structure of Sign Language].* Yleisen kieleitieteen laitoksen julkaisuja 12, University of Helsinki, Helsinki.

Schick, B. and Gale, E. (1996) The development of syntax in deaf toddlers learning ASL. Paper presented at the *Fifth International Conference on Theoretical Issues in Sign Language Research*, September, Montreal, Canada.

Siedlecki, T. and Bonvillian, J.D. (1993) Location, handshape and movement: Young children's acquisition of the formational aspects of American Sign Language. *Sign Language Studies* 78, 31–52.

Singleton, J., Supalla, S., Litchfield, S. and Schley, S. (1998) From sign to word: Considering modality constraints in ASL/English bilingual education. *Topics in Language Disorders* 18 (4), 16–29.

Strong, M. and Prinz, P. (2000) Is American Sign Language skill related to English literacy? In C. Chamberlain, J. Morford, and R. Mayberry (eds) *Language Acquisition by Eye* (pp. 131–141). Mahwah, NJ: Lawrence Erlbaum.

Supalla, T. (1986) The classifier system in American Sign Language. In C. Craig (ed.) *Noun Classes and Categorization: Proceedings of a Symposium, Eugene, OR, 1983* (pp. 181–215). Amsterdam/Philadelphia: John Benjamins Publishing Co.

Sutton-Spence, R. and Woll, B. (1999) *The Linguistics of British Sign Language: An Introduction.* Cambridge: Cambridge University Press.

Takkinen, R. (1988) Kereemipoikkeavuudet kuuron lapsen viittomakielessä 2 v 3 kk–4 v 4 kk iässä [Chereme variations in the sign language of a deaf child at the age of 2.3–3.4 years]. A case study. Unpublished Master's thesis, University of Helsinki, Helsinki, Finland.

Takkinen, R. (1990) Sign articulation at the age of 2.3–3.4 years. In M. Leiwo and R. Aulanko (eds) *Studies in Logopedics and Phonetics 1* (pp. 233–244). Department of Phonetics, University of Helsinki.

Takkinen, R. (1994) Sign articulation of a deaf boy at the age of 2–3 years, 6 years and 8 years. In I. Ahlgren, B. Bergman and M. Brennan (eds) *Perspectives on Sign Language Usage.* Papers from the *Fifth International Symposium on Sign Language Research* (Vol. 2) (pp. 357–368). University of Durham, England: Isla (International sign language association).

Takkinen, R. (1995) Phonological acquisition of sign language: A deaf child's developmental course from two to eight years of age. Unpublished Licentiate's thesis, University of Helsinki, Helsinki, Finland.

Takkinen, R. (1999) Suomalaisen viittomakielen omaksuminen natiivissa ja ei-natiivissa kieliympäristössä [The Acquisition of Finnish Sign Language in a native and non-native language environment]. Unpublished Report, Department of Finnish, University of Jyväskylä & The Service Foundation for the Deaf, Helsinki.

Takkinen, R., Jokinen, M. and Sandholm, T. (2000) Comparing language and interaction skills of deaf children living in a native and non-native language environment. In *XIII World Congress of the Deaf Proceedings* (Vol. 1) (pp. 342–355). Australian Association of the Deaf, Brisbane, Australia.

Takkinen, R. (2002) Käsimuotojen salat. Viittomakielisten lasten käsimuotojen omaksuminen 2–7 vuoden iässä [The secrets of handshapes: The acquisition of handshapes by native signers at the age of two to seven years]. PhD thesis, Kuurojen Liitto ry, Helsinki.

Takkinen, R. (2003) Viittomakielen omaksuminen äidinkielisessä ja kuulevassa viittomakieltä käyttävässä ympäristössä [The acquisition of sign language in native and hearing environments in sign language]. *Puhe ja kieli* 23 (3), 151–164.

Tomasello, M. (1995). Joint attention as social cognition. In C. Moore and P. Dunham (eds) *Joint Attention: Its Origins and Role in Development* (pp. 103–130). Hillsdale, NJ: Erlbaum.

Valli, C. and Lucas, C. (1995) *Linguistics of American Sign Language: An Introduction.* Washington, DC: Gallaudet University Press.

Valli, C. and Lucas, C. (2000) *Linguistics of American Sign Language: An Introduction* (3rd edn). Washington, DC: Gallaudet University Press.

Wallin, L. (1994) Polysyntetiska tecken i svenska teckenspråket [Polysynthetic signs in the Swedish Sign Language]. PhD thesis, Stockholm University, Stockhom, Sweden.

Wallin, L. (2000) Two kinds of productive signs in Swedish Sign Language. Polysynthetic signs and size and shape specifying signs. *Sign Language & Linguistics* 3 (2), 237–256.

Zeshan, U. (2004) Hand, head and face – negative constructions in sign languages. *Linguistic Typology* 8 (1), 1–58.

NB: **Bold text** is used when a developmental feature appears in both native and non-native signers, normal text is used when it appears only in native signers.

Appendix 1: Summary of the Developmental Course of Finnish Sign Language

Age	*Vocabulary*	*Phonology*
	Native signers & Non-native signers *Native signers*	*Native signers & Non-native signers* *Native signers*
1 ½	- **nouns, verbs**	- **simple handshapes, movements**
2	- **nouns, verbs, adjectives, pronominal points,** numerals, **adverbs** - **negative derivatives**	- **variations in the handshapes, movements, in the handshape changes and orientation changes** - **difficulties producing two-handed signs**
3	- **nouns, verbs, adjectives, pronominal points, numerals, adverbs, others** - **negative derivatives** - **concept of colour** - **concept of number** - **concept of time**	- **variations in handshapes,** - **difficulties to produce handshape changes and orientation changes,** - **combination of distal and proximal movements is difficult** - **difficulties producing two-handed signs**
4	- **abstract signs** - **super ordinate concepts** - **compounds** - **negative derivatives** - **concept of number and concept of time more versatile**	- **variations in some handshapes,** - **some difficulties combining distal and proximal movements** - **some difficulties producing two-handed signs**
5	- **vocabulary more versatile** - **more abstract signs**	- **phonological parameters are mastered** - **idiolectic variation**

Age	Morphology	Syntax
	Native signers & Non-native signers *Native signers*	*Native signers & Non-native signers* *Native signers*
1 ½		- **expressions of one sign** - **combinations of sign and point** - **combination of two signs**
2	- first signs of inflection	- expressions of 2–4 signs (native); of two signs (non-native) - **affirmative and negative expressions**
3	- compounds - **non-manual expression of negation** - **possessive forms** - simple forms of plurality - numeral derivatives - modification of verbs and adjectives - verb forms incorporating object and subject information - polysynthetic constructions	- expressions of 5–6 signs (native); of 3–4 signs (non-native) - **affirmative, negative and interrogative expressions** - **sign order varies** - grammatical use of space in sentence formation emerges
4	- **compounds** - **possessive forms** - **numeral derivatives** more versatile - more versatile **forms of plurality** - duality forms using polysynthetic signs - **modification of verbs and adjectives** - **verb forms incorporating object and subject information** - **polysynthetic constructions** more versatile	- long and versatile expressions (native); expressions of 5–6 signs (non-native) - **affirmative, negative, interrogative,** and imperative **expressions** - **sign order varies** - **grammatical use of space in sentence formation** (emerges in non-natives)
5	- **numeral derivatives more versatile** - **more versatile forms of plurality and duality** - **modification of verbs and adjectives** - **more versatile verb forms incorporating object and subject information** - **polysynthetic constructions more versatile and expanded**	- **affirmative, negative, interrogative, and imperative expressions** - **sign order varies** - **grammatical use of space in sentence formation** (more versatile in natives)

Chapter 11

Children with Cochlear Implants Acquiring the Finnish Language

EILA LONKA

Introduction

Each year approximately 0.1% of newborn babies are identified with severe hearing loss in Finland (Maki-Torkko *et al.*, 1998). The effects of profound hearing loss on speech production and spoken language development are extensive. Experience of the use of cochlear implants (CI) in the rehabilitation of these children has shown obvious benefits in spoken language development (e.g. Kirk *et al.*, 2002; Peng *et al.*, 2004; Richter *et al.*, 2002). A cochlear implant is an electronic device converting acoustic energy into coded electronic stimuli bypassing the damaged hair cells of the cochlea. Cochlear implants were first developed for use by postlingually deafened adults. Later many prelingually deaf children fitted with CI have also experienced improvements in speech perception and production. Knowledge of the importance of the early period of language acquisition in normally hearing toddlers has resulted in a tendency to fit children with CI under two years of age as a standard clinical treatment in many countries. Early implantation might, in addition, prevent the development of adverse strategies in speech production caused by the difficulty in integrating limited auditory information into the motor control feedback system.

In Finland, the first prelingually deaf child was fitted with a CI in the year 1997. Since then, the number of Finnish CI-children has steadily been growing up to a total of about 140 cases. Criteria for cochlear implant candidacy have changed during the last 10 years. Children are now fitted as young as one year of age, and the criteria for the degree of hearing loss that can be effectively treated with a cochlear implant have been broadened (see also e.g. Copeland & Pillsbury, 2004).

After cochlear implant activation, Finnish children usually attend speech therapy until school age of about 7 years. Altogether, five University

Hospitals (Helsinki, Turku, Tampere, Oulu, Kuopio) are responsible for the rehabilitation of CI-children. Rehabilitation of children with severe hearing impairment usually starts with hearing aid fitting when the child is younger than one year of age, and speech therapists will meet the family on a regular basis. Depending on the response to the hearing aid the child may be fitted with a CI. In Finland cochlear implantation, and subsequent rehabilitation services including speech therapy and follow-up services are financed by The National Health Service. The main emphasis of rehabilitation is the audioverbal method (Estabrooks, 1998). Initially manually coded Finnish and sign language are also used to support conceptual development in the deaf child. The shift to spoken language usually takes place during the three to four years after successful cochlear implant activation.

From Gestures to Speech

Referential vocalisations are usually recognised as a foundation for phonological development and meaningful spoken language (McCune & Vihman, 2001). In CI-children there is a significant association between preverbal skills at 12 months after cochlear implantation and later speech perception performance (Tait *et al.*, 2001). Gradual transition from vocal and manual gestures to speech utterances takes place during the first two to three years of cochlear implant use (e.g. Huttunen *et al.*, 2004).

According to Lederberg (1993) communication between a hearing impaired child and his or her parents breaks down easily because of a lack in coordination. That is why promoting first interactive means of communication such as conversational turns, gaze, shared attention and self-initiation is especially important for a hearing impaired child and her parents (Tait *et al.*, 2000). The most convenient way to follow the development of preverbal skills is video recording and analysis. In a case study by Kohonen (2001) (also Kohonen & Lonka, 2002) it was observed that during the first months of CI-use, the child (Elisa; CI at 2;11) had a great many imitative abilities (Table 11.1). The first steps of auditory awareness were seen in the child's turning to gaze at her speech therapist during the discourse. During the first nine months she attended intensively to the speech movements and rhythm of her speech therapist and tried to imitate them silently. It has been stated that during the silent period the child may develop her auditory-vocal capacity, which later promotes production skills (also Ertmer, 2001). First signs of Elis's successful turn taking were seen when she sustained her gaze at the therapist and then at the play object (also Tait *et al.*, 2001). Later Elisa showed delayed imitation, and first trials of onomatopoeic sounds and target words emerged. These skills might reflect the development of auditory memory. There was a remarkable increase in the variability of

Table 11.1 The development of Elisa's interactive abilities with CI

	Orientation to communication HA 0:9	*Discursion with vocalisations HA 1:1*	*From imitation to initiation HA 1:6*	*Equal conversational partnership HA 1:10*
Imitation	Acts and speech • voiceless articulation • speech rhythm • onomatopoetic sounds	Speech • word trials, words • onomatopoetic sounds	Speech and grammatical morphemes • words • two-word sentences	Change into spontaneous interaction
Turn taking	Passive, under control of speech therapist • occasional eye contact • acts and gestures • vocalisations • replications of the acts of communication partner	More active • structured eye contact • vocalisations + gestures • word + sign • repair strategies	Active • short sentences • fluent turn taking	Fluent communication • initiation • modification • extension
Spontaneous speech production	Preverbal vocalisations • vowel sounds • variations in babbling	Canonical babbling • Word-like utterances	Long babbling sequences • Words • two-word sentences	Growing intelligibility for familiar people

HA = hearing age.

Elisa's vocalisations after the first year of CI-use, and she started to make active initiations during the interaction. Also the means of repair strategies, such as interrupting, arguing and adding new information, developed in the course of CI-use (see Table 11.1).

Phonological Development

Only little is known about the initial stages of phonology in CI-children. Vocalisations usually persist for about 18 months in normally hearing infants suggesting that practice is needed to develop more complex phonological skills (e.g. McCune & Vihman, 2001). In cochlear implant children their motor, neurological, cognitive and linguistic skills might have undergone substantial development before surgery (Ertmer *et al.*, 2003). That is why, in relation to their hearing age, some of these children may develop their phonological skills at an even faster rate than hearing children of comparable chronological age. Ertmer and Mellon (2001), Ertmer (2001) and Ertmer *et al.* (2003) followed 'Hannah's' early oral language skills from 13 to 42 months after CI-activation. At 12 months of CI-use 'Hannah' was reported to use 10 consonant types. 'Hannah's' post-implant speech intelligibility scores developed from 10% (at 24 months) to 67% (at 42 months). Serry *et al.* (1997) reported a development of 54% of consonant targets over the first four years of CI use.

Phonological development was followed in three Finnish-speaking children with cochlear implants during the first four to 12 months of CI-use (Lonka *et al.*, 2004; Olkkola, 2002). Children were fitted with Nucleus 22 SPrint (ACE-strategy, whole array). The follow-up period was ended at the 25-word milestone (Vihman *et al.*, 1986) of each child. In all 6.5 hours of child–parent play interactions were video recorded (JVC GR DVL20) at two-month intervals. Parent–child interactions consisted of activities, such as playing with a traffic carpet and cars, with animals and a cow-house and with dolls. The speech of the children was transcribed using IPA (http://www2.arts.gla.ac.uk/IPA/ipa.html). Word candidates were identified following the procedure devised by Vihman and McCune (1994) based on both phonetic and functional considerations. Only the relevant (correct) words, produced spontaneously by the children were chosen for the analysis. Marginal phones were determined from words occurring once or twice. Parent diaries supported determination of a relevant word. Consonants produced three times during one recording were selected for the paradigm.

Development of wordforms

Two of the three children in Olkkola's (2002) study already had a lexicon of approximately 25 words at the beginning of the study. A cumulative lexicon of 50 words was achieved before one year of

Hearing Age. Children produced some wordforms that are untypical to Finnish. Reduction of disyllabic words to CVC-forms (CVC-words are untypical to Finnish) instead of open CV syllables/CVCV forms (/sama/ [sam] *'same'*, /satu/ [sat] *'fairytale'*, /auto/ [au] *'car'*) were observed quite long after the 25-words stage. Children also systematically shortened disyllabic CVC-CV-words by pronouncing the first syllable only (/pos:u/ [pos] *'piggy'*). Even though children still had problems in producing disyllabic forms, polysyllabic words (V standing for a vowel-like sound) were observed (/sammak:o/ [jam:ak:V] *'frog'*, /varovasti/ [kakoat:i] *'carefully'*).

Phonological features

Some specific features of the consonant development were observed in CI-children compared to normally hearing Finnish children in the corresponding developmental phase (Olkkola, 2002; see also Kulju and Savinainen-Makkonen in this book). During the first six months of CI-use the consonant inventory was smaller. There were omissions of word-initial stops, even in words with one consonant type only (e.g. /pup:e/ [up:e] *'Spot'*), that are the easiest for normally developing children. Word-medial consonants were observed more often than those in the initial position. Word-initial consonant omissions have been shown to be typical to the speech of normally hearing toddlers with the exception of stop omissions (Savinainen-Makkonen, 2000), which were observed in the productions of CI-children, omitting especially /k/. Omissions were also seen in words of one consonant type only. Towards the end of a one-year follow-up, however, postimplant consonant inventories (9–11 consonants) in CI-children showed a close to normal development (Table 11.2). Consonants

Table 11.2 Consonant inventories at the 25-word point in normally hearing children (Kunnari, 2003) and in three children (A, B, C) with cochlear implants

	Kunnari (2003) Mean age 1;6	A-girl HA = 1;3	B-boy HA = 0;9	C-boy HA = 0;6
Inventory size (+marginal)	10	5 (+6)	6 (+4)	3 (+6)
Consonant inventory	p t k m n s h l v j	p m s h l	t d k m n l	t k v v
Marginal		b t n r v j	p s h v	p g n ŋ h l

HA = hearing age.

still missing were /r/ and /d/. The size of the consonant inventory was comparable to that of Hannah reported by Ertmer and Mellon (2001).

Spoken Language Skills

Many of the children born with profound hearing loss fall behind their normally hearing peers in terms of acquisition of spoken language skills. The variability of development of spoken language skills in children with cochlear implants has been suggested to depend on the length of deafness, age at cochlear implant, pre-implant speech/language abilities and communication style in the family (e.g. Nikolopoulos *et al.*, 2004b, 2004c). Children who undergo cochlear implantation have the ability to learn spoken language at faster rates than profoundly deaf children with conventional hearing aids. An early age at CI seems to favour a more normal chronological language development (Geers, 2004; Peng *et al.*, 2004). However, grammatical forms are reported to be more difficult for children with CIs to learn (Nikolopoulos *et al.*, 2004a; Spencer *et al.*, 2003; Svirsky *et al.*, 2002).

For a study of Finnish children with cochlear implants, speech therapists in five audiological departments were asked to evaluate the use of spoken language of the children based on their regular follow-up records. Language skills were evaluated according to the quality of spoken expressions (see Table 11.3) and sign language use (see also Brackett & Zara, 1998). The results for 92 children are summarised in Tables 11.3, 11.4 and 11.5.

An overall look at the material shows that, after approximately three years of hearing experience (hearing age = HA) at the mean chronological

Table 11.3 Means (m) and standard deviations (std) of chronological ages, hearing ages and ages at CI for the different language levels (*n* = 92)

	Level of language development											
	SL (*n* = 7)		Ws (*n* = 12)		2-wco (*n* = 13)		3–5 wco (*n* = 18)		Grams (*n* = 24)		AgeE (*n* = 18)	
	m	std	m	std	m	std	m	std	m	std	m	std
Chron. age	11,5	4,3	2,9	1,2	4,0	1,2	7,2	2,8	7,7	2,5	7,4	3,6
Hearing age	4,6	1,6	0,8	0,7	1,4	0,8	3,4	1,8	3,6	2	3,7	2
Age at CI	7	4,4	2	1,2	2,7	1	3,8	1,7	4	2,6	3,7	2,9

SL, sign language as a main mode of communication.
Ws, primarily vocalisations with a few single words.
2-wco, two-word combinations.
3–5 wco, three to five-word combinations.
Grams, simple sentences with emerging grammatical (morphological) features.
Age E, complex sentences corresponding the chronological age.

Table 11.4 The number of children at different levels of spoken language skills in respect to the age at cochlear implant

Language development	Age at cochlear implantation (years)					
	<2;0	2;1 – 3;0	3;1–4;0	4;1–5;0	>5;0	Totals
Sign language	1			2	4	7
Words	8	4		1	1	14
1–2 word combinations	4	5	2	4		15
3–5 word combinations	3	5	4	4	2	18
Grammatical sentences	5	8	4		3	20
Age equivalent	7	5	1	1	4	18
	28	27	11	12	14	92

Table 11.5 Language skills in children having their implants before the age of three (white shading) and after the age of three (grey shading) as compared to cochlear implant use (HA = hearing age).

HA	Level of language development											
	Sign L		Ws		1–2 wco		3–5 wco		Grams		Age E	
<1 year			9	1	5	2		2		3	1	1
1–2 years			1		3		2	1	3	1	4	
2–3 years	1	2	1		2	1	3	2	1	3		
3–4 years							1	2	4	1	2	2
4–5 years		2					1	1	1		3	
>5 years		2					1	2	4	3	2	3
Totals	1	6	11	1	10	3	8	10	13	11	12	6

age of seven years children are achieving developed forms of spoken language (Figure 11.1). However, there is a lot of individual variation in those skills (see also Table 11.3). After three years of cochlear implant use, children produce short sentences and approximately after four years they begin to use some grammatical forms of language (bound morphology such as case and verb endings). Gradually skills comparable to those of

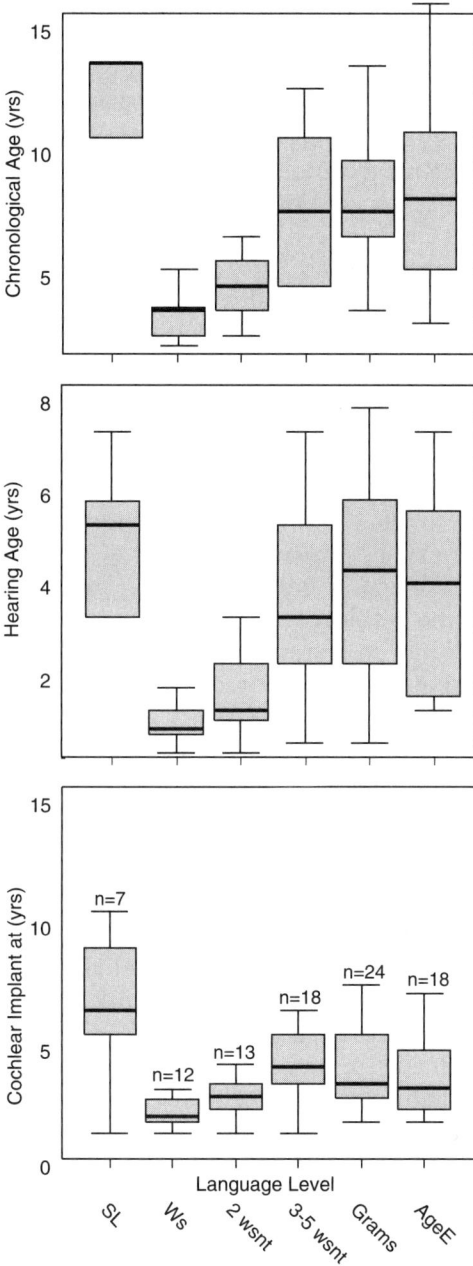

Figure 11.1 Level of language development in respect to children's hearing age, age at cochlear implant and chronological age (medians, quartiles and ranges in boxplots).

hearing peers, such as complex sentences and spoken language as a mode for conversation, emerge.

In several studies the age at cochlear implantation arises as one of the most important factors predicting later language skills (e.g. Kirk *et al.*, 2002; Nikolopoulos *et al.*, 2004b, 2004c). The first years of life are considered to be an accelerated period of language development in normally hearing children (e.g. Locke, 1997). In cochlear implant studies, the three first years of life at CI have been observed to be critical for later language development (Brackett & Zara, 1998; Miyamoto *et al.*, 1999). It is also observed that more and more Finnish children (*n* = 92) are fitted with CI at a young age. The favourable age of two to three for early cochlear implantation in respect to good spoken language skills development is observed in 55 children in this material, 28 of them having their CIs before the age of two (see Table 11.4). Children having their cochlear implants later (after 4 years of age) were already using sign language. Their spoken language development shows a slower tendency. Reasons for that might be that the family prefers sign language, or additional difficulties such language disorder may be present.

In addition to the age at implant, hearing experience also plays an important role in the development of language skills. For a closer look at the age of CI children in respect to cochlear implant use (HA) the 92 children were divided into two groups (Table 11.5; CI before the age of three or later). It was observed that 25 of the 55 children who received their CIs before three years of age had reached excellent language skills (grammatical forms and age equivalent speech) compared to 17 of the later implanted children of whom only six children evidenced age equivalent speech skills. Spoken language skills comparable to chronological age were gradually reached by 12 children implanted before the age of three (Table 11.5). Children having their implants later than three years of age with good language skills but a short hearing experience were those with postlingual deafness. Eleven of the youngest children had used their CIs less than three years and they were still in the initial phase of spoken language development using single words or signs.

The positive influence of early implantation on language development is in agreement with the results of Brackett and Zara (1998), who observed children speaking two-word utterances by one year of hearing age and simple sentences with early grammatical elements by 24–36 months of hearing experience. Miyamoto and his group (1999) observed the advantage of cochlear implantation prior to three years of age for speech perception and production. In this respect Finnish children develop their language skills in a similar way despite the special features of Finnish with its long wordforms and inflectional grammar. Also Huttunen *et al.* (2004) have observed the spoken language development of 18 Finnish CI-children, who produced their first two-word sentences approximately 10 months after cochlear implantation. After five years of implantation speech became the main mode of communication when children reached a 77.5% speech intelligibility rate, which is in accordance with Peng *et al.'s* (2004) results. When the parents were asked to rate children's communication at home a majority of them reported a clear improvement already after one year of CI use (Huttunen *et al.*, 2003).

Receptive and Expressive Language Skills

Developments of receptive and expressive language skills in young cochlear implant children have been followed in several studies using the Reynell (Edwards *et al.*, 1997) scales (e.g. Kirk *et al.*, 2002; Miyamoto *et al.*, 1999, 2003; Richter *et al.*, 2002). Significant ($p < 0.0006$) interaction between age at implantation and length of CI use (Kirk *et al.*, 2002) has been observed in receptive language scores; children implanted prior to three years of age having the highest scores. A child implanted as early as six months of age was observed to achieve Reynell Expressive skills at the rate of his chronological age compared to children implanted late (Miyamoto *et al.*, 2003).

Language development at a slower rate has also been reported. A one year delay was observed in expressive Reynell (Edwards *et al.*, 1997) scores of children fitted with CI prior to two years of age (Manrique *et al.*, 2004). The delay was even greater in children fitted with CI in later years, the number of children studied being 130. Richter *et al.* (2002) describes expressive Reynell scores where the majority (81.1%) of the 106 children were delayed in their speech production by varying degrees, the mean delay being 43,6 months and 25,2 months for the children implanted earlier. Thirteen children reached the age norm, and only seven children evidenced better speech production than the norm.

In her multicase study, Rimmanen (2005) followed the development of receptive language skills in five Finnish children with cochlear implants. The development of Reynell (II: Reynell & Huntley, 1987) scores follows hearing age in three of the children, while the other two evidenced development near to their chronological age (Figure 11.2). After 36 months of hearing experience, children were able to talk on the telephone with a known listener (CAP, Categories of Auditory perception by Archbold *et al.*, 1995). After three to five years of cochlear implant use all these children used morphological forms of spoken language such as tenses, cases, plurals and comparatives.

Discussion

During the first year of life normally hearing children become more and more sensitive to the sounds of their native language (Locke, 1997). Consequently, that helps them in segmenting speech into words and

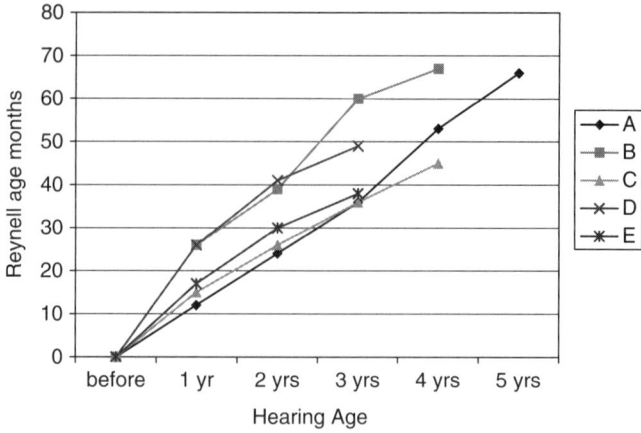

Figure 11.2 Receptive Reynell-test in five (A-E) CI-children (Rimmanen, 2005)

phrases. Early implantation gives a child the possibility to benefit from critical periods of neural development and an opportunity for plastic changes in the auditory pathways (Moore, 2002; Sharma *et al.*, 2004). Early implantation also gives children potential, which we surmise may reduce the spoken language deficits that occur when a child has a profound hearing loss.

A good deal is known about children's acquisition of vocabulary and word combinations. Children are becoming aware of grammatical structures by about two years of age. However, gaining control of the grammatical forms of spoken language is a long process even in normally hearing children (e.g. Locke, 1997; Peters, 1995), and because of this, evaluation of grammatical skills in children with cochlear implants is difficult. So far, children with cochlear implants have been observed to develop their grammatical skills slowly, though the development seems to favour CI at young age (Nikolopoulos *et al.*, 2004a). Even though children with cochlear implants expand their vocabularies they might still be too narrow (nouns, verbs, etc.) for discovering and applying linguistic rules (see Bates *et al.*, 1995; Locke, 1997). An important objective for the children is to achieve skills enabling them to interact, argue and learn academic skills comparable to their hearing peers. However, only little is known about how children with CIs develop in respect to their everyday pragmatic skills. Inscoe (1999) has observed growing pragmatic skills with PPECS (The Pragmatics Profile of Everyday Communication; Dewart & Summers, 1995) in children with cochlear implants.

When more and more children are fitted with cochlear implants additional explanations of the variability and slow spoken language development in some of the children may become available (e.g. Richter *et al.*, 2002; Walzman *et al.*, 2000). For example, oral-motor problems, learning disabilities and language delays will inevitably have an effect on spoken language development (see Walzman *et al.*, 2000). That knowledge is important for developing rehabilitative programs for children using cochlear implants.

In Finland, children with severe hearing impairment have used cochlear implants for a maximum of six to eight years. That is why questions about which kinds of academic skills children with cochlear implants will achieve remain unanswered so far, especially concerning children fitted at a very early age. Children with cochlear implants will have residual hearing problems, which might have an effect on their learning potential. That is why educational needs for children using cochlear implants will require a unique approach to teaching for maximizing their learning experiences (Chute *et al.*, 2003). Educational settings for Finnish children with cochlear implants seem to favor mainstreaming. Only a minority of them attends schools for the hard of hearing or for the deaf.

Finnish children with CI evidence the same kind of overall language development as children from other countries. Early implantation at one to two years of age for children with profound deafness promotes the acquisition a similar level of spoken language skills to age matched hearing peers. That will give new perspectives on the development of reading and academic skills compared to earlier experiences of the development in children with ordinary hearing aids.

Acknowledgements

Parts of this report were supported by the Finnish Cultural Foundation and the Finnish Society of Audiology. The author owes her gratitude to the speech therapists of Audiological Departments for collecting the data of the 92 children with cochlear implants (Finnish University Hospitals of Helsinki, Turku, Tampere, Kuopio and Oulu) and to Kimmo Vehkalahti, PhD, for statistical comments.

References

Archbold, S.M., Lutman, M.E. and Marshall, D. (1995) Categories of auditory perception. *Annals of Otology, Rhinology & Laryngology* 104 (Suppl. 166), 312–314.

Bates, E., Dale, P.S. and Thal, D. (1995) Individual differences and their implications for theories of language development. In P. Fletcher and B. MacWhinney (eds) *The Handbook of Child Language* (pp. 96–151). Oxford: Blackwell.

Brackett, D. and Zara, C.V. (1998) Communication outcomes related to early implantation. *The American Journal of Otology* 19 (4), 453–460.

Chute, P.M. and Nevins, M.E. (2003) Educational challenges for children with cochlear implants. *Topics in Language Disorders* 23 (1), 57–68.

Copeland, B.J. and Pillsbury, H.C. (2004) Cochlear implantation for the treatment of deafness. *Annual Review of Medicine* 55, 157–167.

Dewart, H. and Summers, S. (1995). *The Pragmatics Profile of Everyday Communication Skills in Children*. Windsor: NFER Nelson.

Edwards, S., Fletcher, P.P., Garman, G., Hughes, A., Letts, C. and Sinka, I. (1997) *The Reynell Developmental Language Scales III*. Windsor: NFER-Nelson.

Ertmer, D.J. (2001) Emergence of a vowel system in a young cochlear implant recipient. *Journal of Speech, Language and Hearing Research* 44 (4), 803–813.

Ertmer, D.J. and Mellon, J.A. (2001) Beginning to talk at 20 months: Early vocal development in a young cochlear implant recipient. *Journal of Speech, Language and Hearing Research* 44 (1), 192–206.

Ertmer, D.J., Strong, L.M. and Sadagopan, N. (2003) Beginning to communicate after cochlear implantation: Oral language development in a young child. *Journal of Speech, Language and Hearing Research* 46 (2), 328–340.

Estabrooks, W. (1998) Learning to listen with cochlear implant: A model for children. In W. Estabrooks (ed.) *Cochlear Implants for Kids* (pp. 72–88). Washington: Alexander Graham Bell Association for the Deaf.

Geers, A. (2004) Speech, language, and reading skills after early cochlear implantation. *Archives of Otololaryngology-Head & Neck Surgery* 130, 634–638.

Huttunen, K., Sorri, M. and Välimaa, T. (2003) Parents' views of their childern's habilitation after cochlear implantation. In *Measuring the Immeasurable? Proceedings of a Conference on Quality of Life in Deaf Childern. Nottingham, UK* (pp. 87–96). Oxford: Hughes.

Huttunen, K., Välimaa, T. and Sorri, M. (2004) Development of speech intelligibility after pediatric cochlear implantation. *Abstracts of the 7th European Symposium for Pediatric Cochlear Implantation*, Geneva 2.-5.1004, 52.

Inscoe, J. (1999) Communication outcomes after pediatric cochlear implantation. *International Journal of Pediatric Otorhinolaryngology* 47, 195–200.

Kirk, K.I., Miyamoto, R.T., Lento, C.L., Ying, E., O'Neill, T. and Fears, B. (2002) Effects of age at implantation in young children. *Annals of Otology, Rhinology & Laryngology* 111, 69–73.

Kohonen, R. (2001) Katson, kuuntelen, jäljittelen ja puhun – kuvaus kokleaimplanttia käyttävän lapsen vuorovaikutustaitojen kehittymisestä [I am able to watch, listen, imitate and speak. Development of interactive abilities in a child with cochlear implant]. MA thesis in Logopedics, University of Helsinki, Department of Speech Sciences.

Kohonen, R. and Lonka, E. (2002) Utveckling av preverbala interaktionsfärdigheter hos ett barn med cochlearimplantat [Development of interactive abilities in a child with cochlear implant]. NAS-kongress Helsingfors 26–28.5. 2002.

Kunnari, S. (2003) Consonant inventories: A longitudinal study of Finnish-speaking children. *Journal of Multilingual Communication Disorders* 1 (2), 124–131.

Lederberg, A.E. (1993) The impact of deafness to mother-child and peer relationships. In M. Marschark and M.D. Clark (eds) *Psychological Perspectives on Deafness* (pp. 7–26). Hillsdale, NJ: LEA.

Locke, J.L. (1997) A theory of neurolinguistic development. *Brain and Language* 58, 265–326.

Lonka, E., Olkkola, A., Vikman, S. and Savinainen-Makkonen, T. (2004) CI-children acquiring Finnish phonology. *Abstract and poster presented in the 7th European Symposium on Paediatric Cochlear Implantation*, Geneva 2–5 May 2004.

McCune, L. and Vihman, M. (2001) Early phonetic and lexical development: A productivity approach. *Journal of Speech, Language and Hearing Research* 44 (3), 670–685.

Maki-Torkko, E., Lindholm, P., Väyrynen, M., Leisti, J. and Sorri, M. (1998) Epidemiology of moderate to profound childhood hearing impairments in Northern Finland. Any changes in ten years? *Scandinavian Audiology* 27 (2), 95–103.

Manrique, M., Cervera-Paz, J., Huarte, A. and Molina, M. (2004) Advantages of cochlear implantation in prelingual deaf children before 2 years of age when compared with later implantation. *The Laryngoscope* 114, 1462–1469.

Miyamoto, R.T., Houston, D.M., Kirk, K.I., Perdew, A.E. and Svirsky, M.A. (2003) Language development in deaf infants following cochlear implantation. *Acta Oto-Laryngologica* 123 (2), 241–245.

Miyamoto, R.T., Kirk, K.I., Svirsky, M.A. and Sehgal, S.T. (1999) Communication skills in pediatric cochlear implant recipients. *Acta Oto-Larycologica* 119, 219–224.

Moore, J.K. (2002) Maturation of human auditory cortex: implications for speech perception. *Annals of Otology, Rhinogy & Laryngology* 111, 7–10.

Nikolopoulos, T., Dyar, D., Archbold, S. and O'Donoghue, G. (2004a) Development of spoken grammar following cochlear implantation in prelingually deaf children. *Archives of Otolaryngology-Head & Neck Surgery* 130, 629–633.

Nikolopoulos, T., Dyar, D. and Gibbin, K. (2004b) Assessing candidate children for cochlear implantation with the Nottingham Children's Implant Profile (NChIP): The first 200 children. *International Journal of Pediatric Otorhinolaryngology* 68 (2), 127–136.

Nikolopoulos, T.P., Gibbin, K.P. and Dyar, D. (2004c) Predicting speech perception outcomes following cochlear implantation using Nottingham children's implant profile (NchIP). *International Journal of Pediatric Otorhinolaryngology* 68, 137–141.

Olkkola, A. (2002) Kuulovammaisten, sisäkorvaistutetta käyttävien lasten fonologisen ja leksikaalisen kehityksen piirteitä – kolmen lapsen tapaustutkimus [Fonological and lexical development in three children with cochlear implants]. MA thesis in Logopedics, University of Helsinki, Department of Speech Sciences.

Peng, S.C., Spencer, L. and Tomblin, J.B. (2004) Speech intelligibility of pediatric cochlear implants recipients with 7 years of device experience. *Journal of Speech, Language, and Hearing Research* 47, 1227–1236.

Peters, A.M. (1995) Strategies in the acquisition of syntax. In P.P. Fletcher and B. MacWhinney (eds) *The Handbook of Child Language* (pp. 462–482). Oxford: Blackwell.

Reynell, J. and Huntley, M. (1987) *Reynell Developmental Language Scales. Second Revision*. Windsor: NFER-Nelson.

Richter, B., Eißele, S., Laszig, R. and Löhle, E. (2002) Receptive and expressive language skills of 106 children with a minimum of 2 years' experience in hearing with a cochlear implant. *International Journal of Pediatric Otorhinolaryngology* 64 (2), 111–126.

Rimmanen, S. (2005) Matkalla kielen omaksumiseen – viiden sisäkorvaistutetta käyttävän lapsen kuulon, puheen ymmärtämisen ja tuottamisen kehitys [Targeting spoken language – development of hearing, speech understanding and production abilities in five children with cochlear implants]. MA thesis in Logopedics, University of Helsinki, Department of Speech Sciences.

Savinainen-Makkonen, T. (2000) Word-initial consonant omissions – a developmental process in children learning Finnish. *First Language* 20, 161–185.

Serry, T.A., Blamey, P.J. and Crogan, M. (1997) Phoneme acquisition in the first 4 years of implant use. *American Journal of Otology* 18 (Suppl.), S122–124.

Sharma, A., Tobey, E., Dorman, M., Baharadwaj, S., Martin, K., Gilley, P. and Kunkel, F. (2004) Central auditory maturation and babbling development in infants with cochlear implants. *Archives of Otolaryngology- Head & Neck Surgery* 130, 511–516.

Spencer, L.J., Barker, B.A. and Tomblin, J.B. (2003) Exploring the language and literacy outcomes of pediatric cochlear implant users. *Ear and Hearing* 24 (3), 236–247.

Svirsky, M., Stallings, L., Ying, E., Lento, C. and Leonard, L. (2002) Grammatical morphologic development in pediatric cochlear implant users may be affected by the perceptual prominence of the relevant markers. *Annals of Otology, Rhinology & Laryngology, Supplement 189* 111 (5), 109–113.

Tait, M., Lutman, M. and Nikolopoulos, T. (2001) Communication development in young deaf children; Review of the video analysis method. *International Journal of Pediatric Otorhinolaryngology* 61, 105–112.

Tait, M., Lutman, M. and Robinson, K. (2000) Preimplant measures of preverbal communicative behavior as predictors of cochlear implant outcomes in children. *Ear and Hearing* 21 (1), 18–24.

Walzman, S.B., Scalchunes, V. and Cohen, N.L. (2000) Performance of multiply handicapped children using cochlear implants. *The American Journal of Otology* 21, 329–335.

Vihman, M.M., Ferguson, C.A. and Elbert, M. (1986) Phonological development from babbling to speech: Common tendencies and individual differences. *Applied Psycholinguistics* 7, 3–40.

Vihman, M.M. and McCune, L. (1994) When is a word a word. *Journal of Child Language* 21, 517–542.

Chapter 12
Speech Intelligibility in Hearing Impairment

KERTTU HUTTUNEN

Introduction

The prevalence of hearing impairments in Finland (Uimonen *et al.*, 1999) corresponds to prevalence figures reported from other western countries (Davis, 1995; Karlsmose *et al.*, 1999). About every seventh Finn (about 780,000 out of a population of 5.3 million) is estimated to have a mean of pure tone thresholds from 0.5 to 4 kHz worse than 20 dB in his/her better ear. Furthermore, as an indicator of a need for (re)habilitation, about every 15th Finn (about 280,000) is estimated to have a mean of pure tone thresholds from 0.5 to 2 kHz equal to or worse than 26 dB. In the United States and Europe, hearing impairment is, after osteoarthritis and hypertension or other cardiac/circulatory system diseases, the third most prevalent chronic condition in persons over 65 years of age (Kramer *et al.*, 2002).

About one Finnish newborn in every 1000 live births has a permanent, bilateral hearing impairment of at least moderate degree (Karikoski & Marttila, 1995; Mäki-Torkko *et al.*, 1998a; Vartiainen *et al.*, 1997). However, a great majority of children's hearing impairments are mild or moderate. When it comes to the *aetiology of hearing impairments in Finland*, roughly half of all hearing impairments and a majority of early childhood hearing impairments are genetic in origin, although in many hereditary cases the exact inheritance pattern has remained unknown (Mäki-Torkko *et al.*, 1998b; Parving *et al.*, 1998). As the consanguinity rate in Finland is low, the relatively strong founder effect and genetic drift is explained by national and regional isolation in the history of the country. Therefore, compared to many other countries, the Finnish gene pool is rather narrow, with some 40 inherited diseases that are found only in Finland or are overrepresented in Finland (Norio, 2003; Peltonen *et al.*, 1999). Syndromes that belong to the Finnish disease heritage and cause hearing impairments are Usher syndrome type III, which is manifested in progressive impairment of both hearing and vision (Pakarinen *et al.*, 1995), and infantile-onset spinocerebellar ataxia (IOSCA), a rare disease with a progressive neurological disorder and hearing impairment (Kallio & Jauhiainen, 1985; Nikali *et al.*, 1995). Both of these diseases have been traced back to the time of so-called late settlement (areas in Finland populated in the 1500s and thereafter).

Like elsewhere in Europe, mutation in the GJB2 gene encoding the connexin 26 protein accounts for a considerable part of children's prelingual non-syndromic, sensorineural hearing impairments (Löppönen *et al.*, 2003). Due to high-level prenatal and neonatal care, perinatal aetiology causes less than 10% of early childhood hearing impairments in Finland. The share of postnatal complications such as infections and ototoxic drugs is of approximately the same magnitude (Mäki-Torkko *et al.*, 1998a; Vartiainen *et al.*, 1997). Nowadays, because of the implementation of universal vaccination programmes, maternal rubella and early childhood meningitis caused by Haemophilus Influenzae type b have practically been extinguished in Finland (Mäki-Torkko *et al.*, 1998b; Peltola *et al.*, 1994).

The main cause of hearing impairments in adults is presbyacusis, hearing impairment due to ageing. Hearing impairments that emerge in the working age population are usually of hereditary origin and/or are caused by noise exposure, diseases like otosclerosis and Meniere's disease, and infections.

Speech intelligibility is an important, but complex and variable phenomenon to measure

In speech production, intelligibility – the ability of a speaker to formulate messages in a clear and understandable way – is a part of a speaker's communicative competence, and necessary for the successful use of spoken language (Connolly, 1986; Kent, 1992). Samar and Metz (1991: 699) define speech intelligibility as 'comprehensibility of the specifically linguistic information encoded by a speaker's utterances'. Naturally, the degree of intelligibility varies even within the same speaker – listener dyads and is dependent on, for example, the cooperation of both communication partners. Therefore, understandability of speech can also be seen as the degree to which the speaker's intended message is recovered by the listener at a given moment. If not defined and operationalised properly, intelligibility may be difficult to distinguish from the terms of total impression (Preminger & Van Tasell, 1995), pleasantness (Ellis & Pakulski, 2003), and acceptability (Whitehill, 2002).

Speech intelligibility is measured and followed up in all major areas of speech and language therapy and is included in many critical clinical decisions; it is measured when the severity of a communication disorder is defined, when explanations for interaction problems are sought and when decisions are made on the need of intervention. Assessment of the understandability of speech forms an integral part of the planning of therapy and of monitoring the progress in therapy, and it is also used to compare different speech training methods (Gordon-Brannan & Hodson, 2000; Huttunen, 1996). As an important measure of outcome, speech intelligibility is also used indirectly for medicolegal purposes such as making decisions on care allowances.

Many factors influence the assessment of speech intelligibility

As speech intelligibility is related to the core pragmatic abilities and mastery of spoken language, one would expect its assessment to be ideally realised in an everyday context and by interlocutors who know the speaker well. However, this is usually not viable or even preferred. Speaker and disorder familiarity has been seen as a confusing, extraneous factor, as it leads to the overestimation of speech intelligibility to strangers (Markides, 1983: 112). A pragmatic basis for assessment has high face validity together with high ecological and content validity, but compromised reliability, as familiarity with speech features typically related to the communication disorder in question and personal familiarity with the child or adult being assessed affect the result.

Speaker familiarity is one example illustrating the fact that speech intelligibility is a far from stable phenomenon; within a single speaker it is subject to change due to emotional state, vigilance/fatigue, complexity of the message, formality requirements of the interaction situation, background noise requiring to speak more loudly, and so forth. If the degree of comprehensibility of speech varies within the same speaker, so does the speech reception ability of a listener, again, because of various intrinsic and extrinsic factors. The same speaker with reduced speech intelligibility probably becomes better understood by family members (Flipsen, 1995) and professional clinicians or teachers (Huttunen, 1997; Monsen, 1981; McGarr, 1983) than by laymen. Consequently, the same speaker has a different degree of speech intelligibility in different situations and with different listeners or communication partners. Furthermore, interaction between assessment procedure (Most & Shurgi, 1993), speech material (e.g. different predictability of words, isolated words or words in sentences) and listener experience has been reported (Huttunen, 1997; McGarr, 1983). Because of the different languages in question, results from various studies (Huttunen, 1997; McGarr, 1981, 1983; Sitler *et al.*, 1983) are difficult to compare with each other. All these phenomena make assessment of speech intelligibility a challenging task both in clinical settings and in scientific research.

Speech intelligibility can be assessed by various methods

The ability of listeners to recognise open-set words, sentences and messages (percent correct score based on, preferably, a continuous-speech sample) has been seen as the most valid method of assessing speech intelligibility (Kent *et al.*, 1994). However, this method often requires recording of speech samples and, being laborious and time-consuming, it is not very practical in many hectic clinical situations. Instead, the use of closed-set item identification (transcription of phonemes, words or sentences spoken from a list in a random order) is often quicker. A problematic feature often associated with closed-set item identification is the fact that the listener easily gets accustomed to the item lists used. Among closed-set identification methods, automatic speech recognition utilising neural networks (Metz *et al.*, 1992) may not yet enhance the reliability of measurements of speech intelligibility, at least not in children and in communication disorders where the features of speech production may be notably unstable.

Different rating procedures (usually equally appearing interval scaling or percentage estimation procedures) have been used as the core methods in measuring overall speech intelligibility in clinical settings. Various discrete rating scales are widely used, and although they have been criticised for their midscale insensitivity, for not having the analytic potential to explain intelligibility deficits and also for lacking sufficient structural and criterion validity (Samar & Metz, 1991) when compared to word identification tests, they have been found to have good overall intrarater and interrater reliability (Allen *et al.*, 2001; Doyle, 1987; Samar & Metz, 1988; Subtelny, 1977). Direct magnitude estimation scaling (Ellis & Pakulski, 2003; Fucci *et al.*, 1990; Schiavetti *et al.*, 1981) has attracted some interest, too.

Use of the Visual Analogue Scale (VAS), a 100 mm long continuous scale (see reviews in, e.g. McCormack *et al.*, 1988, and Wewers & Lowe, 1990), has also recently been introduced in the assessment of speech intelligibility (e.g. Huttunen & Sorri, 2004; Keunig *et al.*, 1999). It seems to be a promising tool in perceptual assessment of speech comprehensibility. In a study by Huttunen and Sorri (2004), the reliability and validity of a horizontal VAS scale and a scale based on verbal descriptors (poor, pass, fair, good) were analysed in the assessment of speech intelligibility using item identification (percent correct score) as a criterion variable. Altogether 51 Finnish children with a mild to profound early childhood hearing impairment served as speakers in a picture naming task. The children were four to 17 years old; almost all of them used hearing aids binaurally, and 65% of them used speech as their main communication mode. Eighty-five university or polytechnic students (inexperienced in listening to the speech of children with a hearing impairment) were divided into 17 panels of five listeners each. They listened to audio recordings of four children, of whom one served as a reference speaker and the others represented low, moderate or high intelligibility (one from each of these groups). The listeners were asked to write down the words the children spoke (in a random order) and evaluate their speech intelligibility on a VAS scale and, after

that, on a scale with verbal descriptors. In contrast to many other valida-
tion studies (Bradley & Porter, 1985; Kelly *et al.*, 1986; Schiavetti *et al.*, 1981;
Subtelny, 1977), the listeners rated exactly the same speech productions
with all three different assessment procedures. Finally, the raters were
asked to specify the features of speech (if any) they thought reduced the
speech intelligibility of the child in question. The design of the listening
test is illustrated in Figure 12.1.

The reliability coefficients (Cronbach's alpha) of inter-rater reliability
were 0.99 (percent correct score), 0.98 (VAS score) and 0.96 (scale with
verbal descriptors). When the VAS speech intelligibility ratings were
compared with the percent correct scores, correlations between the different measures varied by degree of hearing impairment from 0.47 to 0.89
and were best in speech samples obtained from children with a mild or
profound hearing impairment. When all degrees of hearing impairment
were taken into account, the VAS and the rating scale with verbal descriptors correlated strongly both with item identification and with each other
(Table 12.1).

Good consistency between the three assessment methods was sustained
for both sexes, various ages and, to a somewhat lesser degree, across the
full range of intelligibility. Namely, although the VAS scores explained 81%
of the variation in the percent correct scores, it was obvious (Figure 12.2)
that the speech samples from the middle range of intelligibility were somewhat underestimated in the VAS scores compared to the values expected
on the basis of the percent correct scores. For example, the 95% confidence

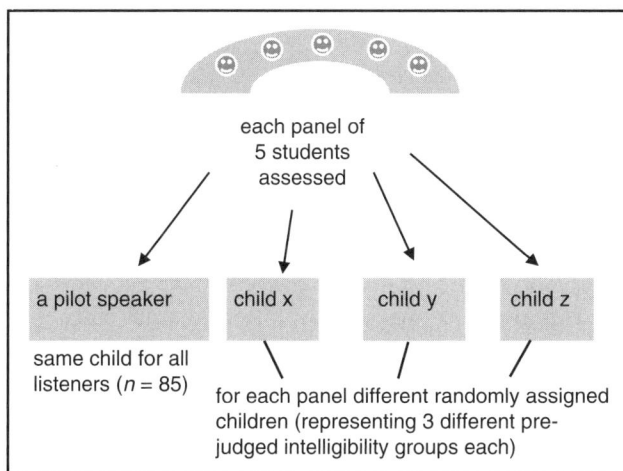

Figure 12.1 Research design of the listening test when comparing a percent correct score, a VAS score and a rating scale with verbal descriptors
with each other

Table 12.1 Correlations between percent correct score and VAS rating (Pearson's coefficient) and rating scale with verbal descriptors (Spearman's coefficient) in speech productions of children with impaired hearing

Speech intelligibility	VAS score	Scale with verbal descriptors
Percent correct score	0.90***	0.78***
VAS score		0.85***

***$p < 0.001$.

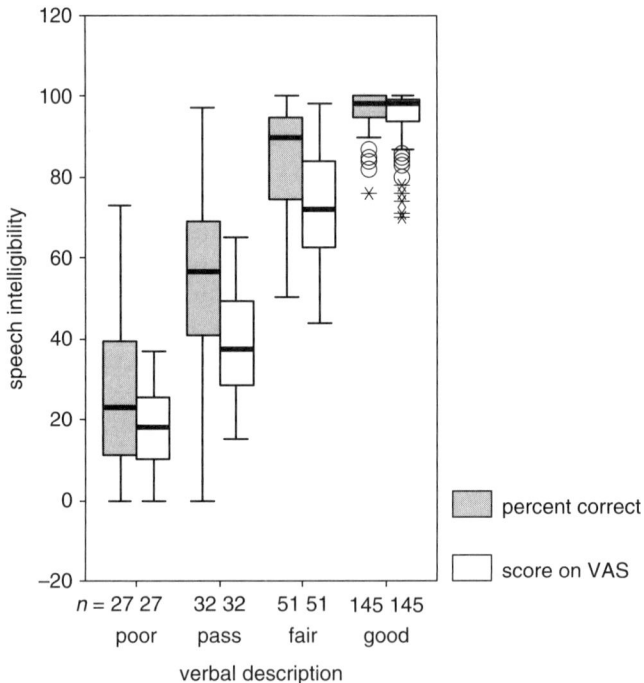

Figure 12.2 Concordance between the VAS and percent correct scores (medians and quartiles represented) plotted against a scale with verbal descriptors. *n* refers to the number of assessments given

intervals of the means obtained with these two methods did not always overlap when speech was moderately intelligible.

It was concluded (Huttunen & Sorri, 2004) that different assessment methods may be used for different purposes. With well-structured speech material specially constructed for intelligibility assessment, item identification methods may be used to trace the linguistic and acoustic-articulatory problems that reduce speech intelligibility. Rating scales on overall speech intelligibility may complement the assessment, as they are simple (easily understood, do not require long training) and relatively easy to administer, and thus suitable for frequent and repeated use with a large amount of data.

In summary, despite some published procedures (Boothroyd, 1985, 1988; Kent *et al.*, 1994; Monsen, 1981; Subtelny, 1977; Weiss, 1982) and research reports on the validity and reliability of various procedures (Allen *et al.*, 2001; Bradley & Porter, 1985; Huttunen & Sorri, 2004; Monsen, 1981; Samar & Metz, 1988; Subtelny, 1977), no simple, internationally accepted tests or procedures are available for measurement of speech intelligibility in different languages and communication disorders. Accordingly, Gordon-Brannan and Hodson (2000: 142) state that 'most clinicians make impressionistic estimates of intelligibility'. According to Kent *et al.* (1994), there may not even be a single way of assessing intelligibility that could be used successfully within all (child) populations. For assessment of children with impaired hearing, equally-appearing interval scaling (Allen *et al.*, 2001; Subtelny, 1977), although criticised (Schiavetti, 1992: 24), and identification tests with a fixed set of materials (Boothroyd, 1985; Monsen, 1981) are the most widely used procedures. It cannot be overemphasised that in clinical work, all procedures used should not only be valid and reliable, but also lead to an index that is easy to communicate to other professionals and to clients/patients and their significant others.

Speech Intelligibility in Children with Hearing Impairment

Speech intelligibility has been seen as the most important single indicator of oral communicative competence in persons with a hearing impairment (Osberger, 1992). The structure of society may influence the importance of speech and hearing ability. Today, many communities are dependent on broad communication networks. Developed countries have entered the phase of information society where literacy, speech communication (and, as a part of it, speech intelligibility) and access to, for example, modern telecommunications, are the basic requirements for participation in society; attaining information, using public services and gaining equality.

Reduced speech intelligibility in childhood hearing impairment not only compromises communicative effectiveness, affects educational choices and later employment (Huttunen & Sorri, 2001), but it may also affect the way the speaker is perceived socially. Personality traits are often evaluated on the basis of the voice characteristics of a person, possibly more so of persons with a speech disorder. For example, in a study by Most *et al.* (1996), listeners evaluated children with reduced speech intelligibility as being cognitively less competent and having more negative personality qualities. Additionally, Ellis and Pakulski (2003) found that judgements of decreased speech intelligibility correlated strongly with increased annoyance as rated by 14 mothers of children with impaired hearing.

Degree of hearing impairment is a major factor that affects speech intelligibility

It is a generally shared finding that the better the hearing level, the better the speech intelligibility of a child (Boothroyd, 1985; Conrad, 1979; Huttunen, 1997, 2000; Markides, 1983; Osberger, 1992; Smith, 1975; Suonpää, 1978). However, the association between hearing ability and intelligibility of speech is usually more consistent in children younger than 13 years of age (Reichstein & Weisel, 1986) and only in mild and moderate hearing impairments. Children with a more severe hearing impairment may represent almost any point in the continuum of intelligibility. According to Doyle (1987), Australian audiologists ($n = 54$) paid attention not only to the degree of hearing impairment, but also to audiogram configuration and pure tone threshold levels at specific frequencies when they made predictions on the future development of children's speech intelligibility. Although Monsen (1978) calculated that approximately 30% to 40% of the variability in speech intelligibility scores of the 37 children he studied was accounted for solely on the average of hearing thresholds of 0.5, 1 and 2 kHz, no consensus has been reached on the correlation between speech intelligibility and average hearing levels at specific frequencies or frequency combinations. The most often cited frequency range of importance is 0.5 to 2 (or 3) kHz. Residual hearing at higher frequencies (over 2 kHz) has been emphasised as well.

In Finland, Suonpää (1978, 1979) collected data from 86 children and adolescents (aged from 11 to 23 years, mean age 17 years) during a picture naming task. The mean pure tone thresholds of the speakers were at around a 90 dB hearing level, and their average speech recognition scores were 32% with hearing aids and 30% without. Only 21 of the subjects had open-set speech recognition ability. Altogether 43 inexperienced listeners identified correctly, on average, 47% of the 30 isolated words spoken by each child/adolescent (Suonpää, 1979; Suonpää & Aaltonen, 1981a). Later, Anttilainen (1987) used the same one to three-syllable words to test, again with an item identification method, the speech intelligibility of 10 to 17-year-olds severely hearing impaired ($n = 10$, their average better ear hearing level over the frequencies from 0.5 to 4 kHz was 90 dB) and profoundly hearing impaired children ($n = 10$, their average better ear hearing level over the frequencies from 0.5 to 4 kHz was 118 dB). The average speech intelligibility of these children was 79% and 29%, respectively.

More recently, Huttunen (2000) studied the speech intelligibility of Finnish hearing impaired children, most of them using their hearing aids regularly. There were seven children with a mild, 17 with a moderate, 13 with a severe and 14 with a profound hearing impairment. The mean pure tone thresholds of these children were at 36 dB, 51 dB, 82 dB and 108 dB hearing levels, respectively. The children were recorded at the average age of nine years (range from 4 to 17 years) during a picture naming task which comprised 62 single, one to four-syllable words depicting everyday objects and events. They used their hearing aids when giving the speech sample. No child in this sample had any concomitant disabilities. The research design of the listening tests was already introduced earlier in this chapter. When the 85 inexperienced listeners had written down the words they had heard the children speak in a random order, it was found that the mean intelligibility scores by grade of hearing impairment were 98 (the 95% confidence interval being 97–99), 96 (95–97), 86 (81–89) and 52 (45–61). The same phenomenon was noted as in many other studies; the rather strong association between the grade of hearing impairment and speech intelligibility was broken at the average hearing threshold level of 85 dB. The intelligibility scores of the children are depicted in Figure 12.3 as a function of their better ear hearing level (averaged over the frequencies of 0.5, 1, 2 and 4 kHz).

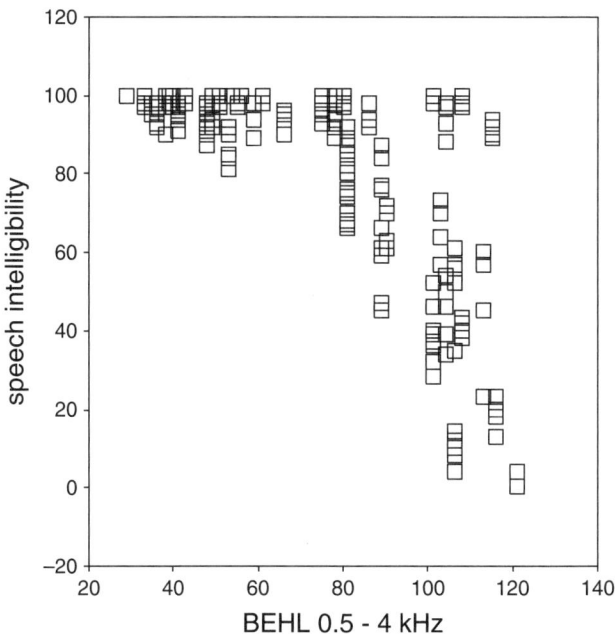

Figure 12.3 Speech intelligibility of 51 Finnish children (most of them using hearing aids regularly) aged 4 to 17 years as a function of better ear hearing levels averaged over the frequencies from 0.5 to 4 kHz

Other factors also influence speech intelligibility

Normally hearing children become more accurate in their speech production between the ages of three and five years (Huttunen & Aikio, 1998; Vance *et al.*, 2005). On the basis of research literature and their own data (47 children studied), Chin *et al.* (2003) estimated that children become fully intelligible by approximately the age of four years. Gordon-Brannan and Hodson (2000) found that about 85% of the speech of typically developing, hearing children (*n* = 48) was intelligible when they produced sentences of the BIT (Beginner's Intelligibility Test) sentence lists at the age of four years. In these researchers' opinion, above four years of age the need for intervention (when using a cut-off point of two standard deviations below the average intelligibility level) is evident if the intelligibility score falls below 66%.

Spoken language acquisition and speech intelligibility in children with a hearing impairment is generally related to their age at ascertainment of the hearing impairment (Markides, 1986; Ramkalawan & Davis, 1992; Smith, 1975; Yoshinaga-Itano, 2000). Early exposure to spoken language is mandatory for propitious development; normally hearing infants have been found to segment words from speech already from the age of approximately seven months (Jusczyk, 1999). The aim of early identification is thus to get the maximum benefit of sensitive periods of auditory, speech and language development. Namely, myelination of the auditory nerve and brain stem is completed already by about the age of six months. Although myelination of the pathway from the brain stem to the auditory cortex continues up to the age of five years (Boothroyd, 1997), auditory deprivation in early infancy, due to a sensorineural hearing impairment, has been found to lead to delayed anatomical and physiological maturation of the central auditory pathway and to be reflected in marked alterations in auditory brainstem responses (Tibussek *et al.*, 2002).

The average age at ascertainment of a hearing impairment was still too high in the 1980s and 1990s both in Finland (median age three years when including all types of hearing impairments) and elsewhere (Billings & Kenna, 1999; Davis & Wood, 1992; Mäki-Torkko, 1998; Mäki-Torkko *et al.*, 1998a). With universal hearing screening of all newborns started in some Finnish hospitals, the situation is expected to change as it has already started to change elsewhere (Harrison *et al.*, 2003). It has to be noted, however, that hearing impairments milder than about 40 dB are not detected with otoacoustic emission screenings. A high-level universal hearing screening programme leads to early identification and early intervention. Yoshinaga-Itano (2000) concluded that the age when children begin to have access to language and communication (either spoken or signed) together with the characteristics of intervention are the primary reasons for better developmental outcomes recently reported.

In the 1970s and 1980s, when hearing aids were practically the only hearing instruments available for compensation of the loss of audibility in the most severe impairments, it was found that development of speech intelligibility may cease quite early. Conrad (1979: 223) criticised especially British schools heavily; despite intensive intervention at that time, the spoken language competence of children with impaired hearing did not proceed as expected. However, this finding may imply more about the limits of auditory capacity that are met, not the effectiveness of intervention itself. Markides (1983) and Monsen (1983) also noticed that the speech intelligibility of children with a severe to profound hearing impairment did not improve much after seven to 10 years of age, and Boothroyd (1985) reported a plateau after the age of 12 years. McGarr (1987) found that the intelligibility of the 80 children taking part in her study reached a plateau at the age of 10 years. However, 16 to 19-year-old Finnish adolescents ($n = 31$) were more intelligible than 11 to 15-year-old children ($n = 25$) in the same school for the hearing impaired (Suonpää, 1978). Since Suonpää did not provide detailed information on the possible hearing level differences between these two age groups, it is difficult to judge whether that could have been the reason for the result or whether we have a real language or speech material dependent finding here.

Nowadays, in the era of cochlear implants, age at implantation is an important factor for facilitation of intelligible speech. The younger the child with a congenital or prelingual profound hearing impairment is when implanted, the better the results usually are (Nikolopoulos *et al.*, 1999). Chin *et al.* (2003) point out that, in addition to younger age at implantation, a variety of factors, like improved hardware and software and improvements in habilitation, have led to increased expectations that children using cochlear implants can catch up with children with normal hearing. Although there may sometimes be fairly large individual variation in results, good speech perception abilities (O'Donoghue *et al.*, 1999), speech as the main communication mode of the child (Archbold *et al.*, 2000), and full or partial mainstream classroom placement (Tobey *et al.*, 2004) have been found to be associated with good speech intelligibility. A hearing impairment caused by intrauterine cytomegalovirus infection seems to indicate poorer than average prognosis for speech intelligibility (Ramirez Inscoe & Nikolopoulos, 2004). As regards genetic factors, the non-syndromic aetiology of a hearing impairment does not, at first glance, seem to affect speech production as such, but, according to Sinnathuray *et al.* (2004), a GJB2 gene-related hearing impairment may, for still unknown reasons, have implications for better outcomes in speech intelligibility after cochlear implantation.

Depending on the age of the child, during the first two years after implantation the child's speech is often unintelligible or contains mainly prerecognisable words (Allen *et al.*, 1998). Five years after implantation two thirds of the children ($n = 29$) in Camels *et al.*'s (2004) study reached the two highest ratings on the five-point SIR (Speech Intelligibility Rating) scale. That is to say that connected speech produced by these children was intelligible either to 'all listeners' or to 'a listener who has a little experience of a deaf person's speech'. Results from Finnish data are in line with studies conducted elsewhere; 18 children with a profound prelingual hearing impairment were found to achieve median speech intelligibility scores (assessment on a VAS scale by children's speech and language therapists) from 46 (one year after activation) to 78 (five years after activation) (Huttunen *et al.*, 2004). In questionnaire responses, the parents of 33 Finnish implanted children expressed their satisfaction with especially the spoken language communicative abilities of their child (Huttunen & Rimmanen, 2004; Huttunen *et al.*, 2005).

When the speech intelligibility of children is concerned, it must be borne in mind that approximately two out of every five children with a hearing impairment also have associated clinical or developmental problems (Fortnum & Davis, 1997), the most common of them being cognitive impairments (learning and attention disorders), visual impairments and neurological problems (motor delays, cerebral palsy, seizures). This has also proven true in Finland (Voutilainen *et al.*, 1988). Naturally, speech intelligibility is often lower when the child has associated problems (Huttunen *et al.*, 2004; Smith, 1975).

Language and speech characteristics are related to speech intelligibility

Since many developmental phenomena are often non-linear and inter-correlated, basic-level correlational analyses do not suffice in this complex field of research. Our knowledge of the characteristics of language and speech affecting speech intelligibility is therefore still quite modest.

As the age of the child is related to his/her linguistic competence, Osberger (1992) reasoned that it is likely that linguistic deficits interact with articulatory and prosodic features. Indeed, the least intelligible speakers have been found to have problems with consonant clusters/sequences, polysyllabic words and more complex syntax and phonology (Monsen, 1978). Overall spoken language development and specifically phonological, lexical, syntactic and morphological deficiencies, together with multiple articulation errors, of Finnish children with a hearing impairment were strongly associated with speech intelligibility in the study by Huttunen (2000: 113). Table 12.2 presents the factors that had statistically significant association with speech intelligibility when multivariate analysis of repeated measurements was applied with age, sex and grade of hearing impairment held constant in the statistical models used.

Table 12.2 Factors related to communication, language, speech and education that were statistically significantly associated with the speech intelligibility of 51 Finnish children

Factor	Increase or decrease in speech intelligibility in %
Main communication mode (compared to speech)	
Speech and signs	−9.7%**
Finnish Sign Language	−44.8%***
Educational setting (compared to full mainstreaming), n = 39, as 12 were not yet in school	
School for the hearing impaired	−16.8%***
Success at school (compared to normal success in a mainstreamed setting), n = 36	
School for the hearing impaired, grade matching age level	−14.9%***
Verbal language development (compared to normal, on the basis of information on patient files)	
Emerging (i.e. very much delayed)	−13.8%***
Lexical, syntactic and morphological development (compared to normal, on the basis of information on patient files)	
Emerging (i.e. very much delayed)	−28.2%***
Articulation errors (compared to normal, on the basis of information on patient files)	
More than three errors	−20.1%***
Phonological processes (per process, compared to those of seven children with a mild hearing impairment, phonological pattern analysis in a picture naming task)	−11.6%***
Duration of vowels (per 10 ms, compared to values of seven children with a mild hearing impairment)	−0.7%***
Duration of words (per 10 ms, compared to values of seven children with a mild hearing impairment)	−0.2%***

$**p < 0.01$, $***p < 0.001$.

When the acoustic features affecting speech intelligibility are explored, the optimal speech data are those derived from the level of single words or meaningless syllables. At the sentence or continuous speech level the acoustic/phonetic features are so intertwined with complex linguistic phenomena that it is usually impossible to detail the effects of single features separately. Segmental features are usually seen as more important than suprasegmental (prosodic) ones (Levitt & Stromberg, 1983; Maassen & Povel, 1985; Markides, 1983; Smith, 1975). The listeners of 51 Finnish children with a mild to profound hearing impairment also detailed many more segmental than prosodic errors when they were asked to list factors reducing the children's intelligibility (Huttunen, unpublished data). However, when studying 8 to 15-year-old children with a profound hearing impairment, Smith (1975) found that children with roughly the same proportion of segmental errors may have speech intelligibility scores that differ from each other by up to 30 percentage points. Furthermore, segmental and prosodic features often strongly correlate with each other.

Poor control of voicing leads children with hearing impairment to replace voiced phonemes with their voiceless cognates (Chin *et al.*, 2001), and improper control of the velum is behind nasal-plosive substitutions. Omissions, vowel and diphthong errors, final consonant errors and adventitious sounds (except those obviously operating as transitional sounds to ease the movement from one place of articulation to another) have been reported to have the greatest negative effect on intelligibility (Levitt & Stromberg, 1983; Markides, 1983; Parkhurst & Levitt, 1978; Smith, 1975). When Parkhurst and Levitt (1978) examined the speech of 40 children, they found that among prosodic features, very long duration and pitch breaks had the greatest negative effect on intelligibility. The importance of correctly produced durations has also been recognised by Metz *et al.* (1985) in the speech of young adults with a congenital severe hearing impairment, and recently by Tobey *et al.* (2003) in the speech of children using cochlear implants. An inappropriate rate of speech, fundamental frequency and variation in pitch and loudness also affect speech intelligibility negatively (Asp, 1975).

In the English language, the role of consonants in speech intelligibility is greater than that of vowels (Tobey *et al.*, 2003). In severe childhood hearing impairments ($n = 30$), the most vulnerable consonants were affricates, fricatives and glides (semi-vowels) (McDermott & Jones, 1984). The Finnish counterparts (all grades of hearing impairments included) have been found to consist of at least fricatives (despite the rather simple fricative paradigm in Finnish). In vowels, open vowel and front-back substitutions and monophthongisation of diphthongs are prevalent in profound hearing impairments (Huttunen, 2000: 78–85; Suonpää & Aaltonen, 1981b).

In the study by Huttunen (2000: 86), consonant place errors occurred clearly more often than manner errors. This finding is consistent with research showing that the place of articulation is not as well identified as voicing and the manner of articulation in speech perception hampered by hearing impairments (Dorman & Hannley, 1985). Compared to normally hearing 15-year-old subjects ($n = 5$), children with a moderate to profound hearing impairment ($n = 44$) had statistically significantly more articulatory and phonological errors combined ($p < 0.0001$). A phonological pattern analysis (Huttunen, 2000: 83, 2001) revealed that most of the speech errors in mild and moderate hearing impairments were phonetic in nature (80% and 57%, respectively), whereas phonological problems were the most prevalent ones in severe and profound hearing impairments. As the picture naming test used comprised one to four-syllable words, it was possible to compare the children's productions by target word length. Given the binary values of 0 (word not identified by the listeners or confused with another word) and 1 (word identified correctly) for the one, two, three and four-syllable words, the average recognition values were 0.77, 0.84, 0.86 and 0.80, respectively. Most of the target words comprised two syllables. The most intelligible words represented syllable types VV-CV (*auto* 'car', *äiti* 'mother'), CVV-CV (*poika* 'boy', *pöytä* 'table'), CV-CV (*nenä* 'nose'), V-CV-CV (*orava* 'squirrel') and, somewhat surprisingly, CVCC-CV-CV (*kynttilä* 'candle') (Huttunen, unpublished data). Consonant substitutions, additions and omissions/reductions, together with vowel substitutions, prolongations and distortions were rather prevalent in all except mild hearing impairment and increased with decreasing hearing ability. Also Hurme and Sonninen (1982, 1985) found that Finnish children with a hearing impairment have difficulty producing correct word durations. Durations are of special importance in Finnish because they may affect word meanings.

Speech Intelligibility in Adults with Acquired Hearing Impairment

Severe to profound hearing impairment acquired in adulthood may sometimes have individually variable effects on speech features. Speech deterioration after an acquired hearing impairment has been explained by the loss of monitoring of speech gestures by audition (Zimmermann & Rettaliata, 1981). According to this rather popular explanation, in the cases of minimal or missing auditory input, monitoring of speech production must be based on (secondary) tactile and kinaesthetic feedback only. Even if loss of the auditory feedback mechanism were a sudden one, speech feature changes usually take place during a longer time span (Zimmermann & Rettaliata, 1981). However, after puberty, kinaesthetic feedback is expected to be so automatised that the role of audition is more a periodical calibrator, not the basic feedback mechanism any more. This theory has been used to explain the phenomenon that after adolescence, speech, especially speech intelligibility, may not always change very much after an acquired profound hearing impairment. However, the role of somatosensory input as a feedback mechanism separate from audition has also been emphasised (Goehl & Kaufman, 1984; Tremblay *et al.*, 2003). It may thus be possible to alleviate speech deterioration via use of (primary) somatosensory information.

Pitch, intonation, speaking rate, nasality, duration of vowels, articulation, voice quality and vocal intensity have been reported to change in adult males with an acquired profound hearing impairment (Leder & Spitzer, 1990). In 12 adventitiously profoundly hearing-impaired adult women, Leder and Spitzer (1993) found the fundamental frequency to be significantly higher, intensity significantly greater, and speaking rate significantly slower than those of 20 normal-hearing control subjects of the same sex and age. As in children, consonants are usually more affected than vowels. However, sustaining vowel qualities may sometimes be difficult as well, as the vocal tract is rather open during production of vowels, providing the speaker with only minimal proprioceptive feedback. That is why vowels have been reported to lose their acoustic features in adolescents and adults after an acquired hearing impairment (Plant, 1984; Schenk *et al.*, 2003). Deterioration of phonological processing skills has also been detected (Andersson & Lyxell, 1999). Despite changes in speech production, reported in many studies, reasonably good intelligibility of speech is maintained after a postlingual acquired hearing impairment (Palethorpe & Watson, 2003). When intelligibility has been degraded, improvements have been noted in the speech of English and Dutch subjects three to 12 months after restoration of hearing with cochlear implantation (Gould *et al.*, 2001; Langereis *et al.*, 1999).

Published Finnish data on the speech intelligibility of adults with a hearing impairment is lacking. Only some indirect information is available on features of speech production of adults who have lost their hearing in adulthood and are now using cochlear implants (Hyvärinen *et al.*, 2002; Naumanen *et al.*, 1998; Salo *et al.*, 2002). After implantation, a slight tendency towards lowering of the fundamental frequency has been reported, especially for male speakers, together with normalised formant values. A more normal vowel quadrilateral would also imply better speech intelligibility, but this has not yet been studied.

Implications for Speech and Language Therapy

Speech intelligibility is a multifactorial phenomenon. Although individual components of intelligibility are not known in detail, and various speech and language features are intertwined, it is generally agreed that segmental aspects are more important than prosodic ones. It has been concluded that improving only prosodic features in speech therapy is not sufficient for gains in speech intelligibility (Stevens *et al.*, 1983). This is not to say that prosodic features would not support intelligibility or be important in the naturalness of speech. In spite of the somewhat minor role of prosodic features in general, the ability to control segment durations is of special importance in the Finnish language, since phonemic quantity is distinctive both for vowels and consonants. Furthermore, a stable phonological system (Huttunen, 2000: 114) and the ability to sustain the correct manner of articulation are possibly more important than the correct place of articulation. However, in planning the content of rehabilitation, much is still dependent on the skills and intuition of the therapist. Gordon-Brannan *et al.* (1992) emphasised well structured, intensive intervention to be supported by a thorough examination and follow-up of hearing, and good amplification. Naturally, with all children mature enough, intervention strategies should include appropriate communication repair strategies to be used when the speech of a child is not understood. Support for language development also supports development of speech intelligibility.

Most children with hearing disorders have a mild or moderate hearing impairment. Therefore, they are able to use their audition (restored with a hearing instrument) in acquiring spoken language and practising speech. For children with a profound hearing impairment (and increasingly also severe, along with implantation criteria being relaxed), cochlear implants have enhanced access to the auditory world. Practising of auditory attention, discrimination and memory (Morgan Barrie, 1995) is therefore of importance in enhancement of speech intelligibility. Namely, for a (still illiterate) child, auditory information (supplemented by speechreading and possibly use of signs) is essential in acquiring the internal representations of phonological, lexical, morphological and syntactical systems of spoken languages.

Despite compensation with hearing instruments, auditory information about the speech of others and the child him/herself is usually not complete in a hearing-impaired child. Therefore, attention needs to be drawn in speech therapy to fine-motor co-ordination of the sets of muscles which control the speech and breathing organs. Intelligibility is enhanced by the distinctiveness of phonemic features and prosody, which, in turn, is based on the consistency of muscle movement patterns.

Planning of therapy is easier when working with adults; adults are able to say what they hear, their linguistic system is fully developed, and their own motivation, self-monitoring skills and cognitive capacity allow for target-oriented training with special techniques (Bernhardt *et al.*, 2003). In adults who speak Finnish, one would expect rather good restoration of articulation of the fricative[s] (which may easily be omitted or lose its quality in profound hearing impairments) after cochlear implantation, as it is reported to be recognised rather well already one month after activation of the implant (Välimaa *et al.*, 2002). Overall, a rather small portion of adults with a hearing impairment are in need of rehabilitative actions for improvement of speech intelligibility.

References

Allen, C., Nikolopoulos, T.P. and O'Donoghue, G.M. (1998) Speech intelligibility in children after cochlear implantation. *The American Journal of Otology* 19 (6), 742–746.

Allen, C., Nikolopoulos, T., Dyar, D. and O'Donoghue, G. (2001) Reliability of a rating scale for measuring speech intelligibility after pediatric cochlear implantation. *Otology and Neurotology* 22 (5), 631–633.

Andersson, U. and Lyxell, B. (1999) Phonological deterioration in adults with an acquired severe hearing impairment. A deterioration in long-term memory or working memory? *Scandinavian Audiology* 28 (4), 241–247.

Anttilainen, K. (1987) Vaikeasti kuulovammaisen lapsen puheen ymmärrettävyys [Speech intelligibility of children with a severe hearing impairment]. In J. Salminen, M. Kortesmaa, M. Lehtihalmes, S. Marna and U. Ström (eds) *Puheterapian vuosikirja 4* (pp. 129–132). Suomen Puheterapeuttiliiton julkaisuja, 15. Helsinki: Finnish Association of Speech Therapists.

Archbold, S.M., Nikolopoulos, T.P., Tait, M., O'Donoghue, G.M., Lutman, M.E. and Gregory, S. (2000) Approach to communication, speech perception and intelligibility after paediatric cochlear implantation. *British Journal of Audiology* 34 (4), 257–264.

Asp, C.W. (1975) Measurement of aural speech perception and oral speech production of the hearing impaired. In S. Singh (ed.) *Measurement Procedures in Speech, Hearing, and Language* (pp. 191–218). Baltimore: University Park Press.

Bernhardt, B., Gick, B., Bacsfalvi, P. and Ashdown, J. (2003) Speech habilitation of hard of hearing adolescents using electropalatography and ultrasound as evaluated by trained listeners. *Clinical Linguistic and Phonetics* 17 (3), 199–216.

Billings, K.R. and Kenna, M.A. (1999) Causes of pediatric sensorineural hearing loss. *Archives of Otolaryngology, Head and Neck Surgery* 125 (5), 517–521.

Boothroyd, A. (1985) Evaluation of speech production of the hearing impaired: Some benefits of forced-choice testing. *Journal of Speech and Hearing Research* 28 (2), 185–196.

Boothroyd, A. (1988) Perception of speech pattern contrasts from auditory presentation of voice fundamental frequency. *Ear and Hearing* 9 (6), 313–321.

Boothroyd, A. (1997) Auditory development of the hearing child. *Scandinavian Audiology* 26 (Suppl. 46), 9–16.

Bradley, K.F. and Porter, S. (1985) A comparison of three speech intelligibility measures of deaf students. *American Annals of the Deaf* 130 (6), 514–525.

Camels, M-N., Saliba, I., Wanna, G., Cochard, N., Fillaux, J., Deguine, O. and Fraysse, B. (2004) Speech perception and speech intelligibility in children after cochlear implantation. *International Journal of Pediatric Otorhinolaryngology* 68 (3), 347–351.

Chin, S.B., Finnegan, K.R. and Chung, B.A. (2001) Relationships among types of speech intelligibility in pediatric users of cochlear implants. *Journal of Communication Disorders* 34 (3), 187–205.

Chin, S.B., Tsai, P.L. and Gao, S. (2003) Connected speech intelligibility of children with cochlear implants and children with normal hearing. *American Journal of Speech-Language Pathology* 12 (4), 440–451.

Connolly, J.H. (1986) Intelligibility: A linguistic view. *British Journal of Disorders of Communication* 21 (3), 371–376.

Conrad, R. (1979) *The Deaf Schoolchild. Language and Cognitive Function*. London: Harper & Row.

Davis, A. (1995) *Hearing in Adults*. London: Whurr.

Davis, A. and Wood, S. (1992) The epidemiology of childhood hearing impairment: Factors relevant to planning of services. *British Journal of Audiology* 26 (2), 77–90.

Dorman, M.F. and Hannley, M.T. (1985) Identification of speech and speechlike signals by hearing impaired listeners. In R.G. Daniloff (ed.) *Speech Science. Recent Advances* (pp. 111–153). London: Taylor & Francis.

Doyle, J. (1987) Reliability of audiologist's ratings of the intelligibility of hearing-impaired children's speech. *Ear and Hearing* 8 (3), 170–174.

Ellis, L.W. and Pakulski, L. (2003) Judgments of speech intelligibility and speech annoyance by mothers of children who are deaf or hard of hearing. *Perceptual and Motor Skills* 96 (1), 324–328.

Flipsen Jr, P. (1995) Speaker-listener familiarity: Parents as judges of delayed speech intelligibility. *Journal of Communication Disorders* 28 (1), 3–19.

Fortnum, H. and Davis, A. (1997) Epidemiology of permanent childhood hearing impairments in Trent Region, 1985–1993. *British Journal of Audiology* 31 (6), 409–436.

Fucci, D., Ellis, L. and Petrosino, L. (1990) Speech clarity/intelligibility: Test-retest reliability of magnitude-estimation scaling. *Perceptual and Motor Skills* 70 (1), 232–234.

Goehl, H. and Kaufman, D.K. (1984) Do the effects of adventitious deafness include disordered speech? *Journal of Speech and Hearing Disorders* 49 (1), 58–64.

Gordon-Brannan, M. and Williams Hodson, B. (2000) Intelligibility/severity measurements of prekindergarten children's speech. *American Journal of Speech-Language Pathology* 9 (2), 141–150.

Gordon-Brannan, M., Hodson, B. and Wynne, M. (1992) Remediating unintelligible utterances of a child with a mild hearing loss. *American Journal of Speech-Language Pathology* 1 (4), 28–38.

Gould, J., Lane, H., Vick, J., Perkell, J.S., Matthies, M.L. and Zandipour, M. (2001) Changes in speech intelligibility of postlingually deaf adults after cochlear implantation. *Ear and Hearing* 22 (6), 453–460.

Harrison, M., Roush, J. and Wallace, J. (2003) Trends in age of identification and intervention in children with hearing loss. *Ear and Hearing* 24 (1), 89–95.

Hurme, P. and Sonninen, A. (1982) Normaalikuuloisten lasten ja aikuisten sekä kuulovammaisten lasten tuottamien KVKV – sekä KVKKV-sanojen kestohahmoista [Duration patterns in Finnish CVCV and CVCCV words as produced by children and adults with normal hearing and by children with hearing impairment]. In A. Iivonen and H. Kaskinen (eds) *XI Fonetiikan päivät – Helsinki 1982* (pp. 39–53). Publications of the Department of Phonetics 35. Helsinki: University of Helsinki.

Hurme, P. and Sonninen, A. (1985) Development of durational patterns in Finnish CVCV and CVCCV words. In P. Hurme (ed.) *Puheentutkimuksen alalta 6* (pp. 3–14). Jyväskylän yliopiston viestintätieteiden laitoksen julkaisuja 1. Jyväskylä: University of Jyväskylä.

Huttunen, K. (1996) Kuulovammaisten puheen ymmärrettävyyden arviointi [Assessment of speech intelligibility of a person with a hearing impairment]. In K. Hyttinen, T. Jääskeläinen, L. Korjus-Julkunen, A. Timonen and P. Toivonen (eds) *Puheterapian uudet suunnat – Logopedinen tutkimus ja kuntoutus tänään.* Suomen Puheterapeuttiliitto ry:n 30-vuotisjuhlajulkaisu (pp. 78–98). Helsinki: Puheterapeuttien Kustannus.

Huttunen, K. (1997) Vibraation käyttöön perustuvan puheterapian vaikutus erittäin vaikeasti kuulovammaisen lapsen puheen prosodiikkaan ja puheen ymmärrettävyyteen [Effect of speech therapy based on the use of vibration on the prosody and speech intelligibility of children with a hearing impairment]. Unpublished Licentiate's thesis, University of Oulu, Oulu, Finland.

Huttunen, K. (2000) Early childhood hearing impairment: Speech intelligibility and late outcome. Acta Universitatis Ouluensis B 35. PhD thesis, University of Oulu, Oulu, Finland.

Huttunen, K. (2001) Phonological development in 4- to 6-year-old moderately hearing impaired children. *Scandinavian Audiology* (Suppl. 53), 79–82.

Huttunen, K. and Aikio, A-R. (1998) Comparison of durations of single words produced by children and adults. In K. Heinänen and M. Lehtihalmes (eds) *Proceedings of the Seventh Nordic Child Language Symposium* (pp. 94–98). Publications of the Department of Finnish, Saami and Logopedics, 13. Oulu: University of Oulu.

Huttunen, K. and Rimmanen, S. (2004) Lasten kuulonkuntoutuksen tuloksia puheterapeutin näkökulmasta [Effectiveness of children's hearing care – the view of the speech and language therapist]. In E. Lehto, M. Hasan and R. Parkas and (eds) *Satakieliseminaari 2004* (pp. 19–30). Helsinki: Kuulonhuoltoliitto.

Huttunen, K. and Sorri, M. (2001) Long-term outcome of early childhood hearing impairments in northern Finland. *Scandinavian Audiology* (Suppl. 52), 106–108.

Huttunen, K. and Sorri, M. (2004) Methodological aspects of assessing speech intelligibility among children with impaired hearing. *Acta Oto-Laryngologica (Stockh)*, 490–494.

Huttunen, K., Rimmanen, S., Vikman, S., Virokannas, N., Sorri, M., Archbold, S. and Lutman, M. (2005) *Parents' views on the quality of life of their children 2 to 3 years after cochlear implantation*, Programme and Abstract Book of the 7th EFAS Congress, June 2005, Göteborg, Sweden, 71.

Huttunen, K., Välimaa, T. and Sorri, M. (2004) Development of speech intelligibility after paediatric cochlear implantation. Paper presented at *Paediatric Cochlear Implantation, 7th European Symposium*, May, Geneva, Switzerland.

Hyvärinen, H., Huttunen, K. and Sorri, M. (2002) Cochlear implantatens inverkan på vokalkvalitet hus vuxendöva [The effect of cochlear implant on the vowel quality of deafened adults]. *Program and Presentations of the 14th Congress of Nordiska Audiologiska Sällskapet*, May 2002, Helsinki, Finland, 93–94.

Jusczyk, P. (1999) How infants begin to extract words from speech. *Trends in Cognitive Sciences* 3 (9), 323–328.

Kallio, A-K. and Jauhiainen, T. (1985) A new syndrome of ophthalmoplegia, hypoacusis, ataxia, hypotonia and athetosis (OHAHA). In V. Colletti and S. D.G. Stephens (eds) *Disorders with Defective Hearing* (pp. 84–90). In M. Hoke (series ed.) *Advances in Audiology* (Vol. 3) Basel: Karger.

Karikoski J.O. and Marttila, T.I. (1995) Prevalence of childhood hearing impairment in southern Finland. *Scandinavian Audiology* 24 (2), 237–241.

Karlsmose, B., Lauritzen, T. and Parving, A. (1999) Prevalence of hearing impairment and subjective hearing problems in a rural Danish population aged 31–50 years. *British Journal of Audiology* 33 (6), 395–402.

Kelly, C., Dancer, J. and Bradley, R. (1986) Correlation of SPINE test scores to judge's ratings of speech intelligibility in hearing-impaired children. *Volta Review* 88 (3), 145–150.

Kent, R.D. (1992) Introduction. In R.D. Kent (ed.) *Intelligibility in Speech Disorders. Theory, Measurement and Management* (pp. 1–10). Amsterdam/Philadelphia: John Benjamins Publishing Company.

Kent, R.D., Miolo, G. and Bloedel, S. (1994) The intelligibility of children's speech: A review of evaluation procedures. *American Journal of Speech-Language Pathology* 3 (2), 81–95.

Keunig, K.H., Wieneke, G.H. and Dejonckere, P.H. (1999) The intrajudge reliability of the perceptual rating of cleft palate speech before and after pharyngeal flap surgery: The effects of judges and speech samples. *Cleft Palate and Craniofacial Journal* 36 (4), 328–333.

Kramer, S.E., Kapteyn, T.S., Kuik, D.J. and Deeg, D.J.H. (2002) The association of hearing impairment and chronic diseases with psychosocial health status in older age. *Journal of Aging and Health* 14 (1), 122–137.

Langereis, M.C., Bosman, A.J., van Olphen, A.F. and Smoorenburg, G.F. (1999) Intelligibility of vowels produced by post-lingually deafened cochlear implant users. *Audiology* 38 (4), 206–224.

Leder, S.B. and Spitzer, J.B. (1990) A perceptual evaluation of the speech of adventitiously deaf adult males. *Ear and Hearing* 11 (3), 169–175.

Leder, S.B., and Spitzer, J.B. (1993) Speaking fundamental frequency, intensity, and rate of adventitiously profoundly hearing-impaired adult women. *Journal of the Acoustical Society of America* 93 (4, Part 1), 2146–2151.

Levitt, H. and Stromberg, H. (1983) Segmental characteristics of the speech of hearing-impaired children: Factors affecting intelligibility. In I. Hochberg, H. Levitt and M.J. Osberger (eds) *Speech of the Hearing Impaired. Research, Training, and Personnel Preparation* (pp. 53–74). Baltimore: University Park Press.

Löppönen, T., Väisänen, M.L., Luotonen, M., Allinen, M., Uusimaa, J., Lindholm, P., Mäki-Torkko, E., Väyrynen, M., Löppönen, H. and Leisti J. (2003) Connexin 26 mutations and nonsyndromic hearing impairment in northern Finland. *Laryngoscope* 113 (10), 1758–1763.

Maassen, B. and Povel, D.-J. (1985) The effect of segmental and suprasegmental corrections on the intelligibility of deaf speech. *Journal of the Acoustical Society of America* 78 (3), 877–886.

Mäki-Torkko, E.M. (1998) Childhood hearing impairments and hearing screening. An epidemiological and clinical study of hearing in children and the implementation of the present hearing screening programme for pre-school children in Northern Finland. Acta Universitatis Ouluensis, D 462. PhD thesis, University of Oulu, Oulu, Finland.

Mäki-Torkko, E.M., Lindholm, P.K., Väyrynen, M.R.H., Leisti, J.T. and Sorri, M.J. (1998a) Epidemiology of moderate to profound childhood hearing impairments in northern Finland. Any changes in ten years? *Scandinavian Audiology* 27 (2), 95–103.

Mäki-Torkko, E., Järvelin, M.-R., Sorri, M., Muhli, A. and Oja, H. (1998b) Aetiology and risk indicators of hearing impairments in a one-year birth cohort for 1985–86 in northern Finland. *Scandinavian Audiology* 27 (4), 237–247.

Markides, A. (1983) *The Speech of the Hearing Impaired Children.* Manchester: Manchester University Press.

Markides, A. (1986) Age at fitting of hearing aids and speech intelligibility. *British Journal of Audiology* 20 (2) 165–167.

McCormack, H.M., de Horne, D.J.L. and Sheater, S. (1988) Clinical applications of visual analogue scales: A critical review. *Psychological Medicine* 18 (4), 1007–1019.

McDermott, R.P. and Jones, T.A. (1984) Articulation characteristics and listeners' judgements of the speech of children with severe hearing loss. *Language, Speech, and Hearing Services in Schools* 15 (2), 110–126.

McGarr, N. (1981) The effect of context on the intelligibility of hearing and deaf children's speech. *Language and Speech* 24 (3), 255–264.

McGarr, N.S. (1983) The intelligibility of deaf speech to experienced and inexperienced listeners. *Journal of Speech and Hearing Research* 26 (3), 451–458.

McGarr, N.S. (1987) Communication skills of hearing-impaired children in schools for the deaf. In H. Levitt, N.S. McGarr and D. Geffner (eds) *Language and Communication Skills of Deaf Children* (pp. 91–107). ASHA Monographs 26.

Metz, D.E., Samar, V.J., Schiavetti. N., Sitler, R. and Whitehead, R.L. (1985) Acoustic dimensions of hearing-impaired speakers' intelligibility. *Journal of Speech and Hearing Research* 28 (3), 345–355.

Metz, D.E., Schiavetti, N. and Knight, S.D. (1992) The use of artificial neural networks to estimate speech intelligibility from acoustic variables: A preliminary analysis. *Journal of Communication Disorders* 25 (1), 43–53.

Monsen, R. (1978) Toward measuring how well hearing-impaired children speak. *Journal of Speech and Hearing Research* 21 (2), 197–219.

Monsen, R.B. (1981) A usable test for the speech intelligibility of deaf talkers. *American Annals of the Deaf* 126 (7), 845–852.

Monsen, R.B. (1983) The oral speech intelligibility of hearing-impaired talkers. *Journal of Speech and Hearing Research* 48 (3), 286–296.

Morgan Barrie, R. (1995) Observing and assessing auditory skills in children. In S. Wirz (ed.) *Perceptual Approaches to Communication Disorders* (pp. 17–38). London: Whurr.

Most, T. and Shurgi, M. (1993) The effect of listener's experience on the evaluation of intonation contours produced by hearing-impaired children. *Ear and Hearing* 14 (2), 112–117.

Most T., Weisel, A. and Lev-Matezky, A. (1996) Speech intelligibility and the evaluation of personal qualities by experienced and inexperienced listeners. *Volta Review* 98 (4), 181–190.

Naumanen, T., Lindholm, P., Vilkman, E. and Sorri, M. (1998) Speech production after multichannel cochlear implantation in Finnish-speaking postlingually deafened adults. In Ph. Dejonckere and H.F.M. Peters (eds) *Communication and its Disorders: A Science in Progress.* Proceedings, 24th Congress International Association of Logopedics and Phoniatrics, August 1998, Amsterdam, The Netherlands, Vol II (pp. 899–902). Nijmegen: Nijmegen University Press.

Nikali, K., Suomalainen, A., Terwilliger, J., Koskinen, T., Weissenbach, J. and Peltonen, L. (1995) Random search for shared chromosomal regions in four affected individuals: The assignment of a new hereditary ataxia locus. *American Journal of Human Genetics* 56 (5), 1088–1095.

Nikolopoulos, T.M., O'Donoghue, G.M. and Archbold, S. (1999) Age at implantation: Its importance in pediatric cochlear implantation. *Laryngoscope* 109 (4), 595–599.

Norio, R. (2003) Finnish disease heritage I: Characteristics, causes, background. *Human Genetics* 112 (5–6), 441–456.

O'Donoghue, G.M., Nikolopoulos, T.P., Archbold, S.M. and Tait, M. (1999) Cochlear implants in young children: The relationship between speech perception and speech intelligibility. *Ear and Hearing* 20 (5), 419–425.

Osberger, M.J. (1992) Speech intelligibility in the hearing impaired: Research and clinical implications. In R.D. Kent (ed.) *Intelligibility in Speech Disorders. Theory, Measurement and Management* (pp. 233–264). Amsterdam/Philadelphia: John Benjamins Publishing Company.

Pakarinen, L., Karjalainen, S., Simola, K.O., Laippala, P. and Kaitalo, H. (1995) Usher's syndrome type 3 in Finland. *Laryngoscope* 105 (6), 613–617.

Palethorpe, S. and Watson, C.I. (2003) Acoustic analysis of monophthong and diphthong production in acquired severe to profound hearing loss. *Journal of the Acoustical Society of America* 114 (2), 1055–1068.

Parkhurst, P.G. and Levitt, H. (1978) The effect of selected prosodic errors on the intelligibility of deaf speech. *Journal of Communication Disorders* 11 (2–3), 249–256.

Parving, A., Admiraal, R.J.C., Apaydin, F., Arslan, E., Davis, A., Dias, O., Fortnum, H., Grisanti, G., Gross, M., Hess, M., Konradsson, K., Lina-Granade, G., Mäki-Torkko, E., Newton, V.E., O'Donovan, C., Orzan, E., Sorri, M., Stephens, D., Tsakanikos, M.D., Waagenaar, M. and Welzl-Müller, K. (1998) Epidemiology of hereditary hearing impairment in childhood – preliminary estimates from the European Union. In D. Stephens, A. Read and A. Martini (eds) *Developments in Genetic Hearing Impairment* (pp. 35–42). London: Whurr.

Peltola, H., Heinonen, O.P., Valle, M., Paunio, M., Virtanen, M., Karanko, V. and Cantell, K. (1994) The elimination of indigenous measles, mumps, and rubella from Finland by a 12-year, two-dose vaccination program. *The New England Journal of Medicine* 331 (21), 1397–1402.

Peltonen, L., Jalanko, A. and Varilo, T. (1999) Molecular genetics of the Finnish disease heritage. *Human Molecular Genetics* 8 (10), 1913–1923.

Plant, G. (1984) The effects of acquired profound hearing loss on speech production. *British Journal of Audiology* 18 (1), 39–48.

Preminger, J.E. and van Tasell, D.J. (1995) Quantifying the relation between speech quality and speech intelligibility. *Journal of Speech and Hearing Research* 38 (3), 714–725.

Ramirez Inscoe, J.M. and Nikolopoulos, T.M. (2004) Cochlear implantation in children deafened by cytomegalovirus: Speech perception and speech intelligibility outcomes. *Otology and Neurotology* 25 (4), 479–482.

Ramkalawan, T.W. and Davis, A.C. (1992) The effects of hearing loss and age at intervention on some language metrics in young hearing-impaired children. *British Journal of Audiology* 26 (2) 97–107.

Reichstein, J. and Weisel, A. (1986) Hearing tresholds as predictors of speech production performance. *Scandinavian Audiology* 15 (4), 223–226.

Salo, S., Peltola, M.S., Aaltonen, O., Johansson, R., Lang, H.A. and Laurikainen, E. (2002) Stability of memory traces for speech sounds in cochlear implant patients. *Logopedics, Phoniatrics, Vocology* 27 (3), 132–138.

Samar, V.J. and Metz, D.E. (1988) Criterion validity of speech intelligibility rating-scale procedures for the hearing impaired population. *Journal of Speech and Hearing Research* 31 (3), 307–316.

Samar, V.J. and Metz, D.E. (1991) Scaling and transcription measures of intelligibility for populations with disordered speech: Where's the beef? *Journal of Speech and Hearing Research* 34 (3), 699–702.

Schenk, B.S., Baumgartner, W.D. and Hamzavi, J.S. (2003) Effects of loss of auditory feedback on segmental parameters of vowels of postlingually deafened speakers. *Auris Nasus Larynx* 30 (4), 333–339.

Schiavetti, N. (1992) Scaling procedures for the measurement of speech intelligibility. In R. Kent (ed.) *Intelligibility in Speech Disorders* (pp. 11–34). Amsterdam: John Benjamins Publishers.

Schiavetti, N., Metz, D.E. and Sitler, R.W. (1981) Construct validity of direct magnitude estimation and interval scaling of speech intelligibility: Evidence from a study of the hearing impaired. *Journal of Speech and Hearing Research* 24 (3), 441–445.

Sinnathuray, A.R., Toner, J.G., Clarke-Lyttle, J., Geddis, A., Patterson, C.C. and Hughes, A.E. (2004) Connexin 26 (GJB2) gene-related deafness and speech intelligibility after cochlear implantation. *Otology and Neurotology* 25 (6), 935–942.

Sitler, R.W., Schiavetti, N. and Metz, D.E. (1983) Contextual effects in the measurement of hearing-impaired speakers' intelligibility. *Journal of Speech and Hearing Research* 26 (1), 30–34.

Smith, C. (1975) Residual hearing and speech production in deaf children. *Journal of Speech and Hearing Research* 18 (4), 795–811.

Stevens, K.N., Nickerson, R.S. and Rollins, A.M. (1983) Suprasegmental and postural aspects of speech production and their effect on articulatory skills and intelligibility. In I. Hochberg, H. Levitt and M.J. Osberger (eds) *Speech of the hearing impaired. Research, Training, and Personnel Preparation* (pp. 35–51). Baltimore: University Park Press.

Subtelny, M.J. (1977) Assessment of speech with implications for training. In F. Bess (ed.) *Childhood deafness: Causation, Assessment and Management* (pp. 183–194). New York: Grune & Stratton.

Suonpää, J. (1978) Vaikeasti kuulovammainen koululainen. Tutkimus Turun kuulovammaisten koulun oppilaiden kuulo- ja tasapainoelimen toiminnasta sekä kielellisestä kehityksestä [Research on the function of the hearing and balance organ of pupils in the school for the hearing impaired in Turku]. PhD thesis, Korva-, nenä- ja kurkkutautien klinikka. Turku: University of Turku.

Suonpää, J. (1979) Communicative skills of deaf children in relation to their physical and socio-psychological characteristics. *Nordisk Tidskrift for Logopedi och Foniatri* 4 (1), 55–62.

Suonpää, J. and Aaltonen, O. (1981a) Intelligibility of vowels in words uttered by profoundly hearing-impaired children. *Journal of Phonetics* 9 (4), 445–450.

Suonpää, J. and Aaltonen, O. (1981b) Phonological vowel system of the profoundly hearing impaired children. *Nordisk Tidskrift for Logopedi och Foniatri* 6 (2), 36–43.

Tibussek, D., Meister, H., Walger, M., Foerst, A. and von Wendel, H. (2002) Hearing loss in early infancy affects maturation of the auditory pathway. *Developmental Medicine and Child Neurology* 44 (2), 123–129.

Tobey, E.A., Geers, A.E., Brenner, C., Altuna, D. and Gebbert, G. (2003) Factors associated with development of speech production skills in children implanted by age five. *Ear and Hearing* 24 (1 Suppl.), 36S–45S.

Tobey, E.A., Rekart, D., Buckley, K. and Geers, A.E. (2004) Mode of communication and classroom placement impact on speech intelligibility. *Archives of Otolaryngology, Head and Neck Surgery* 130 (5), 639–643.

Tremblay, S., Shiller, D.M. and Ostry, D.J. (2003) Somatosensory basis of speech production. *Nature* 423 (6942), 866–869.

Uimonen, S., Huttunen K.H., Jounio-Ervasti, K. and Sorri M.J. (1999) Do we know the real need for hearing rehabilitation at the population level? Hearing impairments in the 5- to 75-year-old cross-sectional Finnish population. *British Journal of Audiology* 33 (1), 53–59.

Vance, M., Stackhouse, J. and Wells, B. (2005) Speech-production skills in children aged 3–7 years. *International Journal of Language and Communication Disorders* 40 (1), 29–48.

Vartiainen, E., Kemppinen, P. and Karjalainen, S. (1997) Prevalence and etiology of bilateral sensorineural hearing impairment in a Finnish childhood population. *International Journal of Pediatric Otorhinolaryngology* 41 (2), 175–185.

Voutilainen, R., Jauhiainen, T. and Linkola, H. (1988) Associated handicaps in children with hearing loss. *Scandinavian Audiology* (Suppl. 30), 57–59.

Välimaa, T.T., Määttä T.K., Löppönen, H.J. and Sorri, M.J. (2002) Phoneme recognition and confusions with multichannel cochlear implants: Consonants. *Journal of Speech, Language, and Hearing Research* 45 (5), 1055–1069.

Whitehill, T.L. (2002) Assessing intelligibility in speakers with cleft palate: A critical review of the literature. *Cleft Palate and Craniofacial Journal* 39 (1), 50–58.

Weiss, A.D. (1982) *Weiss Intelligibility Test.* Tigard, OR: CC Publications.

Wewers, M.E. and Lowe, N.K. (1990) A critical review of visual analogue scales in the measurement of clinical phenomena. *Research in Nursing and Health* 13 (4), 227–236.

Yoshinaga-Itano, C. (2000) Successful outcomes of deaf and hard-of-hearing children. *Seminars in Hearing* 21 (4), 309–326.

Zimmermann, G. and Rettaliata, P. (1981) Articulatory patterns of an adventitiously deaf speaker: Implications for the role of auditory information in speech production. *Journal of Speech and Hearing Research* 24 (2), 169–178.

Part 5
Voice Disorders

Chapter 13

Experiences from Six Years of Screening for Voice Disorders Among Teacher Students

SUSANNA SIMBERG and EEVA SALA

Introduction

The importance of the voice as an occupational tool in a number of professions today is unambiguous. During the last decades there has been increasing interest in studies associated with occupational voice disorders. A review by Vilkman (2004) shows that these studies cover a broad field of research conducted in several disciplines and that Finnish researchers have been some of the pioneers in this area.

The teaching voice has been of special interest in several studies conducted in different parts of the world. The results of these studies show that teachers frequently report voice problems (for a review see Mattiske *et al.*, 1998). In fact, vocal symptoms and voice disorders among teachers seem to be increasing. The results of a study by Simberg *et al.* (2005) employing a questionnaire showed that the number of teachers reporting two or more vocal symptoms occurring weekly or more often had increased from 5% to 20% during a 12 year period. As main background factors for this the teachers reported an increase of restless pupils and larger groups of children taught in the classes. Results of another study (Sala *et al.*, 2001) using the same questionnaire, but in which all participants also underwent a phoniatric examination, revealed that those who reported two or more frequently occurring vocal symptoms often had an organic voice disorder.

The impact of voice disorders in professions where the voice is an occupational tool is two-fold. Voice disorders not only have a negative effect on the quality of life of those who suffer from them (Ma & Yiu, 2001; Roy *et al.*, 2004a; Smith *et al.*, 1996; Yiu, 2002), but they also burden society with additional health care expenses (Verdolini & Ramig, 2001). Voice problems negatively affect job performance, and about 20% of teachers are reported to miss workdays because of voice problems (Roy *et al.*, 2004a; Sapir *et al.*,

1993; Smith *et al.*, 1997). This, of course, increases expenses for society. Another negative effect of voice disorders in teachers may be that a dysphonic voice adversely affects children's processing of spoken language (Morton & Watson, 1998; Rogerson & Dodd, 2005).

The primary risk factors for voice disorders in persons who work in vocally demanding occupations are the need for prolonged voice use and factors in the working environment that can affect voice production (Sala *et al.*, 2001; Vilkman, 2000, 2004). Such environmental factors are background noise, poor acoustic conditions and poor air quality (e.g. Morton & Watson, 1998; Pekkarinen & Viljanen, 1991; Vilkman, 1996; Vintturi *et al.*, 2003). Several authors have addressed the importance of prevention of voice disorders among those who work in vocally demanding occupations (e.g. Buekers *et al.*, 1995; De Bodt *et al.*, 1998; Fritzell, 1996; Morton & Watson, 2001; Roy *et al.*, 2004a; Russell *et al.*, 1998; Sapir *et al.*, 1993; Smith *et al.*, 1997; Verdolini & Ramig, 2001; Yiu, 2002). The issue of preventative voice care is of utmost importance with regard to students studying for such occupations.

There are some epidemiological studies concerning voice disorders and vocal symptoms in students studying for vocally demanding occupations. These studies show that voice problems are common among such students (Sapir, 1993; Simberg *et al.*, 2000; Timmermans *et al.*, 2002, 2003; Winkworth & McCabe, 2001; Yiu, 2002). These results suggest that students should preferably receive information on voice related issues and voice training during their studies. In some teacher training schools it is standard practice that all students undergo a voice examination (Orr *et al.*, 2002), but these measures probably vary significantly between different schools and countries. According to Morton and Watson (2001), primary school teachers in the United Kingdom do not receive any statutory training in voice care. This also seems to be the case in the Netherlands (Buekers, 1998). In Sweden, the educational programme for preschool teachers offers limited or no voice training (Södersten *et al.*, 2002). In Finland, too, issues relating to voice receive little attention in educational programmes for teachers. Most students at Finnish universities take part in a compulsory course (one to two credits) in communication skills. However, the content of the course varies in different universities, and information about ergonomic factors in vocal behaviour is not necessarily included at all, not even for those who are preparing themselves for careers as teachers.

Development of a Voice Screening Test

Marge (1991) mentions two types of prevention of voice problems, that is, primary and secondary prevention. Primary prevention refers to the elimination of something that might cause a voice disorder, for example, to stop smoking or to eliminate poor acoustic conditions so as to prevent future voice disorders. Secondary prevention involves early detection and treatment of voice disorders. As one component of secondary prevention Marge (1991) mentions screening for voice disorders. One massive form of voice screening of prospective students in vocally demanding occupations, such as teaching, acting, singing and similar occupations, took place in the former German Democratic Republic over several decades (Seidner & Wendler, 2001). All candidates for these occupations were required to undergo voice and speech examinations before they were accepted into the educational programmes and were assessed as 'fit' or 'unfit'. If the condition was classified as treatable, the person received treatment and attended a follow-up examination where the suitability for the occupation was re-evaluated. More recently, Buekers (1998) has suggested measuring vocal performance in order to assess suitability for a vocally demanding profession. However, measuring vocal performance in order to exclude students from teacher education because of their current or possible future voice disorders is a rather radical suggestion, especially since the results of several studies show that voice training for students is beneficial (e.g. Broaddus-Lawrence *et al.*, 2000; Sabol *et al.*, 1995; Södersten & Hammarberg, 1993; Timmermans *et al.*, 2004). Additionally, prediction of voice problems does not seem to be uncomplicated. A longitudinal study by De Bodt *et al.* (1998) investigating whether voice problems among teachers could be predicted, showed that the vocal endurance test used in their study was not adequate for this purpose. According to the authors, a combination of laryngeal examination, measurement of maximum phonation time and a perceptual examination of voice quality could be used as a preventative measure in order to identify and help students at risk of voice disorders. Still, it appears that there are no recent, detailed descriptions of simple voice screening tests used as a routine for students studying for vocally demanding occupations.

The screening procedure described in this chapter was initiated by a study on the prevalence of voice disorders, covering all teacher students at the Department of Teacher Education at the University of Turku, Finland, in 1997. The results of that study showed that about 20% of the students participating had a voice disorder and that most of the disorders were organic; that is, there were visible findings on the vocal folds (Simberg *et al.*, 2000). Students who have voice disorders should preferably be offered voice therapy at an early stage. Accordingly, a voice screening test to identify such students was developed. Regular voice screening for teacher students has now been performed since 1999.

The questionnaire

In the study concerning the prevalence of voice disorders among teacher students (Simberg *et al.*, 2000) the 226 students participating completed a questionnaire and their voices were perceptually assessed by a speech therapist. The questionnaire consisted of 16 main groups of questions with multiple-choice sub questions (in total 80 questions). The questionnaire was designed to provide information about the prevalence of vocal symptoms. Questions about respiratory tract health problems, previous voice problems, hobbies such as singing and sports, and time spent in pubs or discotheques were also included. For the screening test, which consists of a questionnaire concerning vocal symptoms and a perceptual assessment of voice quality made by nurses, only the questions that turned out to be the most effective eliciting information about voice disorders were included. In Simberg *et al.*'s (2000) study background factors contributing to voice disorders did not associate with the laryngeal status of the subjects. The purpose of the screening test was to find students who have voice disorders, not to explore the possible background factors contributing to them. Since those subjects who had reported frequently occurring vocal symptoms often had an organic voice disorder, the questionnaire used in the screening test included the questions concerning the following vocal symptoms: (1) throat clearing or coughing, (2) the voice becomes low (low pitched) or hoarse without a cold, (3) the voice becomes strained or tires, (4) voice breaks while talking, (5) a sensation of pain or lump in the throat, (6) difficulty in being heard and (7) loss of voice (see the Appendix). A question about the occurrence of morning hoarseness was also included. The students were asked to report the vocal symptoms that had occurred *during the past year* and the frequency alternatives for the occurrence of vocal symptoms are (1) every day or most days, (2) weekly or most weeks, (3) monthly or most months, (4) less often, (5) only periodic symptoms and (6) no symptoms.

Perceptual assessment of voice quality

The perceptual assessment of voice quality in the study concerning the prevalence of voice disorders among teacher students by Simberg *et al.* (2000) was performed by a speech therapist. The main parameter used for the assessment was the overall degree of dysphonia or Grade (Hirano, 1981). The assessment was made using a visual analogue scale (VAS) which has been in common use in perceptual evaluation of voice quality since the beginning of the 1990s (Bless & Hicks, 1996). A score on 34 mm or higher on a 100 mm long VAS was chosen as the cut-off point between normal and deviant voice quality. This criterion was based on a pilot study carried out by two senior speech therapists listening to recordings of normal and disordered voices and evaluating them on a VAS. A closer analysis of the results from that study by plotting the evaluations for the parameter Grade of 226 students in rank order showed that the graph exhibited an 'elbow' with a rather abrupt discontinuity at 38.5 mm (Simberg *et al.*, 2001). This method has been used in some studies for evaluating voice quality and can be used to separate normal from deviant values in a particular population (Sederholm, 1995; Sederholm *et al.*, 1993). Since the purpose of the voice screening test was to find students with voice disorders at an early stage, a score of 35 mm was set as a cut-off point in the screening test.

In the study evaluating the screening test (Simberg *et al.*, 2001) two nurses and one speech therapist assessed the subjects' voice quality using all the GRBAS parameters, that is, Grade, Rough, Breathy, Asthenic and Strained (Hirano, 1981). For the screening test the nurses at the Student Health Service Center received brief training in the assessment of voice quality. The training consisted of a one hour lecture informing them about the most common voice disorders and vocal symptoms, including listening to voice samples of disordered voices and practising the use of the VAS used for the perceptual assessment. The lecture was followed by two test sessions separated by an interval of one week. In these sessions the nurses listened to tape recordings of 10 normal and 11 abnormal voices and made an assessment using the scale. The results of the study evaluating the screening test indicated that a nurse in a health care setting who had received a brief orientation in the assessment of voice quality could reliably perform a perceptual evaluation of overall degree of dysphonia, Grade (Simberg *et al.*, 2001). Since the results of that study showed that the highest inter- and intra-judge correlation in the perceptual assessment was for that parameter it was chosen for the voice screening test that has been used since 1999. Other authors (e.g. De Bodt *et al.*, 1997; Dejonckere *et al.*, 1993) have also found that Grade has the best inter-judge correlation. According to Kent (1996), different types of errors and variability are common in perceptual evaluations. Thus, he suggests that judging only one parameter is probably easier than judging several. This was also the opinion of the nurses during the training sessions and they considered Grade as the easiest parameter to comprehend.

Since 1998, when the screening test was developed, the training for the nurses to perform the perceptual assessment has been repeated twice at the Student Health Service Center in Turku. In the screening test, the perceptual assessments are performed in a live situation during a normal conversation and a short reading task of 77 words. The nurses are instructed to refer all students who score *35 mm or above* for overall degree of dysphonia on the VAS for a phoniatric examination. Additionally, if a student reports *two or more vocal symptoms occurring weekly or more frequently* during the past year, she/he should be referred for a phoniatric examination even if voice quality is normal.

Results from Six Years of Screening for Voice Disorders

Between 1999 and 2004 a total of 455 students from the Department of Teacher Education at the University of Turku took part in the voice screening test. These students were studying in order to become teachers in preschools, in comprehensive schools and upper secondary schools. All of them were first-year students, and they took part in the voice screening test at the beginning of their first semester at the university when attending a physical examination that is offered to all first-year students at the Student Health Service Center. The examination was voluntary, and approximately 77% of all the students at the Department of Teacher Education from 1999 to 2004 took part in the test. Completing a question-naire and the assessment of the student's voice took about five minutes of the half-hour that was reserved for the physical examination of each student.

The mean age of the 455 students participating in the screening test from 1999 to 2004 was 21.5 years (range 18–38 years). Three-hundred and eighty-four (84%) of the students were female.

Reported symptoms and perceptual evaluation of voice quality

As to the reported symptoms, 63% of the students reported no symptoms, 16% reported one symptom and 21% reported two or more symptoms occurring weekly or more often (Table 13.1).

The most common symptom was *throat clearing or coughing*, which was reported by 21% of the students. Eleven percent reported *voice becomes strained or tires*, 9% reported *voice becomes low or hoarse without a cold* and 8% reported *sensation of pain or lump in the throat*. Six percent of the students reported frequently occurring *voice breaks* and 4% reported *difficulty in being heard*. Only one subject reported *loss of voice* occurring weekly or more often (Table 13.2). One-hundred and seventeen (26%) of the students reported morning hoarseness occurring weekly or more often. The mean of the nurses' score for overall degree of dysphonia on the VAS for all students was 27 mm, ranging from 3 to 61 mm.

A total of 133 (29%) of the 455 students were referred for phoniatric examination. Of these, 118 were females. Thirty-five students were referred

Table 13.1 Number of students reporting no symptoms, one symptom and two or more symptoms occurring weekly or more often

	n	%
No symptoms	287	63
One symptom	74	16
Two or more symptoms	94	21

Table 13.2   Number of symptoms occurring weekly or more often ($n = 455$)

Symptom*	n	%
Throat clearing or coughing	94	21
Voice becomes strained or tires	48	11
The voice becomes low or hoarse without a cold	42	9
Sensation of pain or lump in the throat	38	8
Voice breaks	26	6
Difficulty in being heard	20	4
Loss of voice	1	0.2

*Please note that some students may have reported several symptoms.

for the examination because they reported two or more frequently occurring symptoms even if their voice quality was assessed as normal by the nurses, while 39 students were referred because of deviant voice quality. The students who had scored 35 mm or more on the VAS reported significantly more frequently occurring symptoms. Of the 133 students, 22 reported no frequently occurring vocal symptom and 17 reported one symptom, while 59 were referred for the examination because they had both scored 35 mm or more on the VAS and had reported two or more frequently occurring symptoms (Table 13.3).

Table 13.3   The mark on the VAS and the number of subjects reporting symptoms occurring weekly or more often during the past year; VAS below 35 mm ($n = 356$) and VAS 35 mm or more ($n = 98$)

The mark on the VAS	No symptoms	One symptom	Two or more symptoms
VAS <35 mm	264 (74%)	57 (16%)	35 (10%)
VAS 35 mm or more	23 (23%)	17 (17%)	59 (60%)

$x^2(2) = 126.875, p < 0.001$.

The phoniatric examination

The phoniatric examination comprised indirect laryngoscopy with mirror, anterior and posterior rhinoscopy, and inspection of the pharynx for signs of infection. The same equipment (Welch Allyn Lumi View REF 20501) was used for all subjects. In assessing laryngeal status, signs of erythema and oedema both in the vocal folds and in the hypopharynx were rated separately on a four-point scale (0 = no, 1 = mild, 2 = moderate and 3 = abundant). Values from zero to one were interpreted as normal. If both erythema and oedema were rated 2 or 3, the status was defined as laryngitis (Sala *et al.*, 1996). Indications of vocal nodules, polyps, and minor changes such as signs of swelling between the frontal two-thirds of the vocal folds were also noted. The students who reported two or more weekly or more frequently occurring vocal symptoms and/or deviant voice quality judged by the phoniatrician, but had no organic findings in the vocal folds, were defined as having a functional voice disorder.

If the students had a cold they were asked to postpone the appointment. Of the 133 students referred to the phoniatric examination, 93 attended. Eighty-three were female. The results of the phoniatric examination showed that the most common diagnosis were functional voice disorder (43 students) and chronic laryngitis (41 students), while five students had minor findings, three had vocal nodules and one had sulcus vocalis (Table 13.4).

Of the 93 students attending the phoniatric examination, all who had a functional voice disorder, minor findings and vocal nodules were referred to voice therapy. Additionally, 28 of those who had laryngitis were referred to voice therapy. Most of the subjects who had chronic laryngitis received medication for reflux. These students reported morning hoarseness in combination with frequently reported symptoms of throat clearing and sensation of pain or lump in the throat, which have been associated with laryngopharyngeal reflux (e.g. Koufman *et al.*, 1996). In a study of the prevalence of laryngeal pathologies in a treatment-seeking population by Coyle *et al.* (2001), reflux laryngitis was the most frequent diagnosis, and this also seems to be a common cause of voice disorders in students. Voice disorders that might be caused by laryngopharyngeal reflux should, of course, be properly examined and treated, and about half of all the students who attended the phoniatric examination were offered at least one follow-up appointment.

Table 13.4 The diagnoses made by the phoniatrician (*n* = 93) and the frequency of findings (%) in the whole population (*n* = 455).

Diagnose	*n*	% of the whole population (*n* = 455)
Functional voice disorder	43	9
Chronic laryngitis	41	9
Minor finding	5	1
Vocal nodules	3	0.7
Sulcus vocalis	1	0.2

Some data on the students who did not attend the phoniatric examination

Of the 133 students referred to the phoniatric examination, 40 did not attend. Thirty-five of these students were female. As to gender and age, these students did not differ from those who attended the examination.

Thirteen of the 40 students were referred to the phoniatric examination because they reported two or more frequently occurring symptoms even if their voice quality was assessed as normal by the nurses, while 13 students who reported no or one symptom were referred to the examination because of deviant voice quality. Fourteen students scored 35 mm or more on the VAS and reported two or more frequently occurring vocal symptoms. Twenty-one students who attended the phoniatric examination had normal voice quality but reported two or more frequently occurring symptoms, and 25 students who reported no or one symptom were referred to the examination because of deviant voice quality. Forty-five students who attended the examination scored 35 mm or more on the VAS and reported two or more frequently occurring vocal symptoms (Table 13.5). As to the reported symptoms, there were no significant differences between those who did not attend the phoniatric examination and those who did.

As to the voice quality assessed by the nurses during the screening test, it seems that the students who did not attend the phoniatric examination had in general a somewhat better voice quality than those students who attended the examination. There was a significant difference [$t(131) = 2.698$, $p = 0.008$] between the mean of the nurses mark on the VAS for the perceptual evaluation between the two groups of students. The mean was lower in the group who did not attend the examination (35.1 mm, SD = 7702, $n = 40$) than in the group that attended the examination (39.33 mm, SD = 8537, $n = 93$).

Table 13.5 The perceptual evaluation made by the nurses on the VAS (<35 mm and ≥35 mm) and the number of subjects reporting symptoms occurring weekly or more often during the past year, data from the students who chose not to attend the phoniatric examination ($n = 40$) and those who attended it ($n = 93$)

	Students who did not attend the phoniatric examination ($n = 40$)		Students who attended the phoniatric examination ($n = 93$)	
Perceptual evaluation	*No or one symptom*	*Two or more symptoms*	*No or one symptom*	*Two or more symptoms*
VAS < 35 mm[1]	0	13 (33%)	2 (2%)	21 (23%)
VAS ≥ 35 mm[2]	13 (33%)	14 (35%)	25 (27%)	45 (48%)

[1]Fisher's exact test, $p = 0.525$, n.s.
[2]Fisher's exact test, $p = 0.354$, n.s.

Practical Implementations and Recommendations

The voice screening test for students studying in order to become teachers in preschools, in comprehensive schools and in upper secondary schools has now become a routine at the Student Health Service Center in Turku. The aim of screening for voice disorders among teacher students has been to enable health care personnel to select students for phoniatric examination and voice therapy. The screening test takes five minutes to complete, and thus does not require many resources. The sensitivity of the test has not been investigated, and only those students who have deviant voice quality and/or report two or more vocal symptoms occurring weekly or more often, are referred to the phoniatric examination. It is of course possible that students with laryngeal pathologies can be among those who are not referred to the examination. A study by Elias *et al.* (1997) revealed abnormal laryngeal findings in more than half of the subjects in a population of 65 professional singers without voice complaints. Another study showed a high incidence of reflux laryngitis and vocal fold cysts in a population of 13 singing teachers without voice complaints (Heman-Ackah *et al.*, 2002). Conceivably, the screening test may not be sensitive enough to detect some students who might have laryngeal pathologies. However, this possibility has only minor practical consequences because the students with possible pathologies neither have deviant voice quality nor report frequently occurring vocal symptoms. From a practical point of view, this could be interpreted to mean that they do not have a voice disorder.

Almost one-third of the students referred to phoniatric examination between 1999 and 2004 chose not to attend it. Students whose voice problems have been detected in a screening test are not necessarily motivated to participate in clinical examinations, at least if they do not feel that they have voice problems. Thus, it is understandable that students, who regard their voice quality as normal or who experience no vocal symptoms choose not to attend a medical examination. We do not know why 14 students who scored 35 mm or more on the VAS and had reported two or more frequently occurring vocal symptoms chose not to attend the phoniatric examination. A study by Simberg *et al.* (2004) showed that teacher students did not seem to be very concerned about their vocal symptoms. In that study, the questionnaire included a question inquiring whether the vocal symptoms had an effect on the student's mood. Of the 175 students participating, 74 reported one or more frequently occurring symptoms but only eight students indicated that vocal symptoms affected their mood much or very much. The question inquiring whether the vocal symptoms had an effect on the student's mood was not a very exact one, as it does not necessarily address the degree of concern. However, the results of a study by Yiu (2002) indicate that vocal concerns had much less effect on teacher students' emotions and social life than on those of practicing teachers. Teachers have been reported to be statistically overrepresented in treatment-seeking populations (Fritzell, 1996; Titze *et al.*, 1997). Still, they are not necessarily very active in looking for help since several studies show that only a small percentage of teachers who report voice problems seek professional help (Roy *et al.*, 2004b; Russel *et al.*, 1998; Sapir *et al.*, 1993; Smith *et al.*, 1998). The reasons for this have not been explored but practical and financial causes have been suggested (Sapir *et al.*, 1993; Smith *et al.*, 1998). The teacher students who participated in the screening test and were referred to phoniatric examination did not have to pay for it (most of the services provided for university students in Finland are free or almost free of charge for the students). One reason for ignoring to seek early help may be that persons adapt to such adverse vocal symptoms as hoarseness (Sonninen, 1970). Background factors such as vocally demanding leisure time activities were not associated with the occurrence of voice disorders in the study covering first- to sixth-year students (Simberg *et al.*, 2000). This was mainly because most of the participants took part in vocally demanding activities such as coaching children in various athletic activities or as scoutmasters. Thus, it is possible that students, like teachers, might feel that their vocal symptoms are a normal inconvenience (Morton & Watson, 1998; Russell *et al.*, 1998; Sapir *et al.*, 1993), which may explain why they do not seek help at an early stage.

It is, of course, alarming that voice disorders among students studying for a vocally demanding occupation seem to be common. However, the experiences from six years of voice screening indicate that first-year students have less severe voice disorders than those who have studied for several years. The voice disorders detected in 1997, covering first- to sixth-year students were more severe; 19% of the 226 students participating had an organic voice disorder (Simberg *et al.*, 2000). According to the experience of the speech therapist carrying out voice therapy for the students at the Student Health Service Center, the voice therapy periods for the first year students have generally been shorter than for the students who had studied for several years. Thus, screening of first-year teacher students for voice disorders seems to be beneficial, and as the first-year students have required shorter voice therapy periods this has freed resources to offer voice therapy for other students studying at the university. If voice screening tests lead to the diagnosis of voice disorders, it hardly needs mentioning that adequate resources for treatment of voice disorders should be available. Despite a small increase, the resources for voice therapy at the Student Health Service Centers in Finland are still limited. Therefore, some of the students with mild voice disorders have been treated in small groups. The outcome of the group voice therapy has been promising (Simberg *et al.*, 2005, 2006).

Based on our experience, we recommend that regular voice screening tests should be offered to students who study for vocally demanding occupations. One possibility might be to train health care personnel in a voice screening procedure to enable them to select students for medical examination and voice therapy. Since vocal symptoms and voice disorders seem to be common among teacher students, voice training programmes should be offered and required for all those who are studying to become teachers. Additionally, access to voice therapy and vocal medical care should be offered to teacher students and other students studying for vocally demanding occupations.

References

Bless, D.M. and Hicks, D.M. (1996) Diagnosis and measurement: Assessing the "WHs" of voice function. In S. Brown, B. Vinson and M. Crary (eds) *Organic Voice Disorders: Assessment and Treatment* (pp. 119–170). San Diego, London: Singular Publishing Group.

Broaddus-Lawrence, P.L., Treole, K., McCabe, R.B., Allen, R.L. and Toppin, L. (2000) The effects of preventive vocal hygiene education on the vocal hygiene habits and perceptual vocal characteristics of training singers. *Journal of Voice* 14 (1), 58–71.

Buekers, R. (1998) Voice performances in relation to demands and capacity. Development of a quantitative phonometric study of the speaking voice. PhD thesis, University of Maastricht.

Buekers, R., Bierens, E., Kingma, H. and Marres, E.H. (1995) Vocal load as measured by the voice accumulator. *Folia Phoniatrica et Logopaedica* 47 (5), 252–261.

Coyle, S.M., Weinrich, B.D. and Stemple, J.C. (2001) Shifts in relative prevalence of laryngeal pathology in a treatment-seeking population. *Journal of Voice* 15 (3), 424–440.

De Bodt, M., Wuyts, F., Van de Heyning, P. and Croux, C.T. (1997) Test-retest study of the GRBAS scale: Influence of experience and professional background on perceptual rating of voice quality. *Journal of Voice* 11 (1), 74–80.

De Bodt, M.S., Wuyts, F.L., Van de Heyning, P.H., Lambrechts, L. and Vanden Abeele, D. (1998) Predicting vocal outcome by means of a vocal endurance test: A 5-year follow-up study in female teachers. *Laryngoscope* 108 (9), 1363–1367.

Dejonckere, P.H., Obbens, C., De Moor, G.M. and Wieneke, G.H. (1993) Perceptual evaluation of dysphonia: Reliability and relevance. *Folia Phoniatrica et Logopaedica* 45 (2), 76–83.

Elias, M.E., Sataloff, R.T., Rosen, D.C., Heuer, R.J. and Spiegel, J.R. (1997) Normal strobovideolaryngoscopy: Variability in healthy singers. *Journal of Voice* 11 (1), 104–107.

Fritzell, B. (1996) Voice disorders and occupations. *Logopedics Phoniatrics Vocology* 21 (1), 7–11.

Heman-Ackah, Y.D., Dean, C.M. and Sataloff, R.T. (2002) Strobovideolaryngoscopic findings in singing teachers. *Journal of Voice* 16 (1), 81–86.

Hirano, M. (1981) Clinical examination of voice. In G. Arnold, F. Winckel and B.D. Wyke (eds) *Disorders of Human Communication 5* (pp. 81–84). Wien: Springer-Verlag.

Kent, R.D. (1996) Hearing and believing: Some limits to the auditory-perceptual assessment of speech and voice disorders. *American Journal of Speech-Language Pathology* 5 (1), 7–23.

Koufman, J., Sataloff, R.T. and Toohill, R. (1996) Laryngopharyngeal reflux: Consensus conference report. *Journal of Voice* 10 (3), 215–216.

Ma, E.P. and Yiu, E.M. (2001) Voice activity and participation profile: Assessing the impact of voice disorders on daily activities. *Journal of Speech, Language and Hearing Research* 44 (3), 511–524.

Marge, M. (1991) Introduction to the prevention and epidemiology of voice disorders. *Seminars in Speech and Language* 12 (1), 49–73.

Mattiske, J.A., Oates, J.M. and Greenwood, K.M. (1998) Vocal problems among teachers: A review of prevalence, causes, prevention, and treatment. *Journal of Voice* 12 (4), 489–499.

Morton, V. and Watson, D.R. (1998) The teaching voice: Problems and perceptions. *Logopedics, Phoniatrics, Vocology* 23 (4), 133–139.

Morton, V. and Watson, D.R. (2001) Voice in the classroom. A re-evaluation. In P.H. Dejonckere (ed.) *Occupational Voice: Care and Cure* (pp. 53–69). Hague: Kugel Publications.

Orr, R., De Jong, F. and Cranen, B. (2002) Some objective measures indicative of perceived voice robustness in student teachers. *Logopedics, Phoniatrics, Vocology* 27 (3), 106–117.

Pekkarinen, E. and Viljanen, V. (1991) Acoustic conditions for speech communication in classrooms. *Scandinavian Audiology* 20 (4), 257–263.

Rogerson, J. and Dodd, B. (2005) Is there an effect of dysphonic teachers' voices on children's processing of spoken language? *Journal of Voice* 19 (1), 47–60.

Roy, N., Merrill, R.M., Thibeault, S., Gray, S.D. and Smith, E.M. (2004a) Voice disorders in teachers and the general population: effects on work performance, attendance, and future career choices. *Journal of Speech, Language, and Hearing Research* 47 (3), 542–551.

Roy, N., Merrill, R.M., Thibeault, S., Parsa, R.A., Gray, S.D. and Smith, E.M. (2004b). Prevalence of voice disorders in teachers and the general population. *Journal of Speech, Language, and Hearing Research* 47 (2), 281–293.

Russell, A., Oates, J. and Greenwood, K.M. (1998) Prevalence of voice problems in teachers. *Journal of Voice* 12 (4), 467–479.

Sabol, J.W., Lee, L. and Stemple, J.C. (1995) The value of vocal function exercises in the practice regimen of singers. *Journal of Voice* 9 (1), 27–36.

Sala, E., Hytönen, M., Tupaselä, O. and Estlander, T. (1996) Occupational laryngitis with immediate allergic or immediate type specific chemical hypersensitivity. *Clinical Otolaryngology and Allied Science* 21 (1), 42–48.

Sala, E., Laine, A., Simberg, S., Pentti, J. and Suonpää, J. (2001) The prevalence of voice disorders among day care center teachers compared with nurses: A questionnaire and clinical study. *Journal of Voice* 15 (3), 413–423.

Sapir, S. (1993) Vocal attrition in voice students: Survey findings. *Journal of Voice* 7 (1), 69–74.

Sapir, S., Keidar, A. and Mathers-Smith, B. (1993) Vocal attrition in teachers: Survey findings. *European Journal of Disorders of Communication* 28 (2), 177–185.

Sederholm, E. (1995) Prevalence of hoarseness in ten-year-old children. *Scandinavian Journal of Logopedics and Phoniatrics* 20 (3), 165–173.

Sederholm, E., McAllister, A., Sundberg, J. and Dalkvist, J. (1993) Perceptual analysis of child hoarseness using continuous scales. *Scandinavian Journal of Logopedics and Phoniatrics* 18 (2), 73–82.

Seidner, W. and Wendler, J. (2001) Phoniatric fitness examinations. Evaluation of long-term experiences. In P.H. Dejonckere (ed.) *Occupational Voice: Care and Cure* (pp. 47–52). Hague: Kugel Publications.

Simberg, S., Laine, A., Sala, E. and Rönnemaa, A-M. (2000) Prevalence of voice disorders among future teachers. *Journal of Voice* 14 (2), 231–235.

Simberg, S., Sala, E., Laine, A. and Rönnemaa A-M. (2001) A fast and easy screening method for voice disorders among teacher students. *Logopedics Phoniatrics Vocology* 26 (1), 10–16.

Simberg, S., Sala, E. and Rönnemaa, A-M. (2004) A comparison of the prevalence of vocal symptoms among teacher students and other university students. *Journal of Voice* 18 (3), 363–368.

Simberg, S., Sala, E., Vehmas, K. and Laine, A. (2005) Changes in the prevalence of vocal symptoms among teachers during a twelve-year period. *Journal of Voice* 19 (1), 95–102.

Simberg, S., Sala, E., Sellman, J., Tuomainen, J. and Rönnemaa, A.-M. (2006) The effectiveness of group therapy for students: A controlled clinical trial. *Journal of Voice* 20 (1), 97–109.

Smith, E., Verdolini, K., Gray, S., Nichols, S., Lemke, J.H, Barkmeier, J., Hove, H. and Hoffman, H. (1996) Effects of voice disorders on quality if life. *Journal of Medical Speech-Language Pathology* 4 (4), 223–244.

Smith, E., Gray, S.D., Dove, H., Kirchner, L. and Heras, H. (1997) Frequency and effects of teachers' voice problems. *Journal of Voice* 11 (1), 81–87.

Smith, E., Kirchner, H.L., Taylor, M., Hoffman, H. and Lemke, J.H. (1998) Voice problems among teachers: Differences by gender and teaching characteristics. *Journal of Voice* 12 (3), 328–334.

Sonninen, A. (1970) Phoniatric viewpoints on hoarseness. *Acta Otolaryngologica* 263, 68–81.

Södersten, M. and Hammarberg, B. (1993) Effects of voice training in normal-speaking women: Videostroboscopic, perceptual, and acoustic characteristics. *Scandinavian Journal of Logopedics and Phoniatrics* 18 (1), 33–42.

Södersten, M., Granqvist, S., Hammarberg, B. and Szabo, A. (2002) Vocal behavior and vocal loading factors for preschool teachers at work studied with binaural DAT recordings. *Journal of Voice* 16 (3), 356–371.

Timmermans, B., De Bodt, M.S., Wuyts, F.L., Boudewijns, G., Clement, G., Peeters, A. and Van de Heyning, P.H. (2002) Poor voice quality in future elite vocal performers and professional voice users. *Journal of Voice* 16 (3), 372–382.

Timmermans, B., De Bodt, M., Wuyts, F. and Van de Heyning, P. (2003) Vocal hygiene in radio students and in radio professionals. *Logopedics, Phoniatrics, Vocology* 28 (3), 127–132.

Timmermans, B., De Bodt, M.S., Wuyts, F.L. and Van De Heyning, P.H. (2004) Training outcome in future professional voice users after eighteen months of voice training. *Folia Phoniatrica et Logopaedica* 56 (2), 120–129.

Titze, I.R., Lemke, J. and Montequin, D. (1997) Populations in the U.S. workforce who rely on voice as a primary tool of trade: A preliminary report. *Journal of Voice* 11 (3), 254–259.

Verdolini, K. and Ramig, L.O. (2001) Review: Occupational risks for voice problems. *Logopedics, Phoniatrics, Vocology* 26 (1), 37–46.

Vilkman, E. (1996) Occupational risk factors and voice disorders. *Logopedics, Phoniatrics, Vocology*, 21 (3), 137–141.

Vilkman, E. (2000) Voice problems at work: A challenge for occupational safety and health arrangement. *Folia Phoniatrica et Logopaedica* 52 (1–3), 120–125.

Vilkman, E. (2004) Occupational safety and health aspects of voice and speech professions. *Folia Phoniatrica et Logopaedica* 56 (4), 220–253.

Vintturi, J., Alku, P., Sala, E., Sihvo, M. and Vilkman, E. (2003) Loading-related subjective symptoms during a vocal loading test with special reference to gender and some ergonomic factors. *Folia Phoniatrica et Logopaedica* 55 (1), 55–69.

Winkworth, A. and McCabe, P. (2001) The vocal process of becoming an actor: Vocal risk profiles of first year acting students. *Paper presented at the Fourth Pan European Voice Conference*, Stockholm, Sweden.

Yiu, E.M. (2002) Impact and prevention of voice problems in the teaching profession: Embracing the consumers' view. *Journal of Voice* 16 (2), 215–228.

Appendix: Questionnaire Concerning Vocal Symptoms

Name _____   Age _____

How often have you had the following vocal symptoms during the past year?

My voice gets strained or tires *(only one answer)*

every day or most days	1
weekly or most weeks	2
monthly or most months	3
less often than above	4
only seasonal symptoms	5
no symptoms	6

My voice gets low or hoarse while talking *(only one answer)*

every day or most days	1
weekly or most weeks	2
monthly or most months	3
less often than above	4
only seasonal symptoms	5
no symptoms	6

I have voice-breaks while talking *(only one answer)*

every day or most days	1
weekly or most weeks	2
monthly or most months	3
less often than above	4
only seasonal symptoms	5
no symptoms	6

I lose my voice for at least a couple of minutes while talking *(only one answer)*

every day or most days	1
weekly or most weeks	2
monthly or most months	3
less often than above	4
only seasonal symptoms	5
no symptoms	6

I have difficulty in being heard *(only one answer)*

every day or most days	1
weekly or most weeks	2

monthly or most months	3
less often than above	4
only seasonal symptoms	5
no symptoms	6

I have to clear my throat or cough while talking *(only one answer)*

every day or most days	1
weekly or most weeks	2
monthly or most months	3
less often than above	4
only seasonal symptoms	5
no symptoms	6

I feel pain or a lump in my throat *(only one answer)*

every day or most days	1
weekly or most weeks	2
monthly or most months	3
less often than above	4
only seasonal symptoms	5
no symptoms	6

Index